Interventional Bronchoscopy
A Clinical Guide

介入支气管镜
临床指南

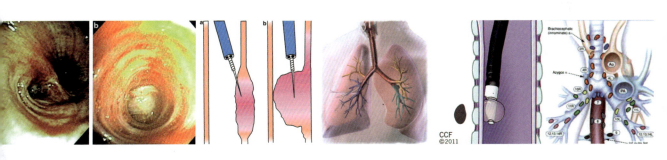

编著　Atul C. Mehta［美］
　　　Prasoon Jain［美］

主译　汪　浩　张哲民
主审　姜格宁

 上海科学技术出版社

图书在版编目（CIP）数据

介入支气管镜临床指南/（美）阿图尔·梅塔（Atul C. Mehta），（美）普瑞森·贾因（Prasoon Jain）主编；汪浩，张哲民主译.—上海：上海科学技术出版社，2017.4

ISBN 978-7-5478-3472-5

Ⅰ.①介⋯　Ⅱ.①阿⋯　②普⋯　③汪⋯　④张⋯　Ⅲ.①支气管镜检-指南　Ⅳ.① R768.1-62

中国版本图书馆 CIP 数据核字（2017）第 040830 号

Translation from the English language edition:
Interventional Bronchoscopy. A Clinical Guide
edited by Atul Mehta and Prasoon Jain
Copyright © Springer Science+Business Media New York 2013
All Rights Reserved

介入支气管镜临床指南
编著　Atul C. Mehta [美]　Prasoon Jain [美]
主译　汪　浩　张哲民
主审　姜格宁

上海世纪出版股份有限公司
上海科学技术出版社　出版
（上海钦州南路71号　邮政编码200235）
上海世纪出版股份有限公司发行中心发行
200001　上海福建中路193号　www.ewen.co
浙江新华印刷技术有限公司印刷
开本787×1092　1/16　印张13　插页4
字数：350千
2017年4月第1版　2017年4月第1次印刷
ISBN 978-7-5478-3472-5/R·1329
定价：128.00元

本书如有缺页、错装或坏损等严重质量问题，
请向承印厂联系调换

内 容 提 要

　　本书是目前国际最新的介入支气管镜临床操作指南，针对目前临床上常见的支气管内镜介入技术及刚刚问世的有巨大临床应用前景的电磁导航等新兴技术，进行了深入的讲解与临床应用指导，满足了国内广大呼吸内镜中心的临床需要。本书作为国外引进版介入支气管镜专著，其优点在于更加偏重临床应用，撰写更简练，表格更清晰易懂，对胸外科、呼吸内科（含肿瘤科及结核科）临床医师和呼吸内镜中心的相关临床工作人员有重要的指导与借鉴价值。

译者名单

主　　审　姜格宁

主　　译　汪　浩　张哲民

副 主 译　顾　晔　杨　洋　刘　继　徐欣楠

参译人员（以姓氏笔画为序）

丁红豆	万紫微	王海峰	史靖涵	包敏伟	边栋亮	朱余明
朱新生	刘小刚	刘鸿程	齐梦凡	李　好	李佳琪	杨　咏
杨　洁	杨　倍	杨　健	杨晨路	励述元	吴　亮	吴　峻
吴　琨	何文新	沈莹冉	宋　楠	张云飞	张凯旋	陈乾坤
范　江	林　磊	金宇星	周　峰	周逸鸣	郑　卉	赵晓刚
赵德平	胡学飞	段　亮	段若望	施　宏	施　哲	姜思明
秦　雄	徐小雄	徐欣楠	郭燕华	黄　威	蒋　雷	谢　冬
谢博雄	靳凯淇	鲍　熠	蔡　健	蔡昊旻	瞿冀琛	

编 者 名 单

主 编

Atul C. Mehta, M.B.B.S. Respiratory Institute, Lerner College of Medicine, Cleveland Clinic, Cleveland, OH, USA

Prasoon Jain, M.B.B.S., M.D., F.C.C.P. Pulmonary and Critical Care, Louis A Johnson VA Medical Center, Clarksburg, WV, USA

参 编 人 员

Fumihiro Asano, M.D., F.C.C.P. Department of Pulmonary Medicine, Gifu Prefectural General Medical Center, Gifu, Japan

John F. Beamis Jr., M.D. Department of Pulmonology, Hawaii Permanente Medical Center, Honolulu, HI, USA

Prashant N. Chhajed, M.D., D.N.B., D.E.T.R.D., F.C.C.P. Lung Care and Sleep Centre, Fortis Hiranandani Hospital, Navi Mumbai, Maharashtra, India

Cliff K. C. Choong, M.B.B.S., F.R.C.S., F.R.A.C.S. Department of Surgery (MMC), The Valley Hospital, Monash University, Melbourne, VIC, Australia

Joseph Cicenia, M.D. Respiratory Institute - Department of Advanced Diagnostic Bronchoscopy, Cleveland Clinic, Cleveland, OH, USA

Yaser Abu El-Sameed, M.B.B.S. Respirology Division, Medicine Institute, Sheikh Khalifa Medical City, Abu Dhabi, UAE

Erik Folch, M.D., M.Sc. Division of Thoracic Surgery and Interventional Pulmonology, Beth Israel Deaconess Medical Center, Harvard Medical School, Boston, MA, USA

Thomas R. Gildea, M.D., M.S. Bronchoscopy, Cleveland Clinic, Respiratory Institute, Cleveland, OH, USA

Sarah Hadique, M.D. Pulmonary and Critical Care Medicine, West Virginia University, Morgantown, WV, USA

Edward F. Haponik, M.D. Pulmonary and Critical Care Medicine, Wake-Forest School of Medicine, Winston-Salem, NC, USA

Cheng He, M.B.B.S., B.Med.Sc., P.G.Dip. Surg.Anat. Department of Surgery (MMC), Monash Medical Center, Monash University, Clayton, VIC, Australia

Arvind H. Kate, M.D., F.C.C.P. Lung care and sleep centre, Fortis Hiranandani Hospital, Navi Mumbai, Maharashtra, India

Sumita B. Khatri, M.D., M.S. Asthma Center, Cleveland Clinic, Respiratory Institute, Cleveland, OH, USA

Noriaki Kurimoto, M.D., F.C.C.P. Department of Chest Surgery, St. Marianna University, Kawasaki, Kanagawa, Japan

Pyng Lee, M.D. Yong Loo Lin School of Medicine, National University of Singapore, Singapore

Division of Respiratory and Critical Care Medicine, National University Hospital, Singapore, Singapore

A. Lukas Loschner, M.D. Section of Pulmonary, Critical Care, Environmental and Sleep Medicine, Carilion Clinic, Virginia Tech Carilion School of Medicine, Roanoke, VA, USA

Adnan Majid, M.D., F.C.C.P. Division of Thoracic Surgery and Interventional Pulmonology, Beth Israel Deaconess Medical Center, Harvard Medical School, Boston, MA, USA

Praveen M. Mathur, M.B.B.S. Pulmonary/CCM Department, Indiana University Hospital, Indianapolis, IN, USA

Sonali Sethi, M.D. Respiratory Institute - Department of Interventional Pulmonary, Cleveland Clinic, Cleveland, OH, USA

Santhakumar Subramanian, M.D., F.C.C.P., I.D.C.C. KG Hospital, Arts College Road, Coimbatore, Tamilnadu, India

译者序

介入呼吸病学是呼吸病学一个新的领域，它着重将先进的支气管镜和胸膜腔镜技术应用到以气管、支气管狭窄至恶性肿瘤所引起的胸腔积液等一系列胸部疾病的治疗，是一门涉及呼吸病侵入性诊断和治疗操作的医学科学和艺术。近年来，随着气管介入技术在国内飞速发展，新设备、新方法层出不穷，无论是呼吸内科还是胸外科医师，都迫切需要了解乃至掌握这些前沿技术来解决临床遇到的实际问题，并开拓创新，持续发展。

本书编者均为当前国际介入呼吸病学相关领域的著名专家学者、技术创始人，或深耕临床工作、主持参与本领域临床指南编写的教授。从介入呼吸病学中的支气管镜着手，分门别类对每一项技术进行详解，同时附有病例与读者分享。国内介入支气管镜技术的开展日益增多，执业医师的视野不断开阔，大量的病例使我们也从学习阶段过渡到参与合作阶段，此时更需要从这些良师益友笔下采撷精华，历练自身，服务患者。

为便于执业医师学习应用，本书内容根据不同种类的诊疗技术进行编排，绘制了大量精美细致的插图，拍摄了清晰的实物照片，图文并茂、深入浅出、条理清晰。本书涵盖了介入呼吸病学中支气管镜技术的传统方法和近年来学界广泛接受的技术，其中不乏一些刚在国内兴起或还未开展的新技术。旨在陈百家之长，学习经典，了解前沿，推广技术开展，推动学科进步。

限于译者水平，中外语言、文化差异及不同国家地区之间的医疗发展差异，翻译难免存在不足，还望读者海涵。同时也希望更多的执业医师加入到介入呼吸病学的大家庭中，集思广益，改写未来！

英文版前言

支气管镜领域正在发生一场变革，过去十年该领域内取得的进展已经成倍地提升了纤维支气管镜诊断和治疗的能力。如今我们可以通过气道内超声从气管壁外部进行观察，也可以通过虚拟支气管镜和电磁导航支气管镜定位到小的外周病变。支气管镜的治疗作用不再局限于缓解肺癌晚期的症状。支气管镜在治疗支气管哮喘、慢性阻塞性肺疾病（COPD）和支气管胸膜瘘中都取得了令人振奋的进展。

支气管镜技术的发展和这个领域知识的更新，没有比这个时代更合适的了。我们正处在一个肺癌世界范围内流行的时代，随着肺癌筛查的普及，我们预计将碰到更多伴有肺结节的患者，而结节可能因为太小，不能通过传统支气管镜技术处理。同时，支气管哮喘和慢性阻塞性肺病持续威胁着全球范围内一部分人的健康。我们相信无论是现在还是将来，先进的支气管镜技术对众多类似患者的诊断和治疗将持续发挥重要作用。

在这本书中，我们邀请了一些国际领先的专家，批判性地回顾了过去十年重要的诊断性和治疗性支气管镜技术。这本书是为呼吸内科医师、住院医师和所有操作诊断性和治疗性支气管镜的医师所写。我们对一些过去几年被主流采纳的新技术提供了全面的观点，分析了这些技术的现状、局限性和未来。

医学领域的任何快速增长都会带来许多相关问题，支气管镜也不例外。我们必须考虑的是新技术是否在提供诊断或改善预后方面比现有的技术更有效，同时新技术的安全问题和局限性必须得到认识。因为大多数新型支气管镜技术都比较昂贵，所以费用问题也要得到解决。目前来看，采用任何高费用技术带来的经济问题都不能忽视。当选择一个费用更高的技术来代替一个现有的低费用技术时，社会和第三方付款人对其经济合理性的要求都越来越高。在全球市场，许多新兴技术因为很难被资源匮乏的社会接受而无法广泛地普及。作者在这本书中已经解决了一些问题，从而指导读者在新技术的应用和卫生资源的分配上做出更加全面、明智的决定。

我们强烈并坚定地感受到支气管镜新技术的出现，但并不表示现有的传统支气管镜技术（如TBBx和传统经支气管针吸活检技术）已经被淘汰或应该被禁止。实际上，新技术的出现提供了一个独特的机会，来改进甚至再定义现有技术的临床作用。我们坚定地相信，有效地使用这些经过时间检验的传统支气管镜技术，在日常支气管镜的临床实践中仍然会发挥重要作用。对每个支气管镜医师来说，在接触更多先进技术前对传统技术的基本原则有全面的了解是基本要求。因此，这本书中相当多的部分用来讲述传统支气管镜技术。

我们真诚地感谢所有在本书中分享了专业知识的作者们。在他们的帮助下，我们尽了最大努力来对这个快速发展的领域提供全面的、先进的综述。我们希望读者能发现这些信息是发人深省的、实用的，并能容易地应用在临床实践中。虽然我们对支气管镜领域现有的进展感到振奋，但是我们真诚地相信这只是开始，最好的尚未来临。

目录

第 1 篇　概述 — *1*

第 1 章　介入呼吸病学：现状和未来方向 — *2*
John F. Beamis Jr. and Praveen M. Mathur

第 2 章　经支气管肺活检 — *13*
Prasoon Jain, Sarah Hadique, and Atul C. Mehta

第 3 章　经支气管针吸活检（TBNA） — *37*
Prasoon Jain, Edward F. Haponik, A. Lukas Loschner, and Atul C. Mehta

第 2 篇　诊断性介入支气管镜 — *57*

第 4 章　径向探头支气管内超声 — *58*
Noriaki Kurimoto

第 5 章　EBUS-TBNA 支气管镜检查 — *66*
Sonali Sethi and Joseph Cicenia

第 6 章　电磁导航支气管镜 — *83*
Thomas R. Gildea and Joseph Cicenia

第 7 章　虚拟支气管镜临床应用 — *94*
Fumihiro Asano

第 3 篇　治疗性介入支气管镜 — *109*

第 8 章　中央气道阻塞的气管镜治疗 — *110*
Sarah Hadique，Prasoon Jain，and Atul C. Mehta

第 9 章　气道支架　　　　　　　　　　　　　　　　　　　*137*
Pyng Lee and Atul C. Mehta

第 10 章　支气管热成形术治疗重症哮喘　　　　　　　　　*145*
Sumita B. Khatri and Thomas R. Gildea

第 11 章　经支气管镜肺减容术　　　　　　　　　　　　　*154*
Cheng He and Cliff K. C. Choong

第 12 章　支气管镜用于治疗支气管胸膜瘘　　　　　　　　*162*
Yaser Abu El-Sameed

第 13 章　支气管镜异物移除　　　　　　　　　　　　　　*174*
Erik Folch and Adnan Majid

第 14 章　支气管镜在咯血中的作用　　　　　　　　　　　*188*
Santhakumar Subramanian, Arvind H. Kate, and Prashant N. Chhajed

第1篇

概 述

Introduction

第 1 章

介入呼吸病学：现状和未来方向

John F. Beamis Jr. and Praveen M. Mathur

本章提要 本章将概述介入呼吸病学在过去 30 多年中的发展，这门学科开始于引入 Nd:YAG 激光进行支气管镜治疗。文中还将提及早期为现代介入呼吸病学打下基础的先行者们。本章将回顾介入呼吸病学目前的实践范围，着重介绍最新用于诊断和对胸部恶性肿瘤进行分期的支气管镜技术。另外还将讨论介入呼吸病学进修的现状以及资格认证和 1 年正规介入呼吸病学进修的需要。

关键词 介入呼吸病学，纤维支气管镜，硬质支气管镜，胸腔镜（内科胸腔镜），支气管内超声，自发性荧光支气管镜，肺癌，导航支气管镜检查，电灼术，冷冻治疗，支架（气道）。

引 言

介入呼吸病学（IP）在过去的 30 年已经演变成胸腔内外科的一种多样化亚专业，它涉及诊断性和治疗性支气管镜、胸腔镜和许多其他表 1.1 中概括的技术。技术上的进步和肺癌在 20 世纪后半叶的流行是刺激介入呼吸疾病发展的主要因素。另外，肺移植在过去的 20 多年成为晚期和终末期肺部疾病的治疗选择，同样刺激了介入呼吸病学领域的研究和发展。肺移植受体为了诊断、对排斥进行随访和治疗气道并发症，需要经历多次支气管镜检查。有人认为如果没有专业支气管镜检查的帮助，肺移植手术不可能成功。

介入呼吸病学不仅仅是手术操作。它常常牵涉对晚期恶性肿瘤、严重中心气道阻塞和胸腔积液引起的呼吸障碍患者的整体管理。比起大多数呼吸内科进修培训和胸外科住院医师培训，介入呼吸病学要求更多的培训和经验。虽然介入呼吸病学的从业者数量在美国和许多其他国家都有所增长，但是他们的分布仍是散在的。许多有需要的患者仍然无法受益于介入呼吸病学。

鉴于这门学科在过去 30 多年取得的发展，本章中我们将回顾介入呼吸病学临床实践和培训的现状，回顾它的历史，并且评价它的未来。

介入呼吸病学的定义

介入呼吸病学于 1995 年在一本专著中被首次定义[1]，在欧洲呼吸协会和美国胸科协会的联合指南中被再次定义[2]。介入呼吸病学被定义为"针对呼吸系统疾病的诊断和侵入性治疗操作的一门科学和艺术。掌握这一门学科，除了要掌握常规的呼吸病学的知识和训练之外，还需要更多专门的训练和更专业的判断"。虽然这个定义已经有 20 多年的历史，介入呼吸病学涉及方法的种类也已经增多，但是它仍然很准确。除了恶性肿瘤的治疗方法外，这里更加强调诊断和使用介入呼吸病学技术治疗良性疾病（如哮喘和气肿）。

表 1.1　介入呼吸病学的组成成分

先进的诊断性支气管镜

　　自发荧光支气管镜[a]；窄带成像；径向支气管内超声[a]；线性支气管内超声引导下经支气管针吸活检[a]；光学相干断层扫描[b]；定位性支气管镜[a]

治疗性支气管镜

　　硬质支气管镜[a]；激光[a]；高频电[a]；氩等离子凝固术[a]；冷冻疗法[a]；放疗；光动力治疗；球囊支气管成形术[a]；支架——硅胶，自膨胀金属支架（覆膜、未覆膜）；异物取出术[a]；支气管热成形术[a]；经支气管镜肺减容术[b]；用于支气管胸膜瘘的气道瓣膜；全肺灌洗术[a]

胸腔检查

　　胸腔镜检查[a]；胸导管留置[a]

危重症检查

　　经皮扩张气管切开术[a]

注：a. 临床可行；b. 只用于研究

介入呼吸病学的发展

先行者

Gustave Killian 医师是一位德国耳鼻喉科医师，他在 1897 年进行了第一例硬质支气管镜手术来移除一位患者主支气管中的一根骨头，首次提供了经喉部进入气管支气管树的方法。Killian 的手术获得世界范围的关注。他的学生中有一位叫 Chevalier Jackson 的匹兹堡耳鼻喉科医师，被认为是"美国支气管食管学之父"[3-5]。Jackson 搬到费城后最终成为那里所有（共 5 所）当地医学院的耳鼻喉科教授。Jackson 设计了硬质支气管镜及其附件，成为以后 100 多年的规范。他取出异物和扩张气道狭窄的技术也经受住了时间的考验。他最大的贡献可能是发展出了一套严格的安全规范，并且他组织的指导性课程已经成为现代介入呼吸病学课程的模范。

胸腔内科作为一个亚学科，它的发展主要是因为 Shigeto Ikeda 医师发明了光导纤维支气管镜，他是东京国家癌症机构的胸外科医师[6]。纤维支气管镜最初被设计为诊断性工具，现在已经证明它在治疗上的宝贵作用[7]。

在 20 世纪，许多新开发的技术都存在借助支气管镜治疗气道疾病的潜力。1920 年 Yankauer 报道了使用支气管镜将镭植入支气管肿瘤内。镭被放在一个胶囊内，胶囊连接到一根可以从口中拉出的绳子上。这个方法虽然有效，但是它让治疗团队暴露在辐射下[8]。来自梅奥诊所的 Neel 和 Sanderson 通过硬质支气管镜下的冷冻疗法或支气管切开术来治疗气道肿瘤[9,10]。Hooper 和 Jackson 描述了最早的气管内电灼术的经验[11,12]。Laforet 等[13]描述了使用二氧化碳激光来治疗气道的一个阻塞性黏液上皮样肿瘤。所有这些治疗支气管内病变的新方法显示了这项技术的前景，但是这些技术还只是掌握在个别专家手中，未被广泛接受。

正如治疗性支气管镜已经有 100 多年的历史，内科胸腔镜作为介入呼吸病学的一个重要技术，也已经发展了 100 多年。一个叫作 Hans-Christian Jacobeus 的瑞典肺内科医师据说在 1910 年进行了第一例胸腔镜手术。他的技术被广泛接纳，作为一种在结核病的抗生素治疗时代之前松解胸膜粘连的方法[14,15]。现在有证据表明在 Jacobeus 之前 50 年有一位爱尔兰的内科医师可能已经探查过胸腔了[16]。当结核的系统性治疗被引入后，胸腔镜手术就明显减少了。

但是，视频技术的改善和微创手术的兴起，使得许多医疗团队将胸腔镜的指征扩大到其他情况，如脓胸、恶性胸腔积液的治疗和胸膜疾病的诊断[17,18]。

介入呼吸病学

20世纪80年代

许多人会将介入呼吸病学开始的时间追溯到20世纪80年代早期，两篇法国的报道描述了利用 Nd:YAG 激光治疗肺癌引起的气道阻塞。Toty 等在 164 例良性和恶性肿瘤源性气道狭窄患者身上进行了激光治疗。最后他们报道了中央气道肿瘤（良性和恶性）的良好治疗结果和通过硬质支气管镜使用激光引起的医源性狭窄。作者觉得激光治疗的主要指征是"用于治疗曾经经过手术和放射治疗的窒息性和难治性癌症[19]"。来自 Marseilles 的 Dumon 等[20] 描述了他们治疗 111 例各种良恶性肿瘤源性气道阻塞患者的经验。治疗效果很好，作者声明"未发生严重并发症"。因为 Dumon 的临床技能和他乐意通过演讲、实践性课程和书面形式和别人分享经验，Marseilles 很快就吸引了许多对治疗性支气管镜技术感兴趣的人。其他欧洲内科医师，其中很多也是 Dumon 的弟子，很快就多了许多激光治疗后的患者[21]。没过多久激光支气管镜术跨越了大西洋传到美国的一些医疗中心[22-25]。

在 20 世纪 80 年代，因为肺癌的持续流行和技术的发展，在欧洲和北美建立了许多激光支气管镜中心。Dumon[26] 和其他人制定出了安全标准。除了对使用硬质支气管镜广泛切除气道肿瘤[27]再次感兴趣外，许多美国支气管镜医师喜欢用纤维支气管镜进行激光治疗[28,29]。

20世纪90年代

在世界范围内使用激光支气管镜 10 年后，我们显然需要其他支气管内治疗方法来对抗肺癌流行引发的对中央气道的影响。用 Nd:YAG 激光凝固中央气道肿瘤，再用硬质或纤维支气管镜技术切除的方法，引起的气道畅通虽然是即时的，却往往又是短期的。伴外在压迫或缺少软骨支撑的患者也不能通过激光来治疗。我们需要其他方法来维持或打开中央气道阻塞，于是重新出现了对腔内放疗的兴趣。对比前几十年原始的放置放射源的方法，最新的使用 I-192 的后装技术被发展出来[30]。曾经的创新家 Dumon 研制出了一种硅胶支架，能够通过硬质支气管镜放置，并且被证明对良恶性肿瘤源性狭窄的长期治疗有价值[31,32]。大量自膨胀金属支架被发明。Wallstents 和 Palmaz 支架[33,34]被证明相对容易通过纤维支气管镜插入，但是它们很多又被镍钛合金做成的 Ultraflex 支架（Boston Scientific，Natick，MA，USA）所代替[35]。

受激光治疗成功的刺激，许多旧技术得到升级，并被证明能成功治疗支气管内疾病。电灼术被证明在有经验人员的操作下和激光治疗效果一样，性价比更高[36-38]。这个技术借助纤维支气管镜使用探头或圈套器。Homasson 和欧洲其他人通过硬质支气管镜使用新的冷冻治疗探头来治疗气道肿瘤[39,40]。Mathur 等引入了能穿过纤维支气管镜工作通道的可弯曲冷冻探头[41]。氩等离子凝固术被证明为另一个凝固和消融支气管内肿瘤的工具[42,43]。所有这些方法成了激光治疗的替代方法，它们的启动成本更低，能通过纤维支气管镜使用。虽然没有研究进行过对比，但是它们的效果在大多数情况下相似。

在 20 世纪 90 年代，北美的呼吸科医师对内科胸腔镜重燃兴趣[44]。微创手术技术上的进步，以及包括 Boutin[45] 和 Loddenkemper[46] 在内的欧洲专家发展出的技术，加深了这种兴趣。虽然这个技术在欧洲非常普遍，但是由内科医师在胸部进行手术的观念在美国引起了很大的争议[47,48]。随着外科胸腔镜手术和内科胸腔镜之间的差别被认可，并且大多数呼吸科医师将从业范围限定为壁层胸膜活检和滑石粉胸膜固定术,这个争议才最终得到解决。

同样在这十年,支气管镜医师知道要治疗晚期肿瘤导致的气道阻塞是困难的,于是开始寻找早期尚能治疗的支气管内肿瘤。Lam 等激动人心的工作表明,重度不典型增生和原位肿瘤区域可以通过荧光纤维支气管镜进行自发性荧光检测[49,50]。不典型增生病灶可以被随访,并可能通过戒烟治疗。侵袭性更强的病灶可以通过各种手段治疗,包括光动力疗法、电灼术和放疗。

支气管内超声成像在 20 世纪 90 年代早期的兴起,在下一个十年将会证明是介入呼吸病学和普遍意义的支气管病学的重大进步。Hürter 和 Hanrath 通过将球囊超声导管穿过纤维支气管镜的工作通道,对气道壁成像来检测侵袭性病变、研究外周病灶和引导支架置入[51]。Shannon 等[52]证明了支气管内超声的这一方法(现称为径向支气管内超声)能对包括血管和淋巴结在内的纵隔结构进行成像,并且能促进 Wang[53]在之前描述过的经支气管针吸活检术。

21 世纪

新世纪带来了径向支气管内超声应用的快速发展。Herth 等[54]概述了使用支气管内超声进行支气管镜治疗的优势。Miyazu 等使用径向支气管内超声来评估早期肺癌对气道壁侵犯的深度,据此决定是进行局部光动力治疗还是手术切除或放疗[55]。Herth 等也表明支气管内超声能用于定位外周肺结节或病灶,它的结果和透视检查获得的结果相似[56]。Kurimoto 等将支气管内超声探头穿过一个导向鞘来改善肺外周病灶取样[57]。在一个对径向支气管内超声诊断外周病灶的系统性综述和荟萃分析中,Steinfort 等提到诊断的特异性为 100%,敏感性为 73%。这些作者总结出虽然这种方法的诊断范围小于 CT 引导下经皮肺穿刺活检,但是支气管内超声引导下经支气管肺活检良好的安全记录"支持用支气管内超声引导下经支气管肺活检对存在肺外周病灶的患者进行最初的检查"[58]。

Olympus 有限公司(Tokyo,Japan)引入的线性支气管内超声支气管镜在胸腔恶性肿瘤的治疗上可能比径向支气管内超声更为重要,因为它实现了动态超声引导下对纵隔和肺门淋巴结的经支气管针吸活检术。这个方法最早由 Krasnik 等[59]报道用于一个小组患者。随后日本的 Yasufuku[60,61]和海德堡/波士顿的 Herth/Ernst[62-64]合作验证了经支气管针吸活检术对大量肺癌患者的诊断。线性经支气管超声引导针吸活检方法改变了肺癌分期的方法,并且已经被证明对诊断其他纵隔和肺门淋巴结疾病同样有效,如淋巴瘤[65]、胸外恶性肿瘤[66]、结节病[67]和结核[68]。在 Adams 等的荟萃分析中,线性经支气管超声引导针吸活检对已知或未知肺癌患者的纵隔淋巴结取样时,其特异性为 100%、敏感性为 88%[69]。另一个 Varela-Lema 等的系统性综述中提到了相似的结果,并提示经支气管超声引导针吸活检能代替纵隔镜检查用于许多病例的肺癌分期[70]。

最近几年,临床上的肺癌已经从中央型病灶变成更多的周围型病灶。这刺激了支气管镜医师研究出方法来诊断周围型肺结节和肿块,改善诊断的结果,相比透视检查和经支气管活检这些经典的技术能有所提高。除了径向支气管内超声外,一些新的导航支气管镜和超薄支气管镜也在这十年产生。Schwarz 等[71]描述了超维支气管系统(superDimen-sion,Inc,Mineapolis,MN),它使用虚拟支气管镜和电磁导航支气管镜来对靶向周围病灶进行取样。克利夫兰诊所使用这个系统对 60 例患者的平均大小为(22.8±12.6)mm 的外周病灶进行取样,报道的阳性率为 74%[72]。Asano 描述了一个虚拟支气管镜定位系统(VBN System,Olympus Medical Systems,Tokyo,Japan)能产生相似的阳性率[73]。Eberhardt 等使用 LungPoint 定位系统(Bronchus Technologies Inc.,Mountain View,CA)引导的超薄支气管镜,对 25 个平均大小为 28 mm 的外周病灶的诊断阳性率为 80%[74]。

良性气道肿瘤和良性气管狭窄的治疗方法

与癌症类似。这十年最主要的发展在于尝试通过介入性支气管镜技术治疗肺气肿和哮喘。但是，治疗哮喘和肺气肿需要新技术。多中心、随机双盲对照试验表明支气管热成形术可以减少哮喘的急性加重和中重度哮喘的卫生服务利用[75,76]。该方法是将一根导管穿过标准纤维支气管的工作通道，利用射频消融能量消融段支气管和亚段支气管的气道平滑肌。这项技术目前已经通过了美国食品药物管理局（FDA）的审核，并作为 Alair 支气管热整形系统销售（Boston Scientific, Natick, MA）。

使用支气管镜治疗严重肺气肿的尝试没有成功。被 National Emphysema Treatment Trial 试验的结果所刺激，许多支气管镜肺减容技术已经被研究出来，包括将瓣膜用于气道阻塞、将可生物降解凝胶用于塌陷肺段、在支气管树和过度膨胀的肺实质之间创造额外的解剖通道。但这些技术中没有一个被证明有充分的疗效或安全性能通过美国食品药物管理局的审批[78]。

介入呼吸病学的培训

20 世纪 80 年代早期，当激光支气管镜被引入的时候，许多美国支气管镜医师来到欧洲学习此项技术，特别是 Marseilles。Dumon 和他早期的弟子很快就开展了课程将他们的经验分享给呼吸科医师们。美国的第一个课程于 1983 年由莱希诊所开展。很快在全美国出现了许多课程。所有这些课程都提供激光治疗的指征、手术的技巧要点和并发症的理论指导，以及非生物模型和动物模型的实践经验[79]。Kvale[80]概述了一个典型的激光支气管镜课程，并表达了对这个新型手术的培训和认证的担忧。在过去的 30 多年里，介入呼吸病学的课程范围已经极大地扩展了。现在的课程包括多种支气管内疗法：激光、电灼术、冷冻治疗、支架和球囊扩张，以及先进的诊断方法：线性、径向支气管内超声和自发性荧光支气管镜。通常利用模拟的方式练习。一些课程也包括了胸腔镜检查和经皮气管切开术。但是，难道一次 2~5 天的课程提供的经验，就能让一个呼吸科医师回去后在患者上进行一个新型手术吗？

在对美国呼吸和危重病医学进修医师培训项目负责人和美国胸内科医师学会成员的问卷调查中，Pastis 等[81,82]报道了美国呼吸科进修医师通常对他们在传统纤维支气管镜方面的培训满意，但是没有足够的"介入性"手术的经验来满足美国胸内科医师学会指南制定的能力标准[83]。他们的欧洲同事通常在进修期间能接触到硬质支气管镜和胸腔镜检查，而大多数美国呼吸和危重病医学进修医师还需要进一步培训来获取操作介入呼吸病学手术的能力。这促进了介入呼吸病学进修培训的发展。美国首个正规的介入呼吸病学进修培训项目由莱希诊所在 1996 年组织。目前在北美有 19 个活跃的介入呼吸病学进修培训项目（表 1.2）。Gildea[84]认为在一个高介入呼吸病学手术量的机构，如克利夫兰诊所，每个进修医师都有接触介入呼吸病学手术的机会，因此不要求有一个独立的介入呼吸病学进修培训项目。与之相反，Feller-Kopman[85]概述了一个正规的 1 年介入呼吸病学进修培训项目的好处，包括接触更多类型和数量的手术、更好的科研机会、人脉，以及一个类似于其他介入性专科（如心脏病学和胃肠病学）的训练过程。作者支持正规的 1 年介入呼吸病学进修培训项目。

Lamb 等近来概述了介入呼吸病学培训的原则和目的。作者强调除了掌握手术技术外，介入呼吸病学进修医师必须在胸腔恶性肿瘤、复杂的气道疾病和胸膜疾病等领域具备一个广阔的知识库，同时具备对各种介入呼吸病学技术以及它们如何应用于良恶性组织的工作知识。2011 年是介入呼吸病学进修培训的里程碑之年，因为这是进修医师通过国家住院医师匹配系统挑选的第一年。它的目标是让介入呼吸病学进修培训最终获得美国毕业后医学教育委员会的认证。在更远的未来可能发展出一个正规的专科执照考试，促进美国医学专业委员会对介入呼吸病学的认可。

表 1.2　目前北美介入性呼吸病学进修单位

- Beth Israel Deaconess Medical Center, Boston, MA
- Cancer Treatment Centers of America, Philadelphia, PA
- Centre Hospitalier de l'University of Montreal, Montreal, QB, CA
- Chicago Chest Center, Elk Grove, IL
- Cleveland Clinic Foundation Respiratory Institute, Cleveland, OH
- Duke University Medical Center, Durham, NC
- Emory University School of Medicine, Atlanta, GA
- Henry Ford Hospital, Detroit, MI
- Johns Hopkins Hospital, Baltimore, MD
- Lahey Clinic, Burlington, MA
- McGill University Royal Victoria Hospital, Montreal, QB, CA
- National Jewish Health, Denver, CO
- Ohio State University, Columbus, OH
- University of Calgary, Calgary, AB, CA
- University of Texas MD Anderson Cancer Center, Houston, TX
- University of Arkansas for the Medical Sciences, Little Rock, AK
- University of Pennsylvania Medical Center, Philadelphia, PA
- Virginia Commonwealth University, Richmond, VA
- Washington University School of Medicine, St Louis, MO

介入呼吸病学的现状

下面的章节会阐明许多介入呼吸病学支气管镜手术在当前实践中的细节。在这里，我们将总结介入呼吸病学在 21 世纪第 2 个十年的发展状况。来自美国胸科学会 / 欧洲呼吸学会[2]和美国胸内科医师学会[83]的指南基于专家们的共识，它们虽然已经有十年的历史，但仍然有效，并且不断反映许多当前实践的情况。

- 虽然激光和其他支气管内治疗为硬质支气管镜注入了活力，但是除了在欧洲外，这个多功能仪器的使用仍然很有限。在美国，标准的呼吸和危重病医学进修培训和心胸外科住院医师进修的项目只提供有限的接触，甚至没有接触这一操作。纤维支气管镜已经成为大多数机构的主要支气管镜治疗方法。虽然在莱希诊所硬质和纤维支气管镜都有使用，但是也已经转向更柔软的支气管镜手术（图 1.1）[87]。最近的英国胸科协会指南回顾了使用纤维支气管镜进行治疗和先进诊断的现有实践[88]。

- 支气管镜下消融术有许多选择：激光、电灼术、放疗、冷冻疗法、氩等离子凝固术。激光仍然是最有效的手段。随着最初的 Nd:YAG 激光被淘汰，许多组改用新的 Nd:YAP 激光，这种激光便携性更好，比 Nd:YAG 激光价格更低，对支气管内肿瘤的凝固效果和前者相似[89]。

- 虽然 Dumon 型号的硅胶支架在治疗外来气道压迫或软骨支撑缺失上经受住了时间的考验，但是这种型号的支架要通过硬质支气管镜置入。Ultraflex® 支架曾经长期是使用最广的自膨胀金属支架，但最近被 AERO® 支架所取代。后

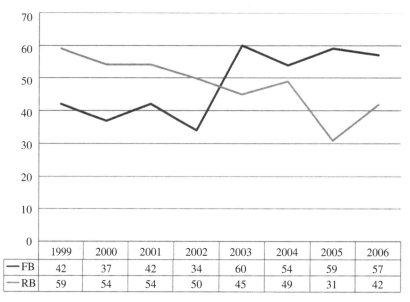

图 1.1 研究期间介入性支气管镜操作的数量更多地趋向于可弯曲纤维支气管镜。FB：硬质支气管镜；RB：纤维支气管镜

者是一种完全由镍钛合金覆盖的自膨胀金属支架（Merit Medical Systems, Inc., South Jordon, UT）。两者都能通过纤维支气管镜置入[90]。

- 尽管在全欧洲以及相对较少的一些美国医疗中心已经有许多优秀经验，但是在美国，内科医师使用胸腔镜仍然是不普遍、不充分的。随着半刚性胸腔镜[91,92]的发展，它的表现和普通的视频纤维支气管镜相似，并且在治疗胸膜疾病方面和硬质设备一样有效[93]。因此，有可能更多的呼吸科医师会将这个安全、高敏感性和高特异性的方法应用到临床实践中。Janssen号召"如今任何处理胸膜疾病的呼吸科医师都应该能操作胸腔镜"[94]。我们响应他的号召。这个手术除了可以处理局部障碍外，Michaud用一个视频[95]描述它应该成为任何介入呼吸病学的一部分，至少处在英国胸科协会2010年指南中的1级推荐[96]。

- 自发性荧光支气管镜是另一个被引入临床实践中却未充分使用的技术。自发性荧光支气管镜在检测气道癌前病灶时表现为敏感性高、特异性不高[97,98]。只有D-Light 1个系统被允许在美国使用（Karl Storz Endoscopy America, Inc., El Segundo, CA）。其他系统可以在欧洲和日本使用。更新的技术，如窄带成像和光学相干断层扫描技术，已经被用来改善自发性荧光支气管镜的特异性。最近的证据表明CT对肺癌的筛查改善了死亡率[99]，这可能会刺激正规的肺癌筛查项目的发展，进而有可能用自发性荧光支气管镜来筛查气道早期病灶。

- 线性支气管内超声很快成为肺癌患者纵隔分期和纵隔淋巴结取样的标准护理方法。虽然大多数支气管镜医师都能够并且应该操作这个方法，但是介入呼吸病学的呼吸科医师好像正率先将支气管内超声整合进每天的实践中。线性经支气管超声引导针吸活检除了用来进行分期外，它正被用来获取肺癌晚期或肺癌复发患者更多的组织，在个性化癌症治疗的新时代指导靶向肺癌治疗[100]。

- 随着肺癌临床就诊的情况从中央型鳞癌转变为以周围型腺癌为主，介入呼吸病学技术被用于诊断外周病灶的频率不断增加。电磁定位、径向经支气管超声引导针吸活检和超薄支气管镜都正在被用于获取外周病灶组织。不同机构偏爱的技术会有差别，它们常常被同时使用。这些技术会和介入放射医师操作的经胸壁针吸活检术竞争。

介入呼吸病学的未来

介入呼吸病学的未来看起来很光明。肺癌在持续流行，其发生率在发达国家只是轻微减少，而在发展中国家正在上升。在可见的未来，患者将会继续因癌性中央气道病灶就诊，要求消融治疗或置入支架。支气管内超声可以用于分期和诊断，并且正在快速地从研究中心引入到社区。介入呼吸病学的设备虽然很贵，但是 Colt 在最近的概述中认为，在地方医院或癌症中心搭建一个介入呼吸病学项目是可行的[100]。关键是在癌症（特别是肺癌）更高发的发展中国家要怎么办。在可见的未来，介入呼吸病学受训人员的志愿帮助和相关产业的慷慨捐助仍是唯一的输送介入呼吸病学到发展中国家的办法。

虽然在 1995 年对介入呼吸病学的定义相对简单，但是要界定是否为介入呼吸科医师仍然是困难的。是那些完成了介入呼吸病学进修培训的人吗？还是参加了几天课程、感觉能够操作支气管内超声和放置自膨胀金属支架的人？或是热情地跟随了一个当地的介入呼吸病学医师，感觉可以设置一个自己工作项目的呼吸和危重病医学毕业生？是来自优秀的学术中心的人，还是来自社区医院的人？抑或是美国支气管病学和介入呼吸病学协会的成员？这是一个重要的需要在未来被定义的问题。可能一个医师资格证书考试能帮助回答这个问题，但是这个答案需要许多年的时间来获得，并且不适用于那些已经在从业的人。

在未来，介入呼吸病学的实践必定会变得更加符合循证医学。大多数介入呼吸病学的医学论文（和大多数本章引用的文章）都来自单机构病例系列。介入呼吸病学研究正在转变为随机对照多中心研究，通常设置了假手术对照组[75,102]。这类研究能最好地为患者服务，并且只会导向医学界内介入呼吸病的改善。

我们很幸运地从一开始就接触到介入呼吸病学的领域，并且见证了这个专科的繁荣和许多新生代的介入呼吸科医师加入这个行列。在过去的 30 多年，我们与来自许多国家的介入呼吸病学从业者合作并成为朋友。介入呼吸病学是一个全球性的专科，它所面对的疾病是全球范围的。在未来，我们必须确认介入呼吸病学提供的护理同样是全球性的。

参考文献

1. Mathur PN, Beamis J. Preface. In: Mathur PN, Beamis J, editors. Interventional pulmonology. Chest Clinics of North America. London: Saunders; 1995. p. ix–xii.
2. Bolliger CT, Mathur PN, Beamis JF, Becker HD, Cavaliere S, Colt H, et al. ERS/ATS statement on interventional pulmonology. European Respiratory Society/American Thoracic Society. Eur Respir J. 2002;19:356–73.
3. Tyson EB. The development of the bronchoscope. J Med Soc N J. 1957;54:26–30.
4. Jackson C. Bronchoscopy: past, present and future. N Engl J Med. 1928;199:759–63.
5. Zolliner F. Gustav Killian: father of bronchoscopy. Arch Otolaryngol. 1965;82:656–9.
6. Ikeda S. Flexible bronchofiberscope. Ann Otol Rhinol Laryngol. 1970;79:916–23.
7. Rand IA, Barber PV, Goldring J, et al. British Thoracic Society guidelines for advanced diagnostic and therapeutic flexible bronchoscopy in adults. Thorax. 2011;66 Suppl 3:iii1–21.
8. Yankauer S. Two cases of lung tumor treated bronchoscopically. N Y Med J. 1922;1922:741–2.
9. Gorenstein A, Neel HB, Sanderson DR. Transbronchoscopic cryosurgery of respiratory strictures. Experimental and clinical studies. Ann Otol Rhinol Laryngol. 1976;85:670–8.
10. Carpenter RJ, Neel HB, Sanderson DR. Cryosurgery of bronchopulmonary structures. An approach to lesions inaccessible to the rigid bronchoscope. Chest. 1977;72:279–84.
11. Hooper RG, Jackson FN. Endobronchial electrocautery. Chest. 1985;87:712–4.
12. Hooper RG, Jackson FN. Endobronchial electrocautery. Chest. 1988;94:595–8.
13. Laforet EG, Berger RL, Vaughan CW. Carcinoma obstructing the trachea: treatment by laser resection. N Engl J Med. 1976; 294:941.
14. Jacobaeus HC. Ü̈ber die Mö̈glichkeit, die Zystoskopie bei

Untersuchung sero¨ser Ho¨hlungen anzuwenden.Mu¨nch med Wschr 1910;57:2090–92.
15. Seijo LM, Sterman DH. Interventional pulmonology. N Engl J Med. 2001;344:740–9.
16. Hoksch B, Birken-Bertsch H, Muller JM. Thoracoscopy before Jacobaeus. Ann Thorac Surg. 2002;74:1288–90.
17. Swierenga J, Wagenaar JPM, Bergstein PGM. The value of thoracoscopy in the diagnosis and treatment of diseases affecting the pleura and lung. Pneumonologie. 1974;151:11–8.
18. Mathur PN, Boutin C, Loddenkemper R. Medical thoracoscopy: techniques and indications in pulmonary medicine. J Bronchol Intervent Pulmonol. 1994;1:228–38.
19. Toty L, Persone C, Colchen A, Vourc'h G. Bronchoscopic management of tracheal lesions using the neodynium yttrium aluminium garnet laser. Thorax. 1981;36:175–8.
20. Dumon JF, Reboud E, Garbe L, et al. Treatment of tracheobronchial lesions by laser photoresection. Chest. 1982; 81:278–84.
21. Cavaliere S, Foccoli P, Farina PL. Nd:YAG laser bronchoscopy: a five year experience with 1,396 applications in 1000 patients. Chest. 1988;94:15–21.
22. McDougall JC, Cortese DA. Neodynium YAG laser therapy of malignant airway obstruction: a preliminary report. Mayo Clin Proc. 1983;58:35–9.
23. Gelb AF, Epistein JD. Laser treatment of lung cancer. Chest. 1984;86:662–6.
24. Kvale PA, Eichenhorn MS, Radke JA, Mika V. YAG laser photoresection of lesions obstructing the central airways. Chest. 1985;87:283–8.
25. Beamis JF, Vergos KV, Rebeiz EE, Shapshay SM. Endoscopic laser therapy for obstructing tracheobronchial lesions. Annals Otol Rhinol Laryngol. 1991;100:413–9.
26. Dumon JF, Shapshay S, Bourcereau J, et al. Principles for safety in application of neodymium-YAG laser in bronchology. Chest. 1984;86:163–8.
27. Cortese DA. Rigid versus flexible bronchoscopy in laser bronchoscopy: Pro rigid bronchoscopic laser application. J Bronchol. 1994;1:72–5.
28. Joyner LR, Maran AG, Sarama R, Yakaboski A. Neodymium-YAG laser treatment of intrabronchial lesions: a new mapping technique via the flexible fiberoptic bronchoscope. Chest. 1985;87:418427.
29. Unger M. Rigid versus flexible bronchoscopy in laser bronchoscopy: pro flexible bronchoscopic laser application. J Bronchol. 1994;1:69–71.
30. Lo TCM, Girschovich L, Lealey GA, Beamis JF, Webb-Johnson DC, Villanueva AG, et al. Low dose rate vs. high dose rate intraluminal brachytherapy for malignant endobronchial tumors. Radiother Oncol. 1995;35:193–7.
31. Dumon JF. A dedicated tracheobronchial stent. Chest. 1990;97:328–32.
32. Diaz-Jimenez JP, Munoz EF, Ballarin JIM, et al. Silicone stents in the management of obstructive tracheobronchial lesions:2-year experience. J Bronchol. 1994;1:15–8.
33. Dasgupta A, Dolmatch BL, AbipSaleh WJ, et al. Self-expandable metallic airway stent insertion employing flexible bronchoscopy: preliminary results. Chest. 1998;114:106–9.
34. Susanto I, Peters JI, Levine SM, et al. Use of balloon-expandable metallic stents in the management of bronchial stenosis and bronchomalasia after lung transplantation. Chest. 1998;114:1330–5.
35. Miyazawa T, Yamakido M, Ikeda S, et al. Implantation of ultraflex nitinol stents in malignant tracheobronchial stenosis. Chest. 2000;118:958–65.
36. Gerasin VA, Shafirovsky BB. Endobronchial electrocautery. Chest. 1988;93:270–4.
37. Van Boxem T, Muller M, Venmans B, et al. Nd:YAG laser vs. bronchoscopic electrocautery for palliation of symptomatic airway obstruction: a cost effective study. Chest. 1999;116:1108–12.
38. Coulter, Mehta AC. The heat is on: impact of endobronchial electrosurgery on the need for Nd:YAG laser photoresection. Chest. 2000; 118:516–21.
39. Homasson JF, Renault P, Angebault M, et al. Bronchoscopic cryotherapy for airway strictures caused by tumors. Chest. 1988;90:159–64.
40. Vergnon JM, Schmitt T, Alamartine E, et al. Initial combined cryotherapy and irradiation for unresectable non-small cell lung cancer: preliminary results. Chest. 1992;102:1436–40.
41. Mathur PN, Wolf KM, Busk MF, et al. Fiberoptic bronchoscopic cryotherapy in the management of tracheobronchial obstruction. Chest. 1996;110:718–23.
42. Crosta C, Spaggiari L, DeStefano A, Fiori G, Ravizza D, Pastorino U. Endoscopic argon plasma coagulation for palliative treatment of malignant airway obstructions: early results in 47 cases. Lung Cancer. 2001;33:75–80.
43. Morice RC, Ece T, Ece F, Keus L. Endobronchial argon plasma coagulation for treatment of hemoptysis and neoplastic airway obstruction. Chest. 2001; 119:781–7.
44. Menzies R, Charbonneau M. Thoracoscopy for the diagnosis of pleural disease. Ann Intern Med. 1991;114:271–6.
45. Boutin C, Viallat JR, Aelony Y. Practical thoracoscopy. Berlin; Heidelberg; New York: Springer; 1991.
46. Brandt HJ, Loddenkemper R, Mai J. Atlas of diagnostic thoracoscopy indications—Technique. New York: Thieme; 1985.
47. Lewis JW. Thoracoscopy: a surgeon's or pulmonologist's domain: pro-pulmonologist. J Bronchol. 1994; 1:152–4.
48. Faber LP. Thoracoscopy: a surgeon's or pulmonologist's domain: pro-surgeon. J Bronchol. 1994;1:155–9.
49. Palcic B, Lam S, Hung J, MacAulay C. Detection and localization of early lung cancer by imaging techniques. Chest. 1991;99: 742–3.
50. Lam S, Kennedy T, Unger M, Miller YE, Gelmont D, Rusch V, et al. Localizarion of bronchial intraepithelial neoplastic lesions by fluorescence bronchoscopy. Chest. 1998;113:696–702.
51. Hürter T, Hanrath P. Endobronchial sonography: feasibility and preliminary results. Thorax. 1992;47:565–7.
52. Shannon JJ, Bude RO, Orens JB, Becker FS, Whyte RI, Rubin JM, et al. Endobronchial ultrasound-guided needle aspiration of mediastinal adenopathy. Am J Respir Crit Care Med. 1996;153:1424–30.
53. Wang K, Brower R, Haponik E, Siegelman S. Flexible transbronchial needle aspiration for staging of bronchogenic carcinoma. Chest. 1983;84:571–6.
54. Herth F, Becker HD, LoCicero J, Ernst A. Endobronchial ultrasound in therapeutic bronchoscopy. Eur Respir J. 2002;20:118–21.
55. Miyazu Y, Miyazawa T, Kurimoto N, Iwamoto Y, Kanoh K, Hohno N. Endobronchial ultrasounography in the assessment of centrally located early-stage lung cancer before photodynamic therapy. Am J Respir Crit Care Med. 2002;165:832–7.
56. Herth FJF, Ernst A, Becker HD. Endobronchial ultrasound-guided transbronchial lung biopsy in solitary pulmonary nodules and peripheral lesions. Eur Respir J. 2002;20:972–4.
57. Kurimoto N, Miyazawa T, Okimasa S, Maeda A, Oiwa H, Miyazu Y, et al. Endobronchial ultrasonography using a guide sheath increases the ability to diagnose peripheral pulmonary lesions endoscopically. Chest. 2004;126:959–65.
58. Steinfort DP, Khor YN, Manser RL, Irving LB. Radial probe endobronchial ultrasound for the diagnosis of peripheral lung

cancer: systematic review and meta-analysis. Eur Respir J. 2011;37:902–10.
59. Krasnik M, Vilmann P, Larsen SS, Jacobsen GK. Preliminary experience with a new method of endoscopic transbronchial real time ultrasound guided biopsy for diagnosis of mediastinal and hilar lesions. Thorax. 2003;58:1083–6.
60. Yasufuku K, Chiyo M, Sekine Y, Chhajed PN, Shibuya K, Iizasa T, et al. Real-time endobronchial ultrasoundguided transbronchial needle aspiration of mediastinal and hilar lymph nodes. Chest. 2004;126:122–8.
61. Yasufuku K, Nakajima T, Chiyo M, Sekine Y, Shibuya K, Fujisawa T. Endobronchial ultrasonography: current status and future directions. J Thorac Oncol. 2007;2:970–9.
62. Herth FJF, Krasnik M, Yasufuku K, Rintoul R, Ernst A. Endobronchial ultrasound-guided transbronchial needle aspiration: how I do it. J Bronchol. 2006;13:84–91.
63. Ernst A, Anantham D, Eberhardt R, Krasnik M, Herth FJF. Diagnosis of mediastinal adenopathy—real-time endobronchial ultrasound guided needle aspiration versus mediastinoscopy. J Thorac Oncol. 2008;3:577–82.
64. Ernst A, Eberhardt R, Krasnik M, Herth FJF. Efficacy of endobronchial ultrasound-guided transbronchial needle aspiration of hilar lymph nodes for diagnosing and staging cancer. J Thorac Oncol. 2009;4:947–50.
65. Steinfort DP, Conron M, Tsui A, Pasricha SR, Renwick WEP, Antippa P, et al. Endobronchial ultrasound-guided transbronchial needle aspiration for the evaluation of suspected lymphoma. J Thorac Oncol. 2010;5:804–9.
66. Navani N, Nankivell M, Woolhouse I, Harrison RN, Munavvar M, Oltmanns U, et al. Endobronchial ultrasound-guided transbronchial needle aspiration for the diagnosis of intrathoracic lymphadenopathy in patients with extrathoracic malignancy: a multicenter study. J Thorac Oncol. 2011;6:1505–9.
67. Tremblay A, Stather DR, MacEachern P, Khalil M, Field SK. A randomized controlled trial of standard vs. endobronchial ultrasonography-guided transbronchial needle aspiration in patients with suspected sarcoidosis. Chest. 2009;136:340–6.
68. Navani N, Molyneaux PL, Breen RA, Connell DW, Jepson A, Nankivell M, et al. Utility of endobronchial ultrasound-guided transbronchial needle aspiration in patients with tuberculous intrathoracic lymphadenopathy. Thorax. 2011;66:889–93.
69. Adams K, Shah PL, Lim E. Test performance of endobronchial ultrasound and transbronchial needle aspiration biopsy for mediastinal staging in patients with lung cancer: systematic review and meta-analysis. Thorax. 2009;64:757–62.
70. Varela-Lema L, Fernandez-Villar A, Ruano-Ravina A. Effectiveness and safety of endobronchial ultrasound-transbronchial needle aspiration: a systematic review. Eur Respir J. 2009;33:1156–64.
71. Schwarz Y, Greif J, Becker HD, Ernst A, Mehta A. Real-time electromagnetic navigation bronchoscopy to peripheral lung lesions using overlaid CT images: the first human study. Chest. 2006;129:988–94.
72. Guildea TR, Mazzone PJ, Karnak D, Meziane M, Mehta AC. Electromagnetic navigation diagnostic bronchoscopy: a prospective study. Am J Respir Crit Care Med. 2006;174:982–9.
73. Asano F. Virtual bronchoscopic navigation. Clin Chest Med. 2010;31:75–85.
74. Eberhardt R, Kahn N, Gompelmann D, Schumann M, Heusel CP, Herth FJF. LungPoint—a new approach to peripheral lesions. J Thorac Oncol. 2010;5:1559–63.
75. Castro M, Rubin AS, Laviolette M, Fiterman J, DeAndrade LM, Shah PL, et al. Effectiveness and safety of bronchial thermoplasty in the treatment of severe asthma: a multicenter, randomized, doubleblind, sham-controlled clinical trial. Am J Respir Crit Care Med. 2010;181:116–24.
76. Wahidi MM, Kraft M. Bronchial thermoplasty for severe asthma. Am J Respir Crit Care Med. 2012; 185:709–14.
77. National Emphysema Treatment Trial Research Group. A randomized trial comparing lungvolume-reduction surgery with medical therapy for severe emphysema. N Engl J Med. 2003;348: 2059–73.
78. Berger RL, DeCamp MM, Criner GJ, Celli BR. Lung volume reduction therapies for advanced emphysema: an update. Chest. 2010;138:407–17.
79. Beamis JF, Shapshay SM, Setzer S, Dumon JF. Teaching models for Nd:YAG laser bronchoscopy. Chest. 1989;95:1316–8.
80. Kvale PA. Training in laser bronchoscopy and proposals for credentialing. Chest. 1990;97:983–9.
81. Pastis NJ, Nietert PJ, Silvestri GA. Variation in training for interventional pulmonary procedures among US pulmonary/critical care fellowships: a survey of fellowship diretors. Chest. 2005;127:1614–21.
82. Pastis NJ, Nierert PJ, Silvestri GA. Fellows' perspective of their training in interventional pulmonary procedures. J Bronchol. 2005;12:88–95.
83. Ernst A, Silvestri GA, Johnstone D. Interventional pulmonary procedures: guidelines from the American College of Chest Physicians. Chest. 2003;123:1693–717.
84. Gildea TR. Is a dedicated 12-month training program required in interventional pulmonology? Con: dedicated training. J Bronchol. 2004;11:65–6.
85. Feller-Kopmn D. Is a dedicated 12-month training program required in interventional pulmonology? Pro: dedicated training. J Bronchol. 2004;11:62–4.
86. Lamb CR, Feller-Kopman D, Ernst A, Simoff MJ, Sterman DH, Wahidi MM, et al. An approach to interventional pulmonary fellowship training. Chest. 2010;137:195–9.
87. Zias N, Chroneou A, Gonzalez AV, Gray AW, Lamb CR, Riker DR, et al. Changing patterns in interventional bronchoscopy. Respirology. 2009;14:595–600.
88. DuRand IA, Barber PV, Goldring J, Lewis RA, Mandal S, Munavvar M, et al. British Thoracic Society guideline for advanced diagnostic and therapeutic flexible bronchoscopy. Thorax. 2011;66: iii1–21.
89. Lee HJ, Malhotra R, Grossman C, Shepherd RW. Initial report of neodymium:yttrium-aluminumperovskite (Nd:YAP) laser use during bronchoscopy. J Bronchol Intervent Pulmonol. 2011;18:229–32.
90. Gildea TR, Downie G, Eapen G, Herth F, Jantz M, Freitag L. A prospective multicenter trial of a selfexpanding hybrid stent in malignant airway obstruction. J Bronchol. 2008;15:221–4.
91. Ernst A, Hersh CP, Herth FJF, Thurer R, LoCicero J, Beamis J, et al. A novel Instrument for the evaluation of the pleural space: an experience in 34 patients. Chest. 2002;122:1530–4.
92. Mohan A, Chandra S, Agarwal D, Naik S, Munavvar M. Utility of semirigid thoracoscopy in the diagnosis of pleural effusions: a systematic review. J Bronchol Intervent Pulmonol. 2010;17:195–201.
93. Khan MAI, Ambalavanan S, Thomson D, Miles J, Munavvar M. A comparison of the diagnostic yield of rigid and semirigid thoracoscopes. J Bronchol Intervent Pulmonol. 2012;19:98–101.
94. Janssen JP. Why do you or do not need thoracoscopy. Eur Respir Rev. 2010;19(117):213–6.
95. Michaud G, Berkowitz DM, Ernst A. Pleuroscopy for diagnosis and therapy for pleural effusions. Chest. 2010;138:1242–6.
96. Rahman NM, Ali NJ, Brown G, Chapman SJ, Davies RJ, Downer NJ, et al. Local anesthetic thoracoscopy: British Thoracic Society pleural disease guideline 2010. Thorax. 2010; 65 Suppl 2:ii54–60.

97. Islam S, Beamis JF. Autofluorescence bronchoscopy. Minerva Pneumol. 2005;44:1–16.
98. Sutedja TG, Venmans BJ, Smit EF, Postmus PE. Fluorescence bronchoscopy for early detection of lung cancer: a clinical perspective. Lung Cancer. 2001;34:157–68.
99. National Lung Cancer Screening Trial Research Team. Reduced lung-cancer mortality with low-dose computed tomographic screening. N Engl J Med. 2011;365:395–409.
100. Bulman W, Saqi A, Powell CA. Acquisition and processing of endobronchial ultrasound-guided transbronchial needle aspiration specimens in the era of targeted lung cancer chemotherapy. Am J Respir Crit Care Med. 2012;185:606–11.
101. Colt HG. Development and organization of an interventional department. Respirology. 2010;15:887–9.
102. Shah PL, Slebos DJ, Cardoso PF, et al. Bronchoscopic lung-volume reduction with exhale airway stents for emphysema (EASE trial): randomised, shamcontrolled, multicentre trial. Lancet. 2011;378(9795):997–1005.

第 2 章
经支气管肺活检

Prasoon Jain, Sarah Hadique, and Atul C. Mehta

本章提要 经支气管肺活检（TBBx）也被称为支气管镜下肺活检，它是纤维支气管镜下最重要的活检方法之一。在大多数病例中，TBBx 在门诊患者意志清醒镇静的状态下进行。TBBx 被用来从肺外周肿块、局限性或弥漫性肺浸润组织中获取标本。这个技术可以用于诊断可疑的肺癌、肺真菌和结核分枝杆菌感染、免疫抑制宿主出现不明原因肺浸润、可疑的肺结节病、肺淋巴管癌病、肺朗格汉斯细胞组织细胞增生症、淋巴管平滑肌瘤病和隐源性机化性肺炎的部分病例。TBBx 对肺移植后评估排斥反应和感染性并发症同样起到重要作用。TBBx 不宜用于特发性肺纤维化的病理学诊断，或者是区分特发性间质性肺炎的组织学分型。它对直径 < 2 cm 的肺结节的诊断率也是次优的。许多最新的技术已经被设计用以改善 TBBx 对孤立肺结节的诊断率，如带导向鞘的径向探头支气管内超声、电磁定位支气管镜和方针支气管镜定位技术。咯血和气胸是 TBBx 最主要的两个并发症，出现在不到 2% 的病例中。每一个支气管镜医师都必须能够进行 TBBx。

关键词 经支气管活检，肺癌，孤立肺结节，肿瘤-支气管关系。

引 言

TBBx 也被称为支气管镜下肺活检，它是纤维支气管镜最重要的应用之一。诊断性的 TBBx 可以避免进行开胸肺活检。虽然这个手术通常是安全的，但是 TBBx 操作时也可能发生严重的、有时甚至是致命的并发症。因此，应该在谨慎的风险—收益分析后再决定是否进行 TBBx。在这一章中，我们将会讨论经支气管活检的技术、临床应用、局限性和并发症。

技 术

TBBx 的操作对每一位支气管镜医师来说都是基本的技能。所有支气管镜医师除了要掌握技术以外，还必须对手术指征、临床应用和手术的局限性有深刻理解。同样，他们也必须准备好治疗手术的早期并发症，如出血和气胸。许多研究证实了在门诊患者意识清醒镇静的状态下进行 TBBx 的安全性[1,2]。

患者评估

在 TBBx 前进行详细的病史询问、体格检查和胸部影像学检查（胸部 X 线片和 CT）是最基本的。手术前应该和患者充分讨论 TBBx 的目的、风险和局限性。患者必须了解这个技术不能确定所有病例的诊断。常规全血细胞计数、凝血功能检查、血生化检查、动脉血气分析、肺功能检测和心电图不要求在手术前进行。是否进行这些检查应该基于个人的临床评估。举个例子，凝血机制的评估适用于有出血性倾向、接受抗凝治疗和由于肝病或肾功能不全导致的高出血风险的患者。

TBBx 的一般禁忌证在表 2.1 中列出。血小板计数低的患者应该在术前接受血小板输注，将血小板计至少增加到 50 000/mm³。我们也碰到一些患者在血小板计数超过 100 万 / mm³ 的情况下出现大出血。恢复凝血机制可能需要给予维生素 K 和新鲜冰冻血浆。没有必要停用阿司匹林[3]，但是有报道说服用氯吡格雷的患者在 TBBx 后出血率比较高[4]。因此，必须在 TBBx 前至少 5~7 天就停止服药。表 2.2 总结了 TBBx 前识别和治疗凝血病的实用方法。

因为尿毒症患者在经支气管活检后有更高的出血风险，所以当怀疑患者存在肾功能不全时要检测血肌酐。根据一个调查，大概一半的支气管镜医师认为尿毒症是经支气管活检的禁忌证[5]。特别是当尿素氮水平 >30 mg/dl 且肌酐水平 >3.0 mg/dl 时，被认为由于相关血小板的功能紊乱可能会增加 TBBx 后的出血风险。比如 1977 年的一个研究报道，45% 的免疫抑制尿毒症患者在支气管镜下肺活检后出现显著出血[6]。更有说服力的结果来自一个小型的回顾性研究，25 例患者中只有一例终末期的肾病患者（4%）有严重出血，另外有 1 例患者（4%）有少量出血[7]。相似地，在 45 例通过经支气管活检评估肺浸润的免疫抑制患者中，没有发现出血风险和肌酐升高的关联[8]。在 TBBx 前 1 小时，通过 30 分钟内静脉输注 0.3 μg/kg 去氨精氨酸加压素可以降低尿毒症患者的出血风险。同样的药物也能通过鼻腔喷雾剂的形式在手术前大概 30 分钟给药，剂量为 3 μg/kg（表 2.2）。

绝大多数支气管镜医师认为肺动脉高压是 TBBx 的绝对或相对禁忌证[5]。但是几乎没有证据表明这类患者在 TBBx 后有高出血风险。比如在一个前瞻性盲法研究中，心电图上肺动脉高压的存在不会增加 TBBx 后出血的风险[9]。但是，这个研究排除了临床上明显肺动脉高压或肺源性心脏病的患者。相似地，在一个回顾性研究中，比起 32 例对照患者，24 例伴有不同严重程度的肺动脉高压患者 TBBx 导致出血

表 2.1 经支气管活检的禁忌证

- 顽固性低氧血症
- 未纠正凝血病（表 2.2）
- 未受控制的心律失常
- 活跃的心肌缺血
- 严重肺性高血压
- 未受控制的支气管痉挛
- 患者无法配合
- 无法控制咳嗽
- 缺乏合适的患者复苏设备
- 异常血小板计数（<5 万 /mm³ 或 >100 万 /mm³）

这一并发症没有显著增加[10]。因为在这个研究中只有少数患者伴有严重的肺动脉高压，所以作者认为 TBBx 对于轻中度肺动脉高压患者是安全的。

放射性检查

对于所有患者，在 TBBx 前，X 线胸片是基本检查。常规胸部 CT 扫描也适用于局部肺浸润和疑似肺癌的患者。在这些病例中，CT 可以显示肺浸润或肿块的位置，以及它们与支气管肺段的关系，这个信息对于 TBBx 会有用[11]。一个研究报道，在人类免疫缺陷病毒感染的患者存在局限性肺浸润时，如果胸部 CT 扫描可以帮助选择活检部位，那么 TBBx 的诊断率会更高[12]。

活检钳

进行 TBBx 时相比小的活检钳，使用大的活检钳能获得更多的肺泡组织。活检标本大小的差异并不总是造成更高整体检出率或并发症[14]。大活检钳存在的问题是它难以在小的外周气道打开尖端，因此减少了获得肺实质目标肺泡标本的可能性[15]。比起同样大小的杯状钳，鳄牙钳能提供更大的肺组织标本。鳄牙

表 2.2 经支气管活检前检测和纠正凝血病的一般规则

病史和体格检查
- 已知出血或凝血障碍
- 鼻出血、点状出血、胃肠道出血、血尿和月经过多的既往史
- 先前手术期间大量出血
- 输血产品
- 肾功能不全
- 肝病
- 血液学恶性肿瘤
- 免疫抑制状态
- 药物：阿司匹林，非甾体类抗炎药（NSAIDs），氯吡格雷（Plavix），噻氯吡啶（Ticlid），普拉格雷（Prasugrel），达比加群酯（Pradaxa），利伐沙班（Xarelto），华法林，普通肝素，低分子量肝素

实验室检查（基于临床评估）
- 血小板计数
- 凝血酶原时间（PT-INR）
- 活化部分凝血活酶时间（aPTT）
- 肾功能
- 肝功能检测

特别推荐[a]
- 只有当 PT-INR<1.5、aPTT<50 秒、血小板计数 >5 万 /mm^3 时，才能进行 TBBx
- 没必要停止阿司匹林或非甾体类抗炎药
- 停止氯吡格雷、噻氯吡啶和普拉格雷 5~7 天
- 停止华法林 3 天，在检查前先检测凝血酶原时间
- 停止普通肝素 6 小时，在检查前先检测活化部分凝血活酶时间
- 停止低分子量肝素至少 12 小时
- 停止达比佳群和利伐沙班 2 天（存在肾衰竭的情况下停止更长时间）
- 如果血小板计数 <5 万 /mm^3 则输血小板，在 TBBx 前立刻检测血小板计数
- 重新考虑是否对尿毒症患者进行 TBBx。如果尿酸 >30 mg/dl、肌酐 >3 mg/dl，给予醋酸去氨加压素片：0.3 μg/kg 溶于 50 ml 生理盐水中静脉注射，持续时间 30 分钟；在检查前 60 分钟开始输液，或 TBBx 前 30 分钟给予 3 μg/kg 经鼻喷雾

注：a. 在停止抗血小板药或抗凝药前先咨询开药的内科医师（如心内科医师）。对使用标准临床指南的部分患者考虑进行过渡性治疗。与患者讨论停止抗凝药的风险

钳的尖端能撕裂组织，而杯状钳的尖端只能切开组织，因此后者获取的活检标本大小会受限制。我们在大多数情况下偏好使用鳄牙钳进行 TBBx。

透视引导

一些检查者在没有透视引导的情况下进行 TBBx[16]。但是，我们建议在透视引导下进行

活检。TBBx时X线透视的使用明显地改善了它对局限性肺浸润和肺肿块的诊断率[17]。在有或没有透视引导的情况下，TBBx对弥漫性肺浸润的诊断率是相似的。然而，在弥漫性肺浸润时，X线透视能帮助支气管镜医师选择活检的不同区域，并允许操作者对肺外周靠近胸膜表面的地方进行活检。另外，X线透视减少了TBBx时气胸的风险。TBBx时使用X线透视的主要缺点在于X线机的配备，还有患者和工作人员会暴露在辐射下[18]。没有证据表明诊断性支气管镜术时的辐射照射对于患者或支气管镜工作人员有任何长期不良作用。X线透视时间能够通过适当的训练和教学来缩短[19, 20]。然而，TBBx可以在没有透视引导的情况下成功操作。这种操作通常用于伴弥漫性肺实质疾病的重症监护患者。

活检技术

其他文献已经回顾过TBBx的技术方面的内容[21,22]。在TBBx前应该先进行彻底的气道检查，因为肺活检后的出血会阻止充分的气道检查。通过局部应用利多卡因和阿片类全身用药来充分控制咳嗽对于最佳的活检手术来说是基本的，并且能减少气胸发生的风险。

活检部位的选择依靠放射学和透视结果。任何情况下都不能在一天内同时对双侧肺进行一样的支气管镜操作，因为会有延迟的双侧气胸的风险。处理局部疾病时，TBBx区域的选择是简单的。但是在弥漫性疾病的情况下，五肺叶疾病选择TBBx的区域需要一些考虑。在后一种情况下，我们偏好对肺的重力依赖区部分进行活检，即右下肺和左下肺。在出血的情况下，血液至少在溢出到其他肺叶前先容纳在这个区域。同时，相比右侧我们更加偏好左侧，因为左侧主支气管长度更长，允许更多血流在溢出到对侧前先聚集。这也预留了更多的时间来识别和处理并发症。从反面来看，我们努力避免对右上肺叶进行活检。这一区域的出血会流向双侧肺，限制了反应的时间。

活检部位选好后，就可以将支气管镜的远端楔入特定的肺段支气管。后续步骤在透视引导下进行。助手被要求通过活检孔将活检钳放入工作通道并向前推进。当活检钳抵达纤维支气管镜远端时通常可以感到轻微阻力，对肺上叶和肺下叶上段进行TBBx时尤其明显。这是因为远侧弯曲段需要弯成一个锐角才能抵达这些肺段。在这种情况下，操作者不应该用过大的力量来推动活检钳，因为这样会破坏设备的内侧通道。操作者反而应该通过放松偏转控制杆减少弯曲段的曲度，并且轻轻地推动活检钳通过远端。虽然这个简单的策略通常会成功，但是它会失去支气管镜的楔形位置。如果这个策略不成功，那么最好的办法是将支气管镜拉回叶支气管或主支气管，并将活检钳向前推动越过支气管镜远端几厘米，让活检钳进入想要进入的亚段支气管。然后可以使用活检钳作为导丝让支气管镜成楔形位置。这个策略让活检钳进入难以抵达的支气管肺段，同时又减少了损伤支气管镜的风险。

为了在透视引导下获取弥漫性肺浸润患者的标本，活检钳要进入肺实质并朝胸膜推进，直到遇到阻力。然后将活检钳往近端拉1.5~2 cm，指示患者进行最大量的深呼吸并屏住气息。这个策略扩张了外周气道，使得活检钳的尖端能敞开。当患者屏住呼吸时，助手会被指示打开活检钳。然后患者被要求呼气，在呼气时活检钳在透视引导下轻轻地向前到达感兴趣区域，并确认活检钳尖端没有超过胸膜边缘。当患者呼吸时，活检钳向前会遇到阻力。这是由于张开的尖端卡在了呼吸道或终末细支气管的分叉处。在这一阶段，助手会被要求关闭活检钳尖端，并将其轻轻地收回。通常肺组织被切下时会有拖拽感。但是，这个感觉不能确保已经取回了好的活检标本。当活检钳被拉回时，操作者应该在透视屏上仔细地观察肺浸润性病变组织的活动。在我们的经验里，TBBx时浸润性病变组织的这种活动强烈提示了病变肺实质的成功取样。肺组织通过自然地撕下呼吸道或终末细支气管获取。拖拽收回活检钳时没必要刻意快速用力地操作。

为了从局部病灶（如肺癌）获得活检组织，活检钳要推进直到抵达肿块边缘（图2.1）。此时可以感到阻力，并且无法再推动活检钳。此时旋转C臂X线透视机来观察透视屏上活检钳和肺肿块相对位置的移动。如果通过这个策略看见活检钳远离肺肿块，那么需要重新摆放活检钳的位置。当透视机旋转时，如果肺肿块和活检钳一起活动，那么活检钳就处于好位置。在确认活检钳和肺肿块相邻后，将活检钳往后拉 0.5~1 cm，要求助手张开活检钳尖端。稳定地将张开的活检钳尖端推向肿块，通过透视屏确认活检钳和肿块之间的接触。合上活检钳并轻轻地后退。呼吸的策略在肺肿块活检时通常不需要。当退出活检钳时，重新通过透视屏观察肺肿块的活动来预计肺肿块的取样是否成功。

尽可能维持楔形位置的同时，对感兴趣区域进行进一步活检。支气管镜维持楔形的目的是使支气管镜的远端周围密封，来填塞出血源并防止血液溢出进入近端气道。在取得所有肺段的活检组织后，谨慎的办法是维持支气管镜的楔形位置至少4分钟（通常出血的时间）。此时不需要进行抽吸。

活检标本的数量

关于经支气管活检标本的最佳数量的信息比较有限。普遍地，大多数弥漫性肺病患者取 4~6 个活检标本就足够了[24]。一个研究表明，第一个标本能提供 53% 的诊断率，第 2 个标本提供 33% 的诊断率[25]。Ⅱ期和Ⅲ期结节病患者取 4~6 个 TBBx 标本能提供最佳诊断率[26]。但是，Ⅰ期结节病患者需要取 10 个活检标本来获取最大诊断率[27]。对于局限性肺外周肿块和肺感染，最少取 6 个标本，可能的话取 10 个标本[28]。在一个大型研究中，局部病灶的诊断率从 1~3 个标本的 23% 增加到 6~10 个标本的 73%[24]。

活检后透视

在手术的最后应该进行透视检查来排除气胸。患者应该在恢复室观察至少 1.5 小时。在临床情况稳定的患者进行单纯 TBBx 后，常规胸片对气胸的诊断率较低，但是它适用于经支气管活检后胸部不适、呼吸困难、大量咯血或不明原因的低氧血症等情况。

标本处理

在灭菌生理盐水中打开活检钳尖端，轻轻地摇晃钳子来采集肺活检标本。可以使用牙签

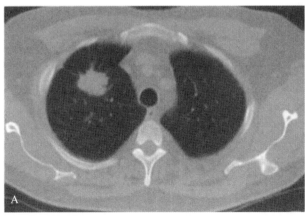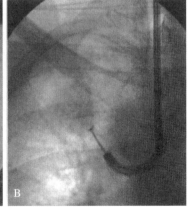

图 2.1　A. 胸部 CT 显示右上叶肺结节；B. 活检钳在透视引导下推进到病灶来获取活检

从活检钳上回收标本。出于控制感染的考虑，应该避免使用针来移动活检标本。获取所有活检标本后，如果用于常规病理检查可以通过含10%福尔马林的容器来转移标本。还需注意的是活检组织离体后应尽可能快地浸到固定液。在可能存在感染的情况下，对于1个或更多组织标本要放在乳酸林格氏液中送往微生物实验室。用于电镜、免疫染色和流式细胞术等特殊研究的活检标本，应该在与接收的病理实验室协商好后再进行采集和运输。

活检标本的质量

TBBx手术时很难去评估活检的质量和充分性。来自TBBx手术的组织碎片大小通常在1~3 mm。由于标本较小，TBBx在评估一些疾病进程时存在固有的局限性。如间质性肺纤维化的病理诊断要求识别肺实质的典型结构改变。

有时候活检得到的组织主要是支气管黏膜，而肺泡组织可能很少甚至没有。这种情况通常发生在对肺近端区域进行TBBx时。当然，很少或没有肺泡组织的活检标本提供不了关于肺实质病理进程的有用信息。有人认为带有肺泡组织的肺活检标本更容易漂浮在10%的福尔马林液体上，并且比起不含肺泡组织的标本，它更能代表病理改变。举个例子，在一个研究中发现，比起不含肺泡组织的标本，含有肺泡组织的TBBx标本更容易漂浮在10%的福尔马林液体上，并且在患有结节病的患者中，包含非干酪性肉芽肿的标本比不含的标本更容易漂浮[29]。但是，漂浮这一现象的实用价值仍然不确定，因为另一个有更多异质性患者数量的研究不能重复这些结果[25]。另外，更近端的活检会导致更多出血，而太远端的活检会增加气胸的风险。

大多数病理医师认为肾活检标本至少要包含5个肾小球才是合格的。而对于TBBx却没有这样的共识。一个组提议TBBx标本包含20个或更多的肺泡才是合格的，因为它比含肺泡少的标本更容易检测出肺部感染[30]。但是，这个观点没有在其他疾病（如肺恶性肿瘤）的诊断上被证实，大多数专家还是相信TBBx的诊断率与获取标本的数量关系更加密切，而不是每个活检标本中肺泡的数量。

经支气管肺活检的临床应用

对各种肺部疾病的合理诊断和治疗都需要进行肺活检。用于诊断的肺组织标本可以通过TBBx、CT引导下的细针抽吸术以及视频辅助的胸腔镜或肺活检手术获取。除了极少的特例，手术肺活检是获取间质性肺病患者肺组织的金标准，但是它有损伤性、价格高、要求全麻和住院治疗。CT引导下的细针抽吸术的使用主要限定在肺外周结节和肿块，该手术获取的标本通常不能够诊断良性疾病的进展。接近1/4的患者会在CT引导下的细针抽吸术后出现气胸，10%的患者需要放置胸导管[31]。相比之下，TBBx的临床应用范围更广，并发症发生率更低，并且手术能在门诊支气管镜室内、患者意识清醒镇静状态下安全操作。支气管镜也最适合获取连续的肺活检组织。

对各种有潜在疾病的异质性患者进行TBBx时存在的诊断率问题，许多大的病例系列分析已经解决[24,32-36]。虽然TBBx在70%~90%的病例中能提供合格的肺标本，但是仍有很大比例的患者无法获得特异性诊断。特异性诊断的整体检出率变化很大，依赖标本的大小、位置、肺浸润的程度和潜在肺部疾病的本质。TBBx的结果也依赖于支气管镜医师的经验和技术。分析关于TBBx的诊断率的文献时要特别小心，因为大多数作者将非特异性纤维化或机化性肺炎病例包括到诊断率中，只有少数作者在对TBBx的标本进行病理分析时使用了更严格的标准。TBBx的非特异结果通常没有帮助，并且会导致错误的临床决策。能够通过TBBx得到明确诊断的肺部疾病列在表2.3中。在弥漫性肺部疾病中，TBBx 更有可能明确结节病和淋巴管癌病等疾病的诊断，而不是肺血管炎和特发性肺纤维化这类弥漫性肺病，因为诊断特发性肺纤维化的基础是低倍镜下的整体结构。TBBx 用于诊断肺朗格汉斯细胞组织细胞增生症和淋巴管平滑肌瘤病是可靠的，但由于取样误差的原因诊断率会比较低。所以，如果在这些情况下有典型的组织学发现，就能够明确诊断，但是如果没有也不能排除诊断。下面会讨论 TBBx 在特定情况下的诊断作用。

肺癌

纤维支气管镜是诊断周围型肺癌最常用的技术。通常为了诊断率的最大化，会在这些患者上联合使用支气管冲洗液细胞学检查、毛刷涂片、TBBx 和 P-TBNA 这些取样技术。根据一个循证评价，纤维支气管镜在 16 例周围型肺癌的诊断中提供了 36%~88%、平均 78% 的诊断结果[37]。TBBx 是诊断周围型肺癌最常用的取样方法。TBBx 对周围型肺癌的诊断率为 17%~77%，平均为 57%。当联合支气管冲洗液细胞学检查和毛刷涂片一起操作时，TBBx 为接近 19% 的患者提供排除诊断[38]。当除了这些取样方法外还进行 P-TBNA 时，TBBx 为 7% 的患者提供排除诊断。

虽然 CT 引导下的细针抽吸术也是可选的诊断方法，纤维支气管镜下 TBBx 能诊断出 30%~40% 的肺上沟瘤[39,40]。TBBx 对淋巴管癌病患者有较高的诊断率[41,42]。虽然 TBBx 诊断转移性肺肿瘤效果的数据有限，但是一项研究表明 12 例患者中只有 2 例（17%）能通过活检获得诊断组织[43]。

TBBx 对肺癌的诊断率随着活检标本数量的增加而上升。在一项研究中，只获取 1~3 个 TBBx 标本时诊断率为 21%，而获取 6~10 个标本时诊断率为 78%[24]。另一项研究中，诊断率从单一标本的 45% 升高到多个标本的 70%[28]。基于这些研究，从这些患者中获取 6~10 个 TBBx 标本时，能得到最佳诊断率。

病灶的大小是最影响支气管镜诊断周围型肺癌敏感性的因素。来自 10 项研究的合并数据表明，直径 <2 cm 病灶的诊断率是 34%，≥2 cm 的病灶诊断率为 63%[37]。因为位于肺外 1/3 的 ≤2 cm 的病灶诊断率较低，一些作者建议使用 CT 引导下的细针抽吸术等替代方法来获取诊断组织[44]。

肿瘤-支气管关系也会影响 TBBx 对周围型肺癌的诊断率。Tsuboi 等检查了 47 例患者手术切除的标本，并识别出 4 种肿瘤-支气管关系的类型：Ⅰ型，支气管在肿瘤内保持通畅；Ⅱ型，支气管在肿瘤内部被截断；Ⅲ型，支气管被压迫、狭窄或被肿瘤代替，但是支气管黏膜

表 2.3 经支气管活检适用的肺部疾病

恶性肿瘤
- 肺癌
- 肿瘤转移

感染
- 肺结核
- 非结核性分枝杆菌感染
- 真菌感染
- 肺孢子虫肺炎
- 病毒感染，如巨细胞病毒性肺炎

急性肺移植排斥反应

机械通气患者中未诊断肺浸润

弥漫性肺病
- 结节病
- 淋巴管癌病
- 肺泡蛋白沉积症
- 肺朗格汉斯细胞组织细胞增生症
- 肺泡微石病
- 淀粉样变
- 淋巴管平滑肌瘤病
- 闭塞性细支气管炎伴机化性肺炎

完整；Ⅳ型，黏膜下和支气管旁肿瘤扩张、纤维化或淋巴结肿大引起近端支气管狭窄[45]（图2.2）。作者还提到超过60%的直径＜3 cm的肿瘤只累及1个支气管，然而接近60%的直径＞3 cm的肿瘤累及3个或更多支气管[45]。高分辨率的胸部CT以其高精确度证明了不同类型肿瘤-支气管关系的存在[46]（图2.3）。

CT上支气管标志是指一个支气管直接通向外周肺肿块或支气管包含在肺肿块的内部而被截断[47]。当这个支气管标志不存在时，支气管镜对外周病灶的诊断率为0~44%；而当它存在时，诊断率为60%~82%[46-50]。比起包括TBBx在内的传统取样方法，P-TBNA术获取Ⅲ型和Ⅳ型肿瘤-支气管关系外周肿块的诊断组织成功率更高[51]。在一项研究中，P-TBNA术获取了26例存在Ⅲ型和Ⅳ型肿瘤-支气管关系的患者中20例（77%）的病灶诊断组织，而TBBx只获取了其中的5例（19%）[48]。P-TBNA术对于存在Ⅲ型和Ⅳ型肿瘤-支气管关系的病灶有更高的成功率，可能和TBNA活检针能穿透错位的支气管壁，或是能绕过变细的和狭窄的支气管段到达肿瘤核心有关，而使用标准的TBBx活检钳就不能（图2.4）。

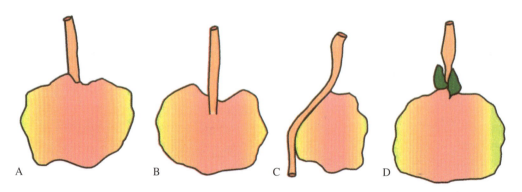

图2.2 肿瘤-支气管关系。A. Ⅰ型：支气管在肿瘤内保持通畅；B. Ⅱ型：支气管在肿瘤内部被截断；C. Ⅲ型：支气管被压迫、狭窄或被肿瘤代替，但是支气管黏膜完整；D. Ⅳ型：黏膜下和支气管旁肿瘤扩张、纤维化或淋巴结肿大引起近端支气管狭窄

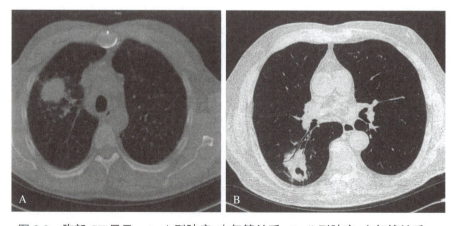

图2.3 胸部CT显示。A. Ⅰ型肿瘤-支气管关系；B. Ⅱ型肿瘤-支气管关系

第1篇 概述

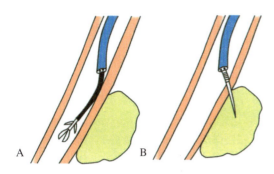

图 2.4　A. 活检钳偏离Ⅲ型肿瘤-支气管关系的病灶；B. 可见经支气管活检针穿透支气管壁，并且从肿瘤获取标本

肺部感染

不可吸收性肺炎

纤维支气管镜通常用来对不可吸收性肺炎进行进一步评估[52]。在这些情况下 TBBx 能提供有用信息。比如说，在一项研究中 TBBx 能为 57% 的患社区获得性肺炎而抗生素治疗失败的患者提供诊断[53]。TBBx 标本能证明是分枝杆菌感染还是真菌感染，还能通过标本组织诊断出其他类似肺炎的情况，如细支气管肺泡癌（原位腺癌）、隐源性机化性肺炎和过敏性肺炎。检查空洞性病变时，能从空洞壁获取活检可以增加检测出潜在肺病变的机会（图 2.5）。

结核病

纤维支气管镜通常用于涂阴肺结核患者。大多数情况下，支气管冲洗液细胞学检查、支气管肺泡灌洗和 TBBx 联合诊断，能使诊断率最大化。TBBx 能快速确诊 17%~60% 的活跃肺结核患者[54-57]，并且对其中 10%~20% 的患者来说这是诊断标本的唯一来源[58-60]。TBBx 也能快速诊断粟粒性肺结核。另外，在很大比例的患者中，TBBx 能诊断出其他类似结核的疾病，如肺癌和真菌性感染。所以，对痰检阴性的肺结核患者进行支气管镜检查时，选择 TBBx 在任何时候都是明智的。

非结核分枝杆菌

非结核分枝杆菌感染比较难明确诊断，因为非结核分枝杆菌会间歇性地出现在痰中。另外，痰中出现非结核分枝杆菌通常更可能认为是呼吸道寄生或污染，而非真的感染[61]。

通常需要纤维支气管镜伴 TBBx 检查来证实这些病例的诊断。根据现有的美国胸科协会/美国感染病协会的指南，在合适的临床背景下，非结核分枝杆菌的诊断要求至少有 1 项下列微生物学指标：①至少 2 个不同的痰标本出现细菌培养阳性；②至少 1 次支气管冲洗液或灌洗液细菌培养检查阳性；③经支气管活检发现肉芽肿样感染、抗酸杆菌染色阳性、非结核分枝

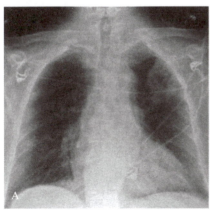 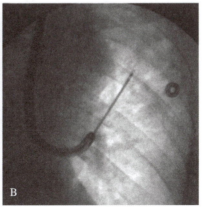

图 2.5　A. 胸部影像显示 1 例免疫抑制患者左上肺叶空洞型病灶；B. 从空洞型病灶壁获取经支气管活检标本

杆菌细菌培养或分枝杆菌组织学特征阳性、1个或多个痰标本或支气管冲洗液非结核分枝杆菌细菌培养阳性[62]。

真菌性感染

支气管冲洗和支气管肺泡灌洗是诊断肺部真菌感染的最有价值的支气管镜方法[63-66]。这些患者额外加上TBBx能轻度改善诊断率[67-69]。任何需要进行纤维支气管镜的时候，我们会常规对疑似肺真菌感染的患者进行TBBx。

免疫抑制宿主中的感染（非HIV）

免疫抑制宿主会受到大范围严重的甚至威胁生命的条件性肺感染。纤维支气管镜下进行支气管肺泡灌洗能提供接近2/3患者的诊断信息，伴随的手术相关并发症最小。虽然支气管肺泡灌洗的诊断价值是明确的，但是在这些患者中采用TBBx替代治疗和改善预后的作用是存在争论的。TBBx能提供15%~68%的伴有肺浸润免疫抑制患者的诊断信息[8,70-80]。不幸的是，TBBx会造成严重的手术相关并发症，这限制了它在这些患者中的应用。

在一个前瞻性研究中，Stover等对97例存在肺浸润的免疫抑制患者进行了支气管镜检查[70]。支气管肺泡灌洗能诊断出92例患者中的61例（66%），而TBBx能诊断出57例患者中的36例（63%），两者联合诊断率为83%。我们对104例存在肺浸润的免疫抑制患者进行了支气管镜检查[8]。对这些患者中的45例进行了TBBx。支气管镜整体检出率是56%。TBBx能提供38%患者的特定诊断。支气管肺泡灌洗和TBBx的联合诊断率（70%）比起单独使用支气管肺泡灌洗的诊断率（38%）更好。在这项研究中，TBBx排除诊断13%的病例，并且比起支气管肺泡灌洗，TBBx更容易检测出免疫抑制宿主中肺浸润的非感染性原因。虽然TBBx手术后31%的患者出现手术相关并发症，但是没有出现手术相关死亡。在一项大型的回顾性研究中，Cazzdori等回顾了他们对142例伴肺浸润的免疫抑制患者进行TBBx的经验[72]。最终结果，TBBx和支气管肺泡灌洗的诊断率分别是68%和36%。只有3例患者出现气胸，1例患者出现出血。

尽管如此，这些患者中TBBx的局限性必须提到。首先，不是所有的研究都表明TBBx对伴有肺浸润的免疫抑制患者的诊断有用。比如在一个回顾性研究中，White等回顾了52例伴肺浸润的骨髓移植患者的支气管镜结果。总共进行了68次支气管镜检查[81]。其中有42次在进行支气管肺泡灌洗外，还进行了TBBx。在这项研究中只有1次额外的诊断是只通过TBBx做的。15%的患者出现并发症。在另一项研究中，71例造血干细胞移植的患者进行了TBBx[82]。82%的患者的病理结果是非特异的。进行检查的患者获得特异诊断的比例<10%。8%的患者出现了并发症。这些数据对伴随肺浸润的骨髓移植患者常规进行TBBx的价值提出了疑问。

另外，大多数需要支气管镜检查的免疫抑制患者都比较危重，并且相关的共存性疾病让他们出现手术相关并发症的风险变高[8]。在许多情况下，出于安全考虑不对这些患者进行TBBx。研究表明TBBx的并发症发生率比支气管肺泡灌洗更高。因此在一些报道中可以清楚地看到，出于安全考虑大多数免疫抑制患者不进行TBBx[83-85]。

同时，对伴有肺浸润的免疫抑制患者进行TBBx时，常常报道出非特异性炎症和纤维化。临床医生分析这些非特异性结果时需要小心。一些作者发现经支气管镜肺活检的非特异性发现对不可治疗的病情有预测价值。例如在一项研究中，在35例进行TBBx的患者中16例（48%）给出了特异性诊断[86]。余下得到非特异性组织学结果的患者大多要么表现出临床上和影像学上的改善，要么存在不可治疗的疾病。作者报道TBBx对可治疗的条件性感染的敏感度为84%、特异性为100%。然而，其他人有不同经历，并且认为对伴有肺浸润的免疫抑制患者进行TBBx的非特异性发现不能排除肺部可治愈性感染和可治疗的非感染性疾病[87]。所以如果在伴有肺浸润的免疫抑制患者中 TBBx 得到非特异性结果，那么进行一个彻底的临床回顾是必要的。这种情况通常考虑进行手术肺活检。报道的手术肺活检对伴有肺浸润的免疫抑制患者的诊断率为 46%~85%[88-96]。对这些患者的手术肺活检可以显示非感染性疾病，如恶性肿瘤、淋巴瘤、药物毒性反应和隐源性机化性肺炎，也可以显示感染性疾病，如卡氏肺孢子虫肺炎、军团菌肺炎、巨细胞病毒性肺炎、侵袭性曲霉病、革兰阴性肺炎、诺卡氏菌病和肺弓形虫病。许多这类疾病可以通过一系列合理治疗得到解决。所以，当 TBBx 无法诊断或患者在经验性治疗后没有改善时，应该考虑进行手术肺活检[97]。

HIV 感染患者中的感染

感染人类免疫缺陷病毒（HIV）的患者出现肺部并发症非常普遍。纤维支气管镜在对 HIV 感染的肺部并发症的诊断和合理治疗上有重要作用[98]。最近随着抗病毒治疗的进步，肺部感染的发生率和诊断性支气管镜检查的需要显著减少。但是在资源匮乏的地区，肺部并发症仍然对伴 HIV 感染的患者造成严重威胁。一个在获得性免疫缺陷综合征流行早期进行的大型回顾性研究表明，91% 的肺部感染可以通过支气管肺泡灌洗和 TBBx 联合诊断[99]。随后的研究报道，支气管肺泡灌洗和 TBBx 联合检查的诊断率为 65%~96%[100-104]。Stover 等对 72 例患获得性免疫缺陷综合征的患者进行支气管肺泡灌洗和 TBBx[100]。支气管镜为 65% 的患者提供了诊断。纤维支气管镜对肺孢子虫肺炎的诊断率为 94%，巨细胞病毒性肺炎为 67%，鸟型结核分枝杆菌感染为 62%。在这个病例系列中，TBBx 比支气管肺泡灌洗更有用的地方在于它对肺孢子虫肺炎的诊断。Broaddus 等报道了 171 例患获得性免疫缺陷综合征的患者在纤维支气管镜下进行支气管肺泡灌洗和 TBBx 的结果[102]。支气管镜的整体检出率为 96%。支气管肺泡灌洗和 TBBx 的诊断率分别为 86% 和 87%。支气管肺泡灌洗和 TBBx 对肺孢子虫肺炎的诊断率分别为 89% 和 93%。TBBx 是 11% 的患者唯一的诊断方法。9% 的患者手术后出现气胸，6% 的患者需要放置胸导管。因为支气管肺泡灌洗有高诊断率，而 TBBx 跟并发症的出现有关，所以作者总结认为支气管镜检查后存在高并发症风险的患者应该避免进行 TBBx。一项卢旺达的研究报道了一些不同的结果，该研究对 111 例伴有不明病因肺浸润的 HIV 感染患者做纤维支气管镜检查，并且进行支气管肺泡灌洗和 TBBx[103]。在这项研究中，支气管肺泡灌洗诊断出 26% 的患者，而 TBBx 诊断出 82% 的患者。对研究中患者最终的诊断 38% 为非特异性间质性肺炎、23% 为肺结核、13% 为肺隐球菌病、9% 为卡波西肉瘤、5% 为肺孢子虫病。16% 的患者的诊断仍然不清楚。TBBx 和支气管肺泡灌洗分别是 74% 的患者和 18% 的患者的唯一诊断来源。13% 的患者出现并发症，其中 5% 的患者出血、8% 的气胸。这个病例系列中支气管肺泡灌洗的低诊出率明显是因为这个研究中患者肺孢子虫病的发生率低。

TBBx 为 58% 的患有 AIDS 相关非霍奇金淋巴瘤的患者提供诊断材料[105]。相比之下，TBBx 在肺卡波西肉瘤中的应用有限，通常需要手术肺活检进行诊断[100,106,107]。在一些报道中，伴肺浸润的 HIV 感染患者基于 TBBx 可以诊断出非特异性间质性肺炎[108,109]。非特异性间质性肺炎的诊断是基于组织学证据，包括弥漫性肺泡损伤、合并肺泡隔慢性炎症和支气管肺泡灌洗液染色、细菌培养或组织病理学检查未发现微生物病原体。许多这类患者在经验性治疗后会表现出临床上和影像学上的改善。

一些检查者质疑伴肺浸润的 HIV 感染患者常规进行 TBBx 的价值[110]。这个结论主要基于一些患者大多患卡氏肺孢子虫肺炎的研究。相反的是，当分析纤维支气管镜用于伴有多种肺部并发症的 HIV 感染患者时，TBBx 明显改善了整体检出率。甚至在卡氏肺孢子虫肺炎中，一些作者发现联合支气管肺泡灌洗和 TBBx 时，纤维支气管镜的诊断率得到显著改善。比如在最近的一项研究中，支气管肺泡灌洗对卡氏肺孢子虫肺炎患者的诊断率为74%，而支气管肺泡灌洗和TBBx的联合诊断率为95%[111]。TBBx同时也增加了纤维支气管镜检查对需接受雾化喷他脒预防患者的诊断率，而支气管肺泡灌洗的诊断率就明显较低[112]。如果可行的话，我们建议纤维支气管镜检查伴有肺浸润的HIV感染患者时同时应用支气管肺泡灌洗和TBBx。

面对支气管肺泡灌洗和TBBx无法诊断的HIV感染患者时，对手术肺活检所处的争议很大。手术肺活检通常用于肺浸润病因未明，或者依据纤维支气管镜的诊断进行对症治疗无效时。在一项研究中，66例符合适应证进行手术肺活检的患者中，只有1例改变了治疗方案[113]。其他研究报道了更理想的结果，对仔细挑选的患者进行手术肺活检后，很大比例的患者改变了治疗方案[114,115]。在一个病例系列中，总共进行42例手术肺活检，其中所有4例没经过支气管镜检查的患者获得有用诊断，18例支气管肺泡灌洗和TBBx无法诊断的患者中13例得到诊断，11例支气管肺泡灌洗无法诊断的患者中8例得到诊断，但是9例依据纤维支气管镜的诊断进行对症治疗后仍然恶化的患者中只有1例得到诊断[116]。基于这些研究，作者不支持对已经接受适当治疗、情况仍然恶化的患者进行手术肺活检。我们强烈建议在决定对这些患者进行手术肺活检前，能有一位HIV医学领域专家的参与。

肺移植

TBBx在肺移植患者的长期治疗中起重要作用。对TBBx在肺移植受体中作用的详细讨论不是本章的范围，读者可以参考最近的综述来了解细节[117,118]。我们简要地强调一些重点。

在许多医疗中心里，虽然传统TBBx通常被用来监测无症状肺移植受体，但是它们的作用仍然有争议。许多研究发现用经支气管肺活检进行监测是一个高诊断率的方法。在一项早期的研究中，43例肺移植受体进行了90次经支气管肺活检监测。57%的检查发现了排斥反应或感染的特定组织学特征[119]。在另一项研究中，在5年里230例肺移植受体进行了836次TBBx检查[120]。19%的检查发现了急性排斥反应、淋巴细胞性细支气管炎或感染的组织学特征。肺移植后4~12月TBBx检查监测急性移植排斥的诊断率为6.1%。另一项研究报道了124例肺移植受体进行的353次支气管镜监测手术的临床作用[121]。据报道，一直到肺移植后1年临床上重视的急性排斥反应仍然有较高的发生率。

与之相反，其他研究没有发现支气管镜监测和TBBx在肺移植受体中的好处[122-124]。比如在一个研究中对比了24例经历支气管镜监测的肺移植受体和23例由于特定临床指征进行支气管镜检查的患者的预后[125]。47例患者总共进行了240次TBBx。支气管镜监测没有检测出任何需要治疗干预的急性排斥反应。两组患者间没有发现呼吸道感染、急性排斥反应、闭塞性毛细支气管炎或生存期上的显著差异。

临床上评估肺移植受体发生可疑的急性排斥反应或肺部感染时，纤维支气管镜和TBBx报道的结果更加理想。实际上，TBBx是诊断可疑急性排斥反应的诊断方法之一[126]。TBBx诊断这种情况的敏感性和特异性分别为94%和90%[127]。大多数移植中心至少获取这类患者6~10个令人满意的经支气管活检标本[128]。

临床上进行支气管镜下TBBx的原因有：第一秒用力呼气容积下降>10%；用力呼气25%~75%肺活量时的平均流速下降>20%；影像学发现浸润；临床疑似感染；呼吸道症状。支气管镜下TBBx对这些患者的诊断率较高，如果根据临床指征进行检查，这种方法的诊断率接近70%[119,129]。除了检测急性排斥反应外，纤维支气管镜下支气管肺泡灌洗和TBBx还是诊断和监测肺移植患者呼吸道感染的重要手段。比如在一个研究中，51%存在临床指征的纤维支气管镜检查和12%的支气管镜监测中诊断出感染[130]。必须提到的是这个研究中对大多数感染的诊断基于支气管镜肺泡灌洗标本。

TBBx也被用来对急性排斥反应治疗后患者进行随访。许多研究表明，尽管早期进行了合适治疗，但是相当多患者仍然出现持续的排斥反应[119,129,131]。在一项研究中，TBBx随访发现26%的患者持续存在急性排斥反应[132]。支气管镜下支气管肺泡灌洗和TBBx也被报道对伴有单个或多个肺结节的患者诊断率为74%[133]。

纤维支气管镜下TBBx同样也适用于慢性排斥反应的患者，但是TBBx检测闭塞性细支气管炎的敏感性较低，而这是慢性排斥反应的特征性组织学改变[134,135]。纤维支气管镜在这些病例中的主要价值在于排除气道并发症、肺部感染和急性排斥反应。TBBx的另一个价值在于预测未来闭塞性细支气管炎综合征的风险。急性排斥反应是明确的闭塞性细支气管炎综合征的危险因素[136]。最近的研究提示，多个经支气管活检发现的最小的急性排斥反应（A1级）也跟发生闭塞性细支气管炎综合征的高风险相关[137]。最近的研究也明确经支气管活检发现的淋巴细胞性细支气管炎是发生闭塞性细支气管炎综合征和死亡的危险因素，并且独立于肺移植受体的急性排斥反应[138]。淋巴细胞性细支气管炎也跟肺移植受体急性细胞性排斥反应的发生和严重程度有关[139]。

机械通气患者中的经支气管肺活检

纤维支气管镜下支气管肺泡灌洗通常用于伴有弥漫性肺浸润的机械通气患者。手术安全，并能为大多数患者提供有用的诊断信息。出于安全考虑，TBBx很少用于机械通气患者。比如在一个前瞻性研究中，147例机械通气患者进行支气管镜检查时只有7例进行了TBBx[140]。现有的数据很少支持TBBx在机械通气患者中的准确临床作用。Papin等在15例需要机械通气的患者中进行了TBBx[141]。TBBx为15例患者中的5例（33%）提供了诊断，并改变了7例患者的治疗。3例患者出现自限性出血，1例患者出现迟发性气胸。Pincus等在13例机械通气患者中进行了TBBx[142]。TBBx明确了13例患者中6例（46%）的特异性诊断。这个检查被认为对所有13例患者的治疗有提示作用。术后2例患者出现气胸。Bulpa等在38例机械通气患者中进行了纤维支气管镜下支气管肺泡灌洗和TBBx[143]。所有研究对象都存在不明原因肺浸润。TBBx能明确74%病例的诊断，更改63%患者的治疗方法。术后的并发症为9例气胸（23%）和4例自发性出血（11%）。在迄今为止最大的病例系列中，O'Brien等报道了71例机械通气患者TBBx的结果[144]。35%的患者得到了特异性组织学诊断，41%的患者改变了治疗方案。TBBx的结果也导致了26%肺移植受体的重要治疗改变。TBBx的结果和对13例患者手术肺活检或尸检获得的结果中的11例相似。术后14%的患者发生气胸。

按照传统，手术肺活检用于诊断不明肺浸润的危重患者。手术肺活检为45%~65%的患者提供诊断信息[145,146]。这些结果导致接近70%的患者出现重要治疗改变。但是，手术肺活检比起TBBx侵犯性更强，并发症发生率至少为20%。在一项研究中，机械通气患者进行手术肺活检的死亡率为8.4%。TBBx可能更安全些，但是也有许多重要的问题需要进一步澄清。TBBx应该作为常规步骤，或是当最初的纤维支气管镜下支气管肺泡灌洗无法诊断时再进行，TBBx的结果是否改变了患者预后？只有通过设计良好的前瞻性研究才能回答这些问题。

弥漫性肺病

结节病

支气管镜下TBBx适用于疑似结节病的患者。在一些报道中，TBBx能诊断出90%~95%的结节病患者[26,147]。TBBx对结节病的诊断率随着影像学分期而改变，Ⅰ期为50%~65%，Ⅱ期为63%~82%，Ⅲ期为80%~85%[148-150]。纤维支气管镜要获得最佳的诊断率，Ⅰ期结节病要获取10个活检标本[27]，Ⅱ期和Ⅲ期要获取4~6个标本[26]。结节病通常会累及支气管黏膜，支气管内活检的诊断率比TBBx增加20%[148,151]。在TBBx加上经支气管针吸活检[148,150,152]或支气管内超声-经支气管针吸活检[153]也能提高支气管镜对结节病的诊断率。

肺朗格汉斯细胞组织细胞增生症

虽然临床特征和高分辨率CT结果能强烈地提示这个诊断，但是疑似肺朗格汉斯细胞组织细胞增生症的患者通常需要组织学确认。手术肺活检仍然是这一诊断的金标准。但是，在一些情况下可以通过TBBx得到的独特组织学特征来明确诊断。报道的TBBx对肺朗格汉斯细胞组织细胞增生症的诊断率为10%~40%[154,155]。肺朗格汉斯细胞组织细胞增生症患者的肺部病变通常散在分布，由此导致的取样误差是TBBx低诊断率的原因。因此，对TBBx没有发现典型的组织学特征不应该下最终诊断，而应该进行手术活检进行进一步评估。对TBBx标本进行CD1a和S100蛋白免疫细胞化学染色，如果朗格汉斯细胞存在，进一步支持诊断。吸烟者会观察到假阳性的免疫细胞化学结果。所以，对这些标记物的染色应该只在组织学检查与肺朗格汉斯细胞组织细胞增生症一致的活检标本中进行[156]。用CD1a抗体对支气管肺泡灌洗液中的朗格汉斯细胞进行染色，如果数量增加>5%也支持肺朗格汉斯细胞组织细胞增生症的诊断[157]。

淋巴血管平滑肌肉增生症

手术肺活检通常用来明确淋巴血管平滑肌肉增生症的诊断[158]。经支气管活检能够诊断部分淋巴血管平滑肌肉增生症病例，但是要小心的是，肺实质中异常增生的平滑肌细胞可能会被解释为纤维化。免疫组化研究表明异常增生的平滑肌细胞HMB-45单克隆抗体染色阳性。TBBx标本雌激素受体和HMB-45染色阳性，强烈支持淋巴血管平滑肌肉增生症的诊断[159,160]。

隐源性机化性肺炎

隐源性机化性肺炎的病理学标志是终末及呼吸性细支气管和肺泡管肉芽组织增生，伴随肺泡的机化和周围间隙的慢性炎症改变[161]。需要胸腔镜或手术肺活检获取大的肺组织标本来明确诊断，并排除其他类似隐源性机化性肺炎的情况[162]。在一些情况下TBBx足以进行诊断[163-165]。Poletti等对32例可疑隐源性机化性肺炎患者进行TBBx[165]。TBBx的敏感性、特异性、阳性预测值和阴性预测值分别是64%、86%、94%和40%。虽然对最理想的方法仍然有争议，但是一些该领域的权威专家建议患者在接受侵犯性更强的方法前先进行TBBx[166]。然而，如果行TBBx后诊断仍不明确，或是口服糖皮质激素效果不明显时，则必须进行手术肺活检。

过敏性肺炎

过敏性肺炎基本上是一个临床诊断，不需要常规的组织学检查确认。偶尔出现全面的临床评估后仍然不能明确诊断的情况时，可以进行肺活检。亚急性过敏性肺炎常见的组织学三联征是细胞性细支气管炎、慢性炎症细胞的弥漫性间质浸润和形成欠佳的散在非坏死性肉芽肿。这些结果通过手术肺活检能得到最好的证明[167]。但是，TBBx能够对一些急性[168]和亚急性过敏性肺炎[169]的病例提供诊断标本。慢性过敏性肺炎不容易通过TBBx诊断[156]。

其他

经支气管活检是疑似淋巴管癌病的诊断方法之一[41,42,170]。在患肺泡蛋白沉积症的患者中，TBBx可以发现典型的肺泡蛋白沉积症阳性肺泡浸润[171]。相似地，TBBx是诊断弥漫性肺淀粉样变的初始步骤[172]。TBBx能够为疑似类脂性肺炎和肺泡微石症的患者提供诊断材料[173]。

经支气管活检的局限性

弥漫性肺病的低诊断率

在大多数弥漫性肺病的情况下，TBBx的非特异性结果不能得出确定的病理学诊断[174]。一个普遍的例子是特发性肺纤维化，它的病理性诊断主要基于活检标本的结构紊乱，而这个结果无法通过TBBx确认。一项研究回顾了22例特发性肺纤维化患者的TBBx结果,判断普通型间质性肺炎的诊断是否成立[175]。除了1例患者外,几乎所有手术肺活检后的患者都诊断为普通型间质性肺炎。在检查许多单个患者的TBBx标本后,检查者报道22例患者中的7例(30%)可以通过TBBx诊断。但是,这个研究存在严重缺陷,因为分析的病理医师已经知道了手术肺活检的结果。在一项更早的研究中,Wall等对33例患弥漫性浸润疾病、而经支气管活检结果非特异或无法诊断的患者进行了手术肺活检[176]。手术肺活检提供了92%的患者的特异性诊断。手术活检标本和TBBx的结果没有关联。比如,21例TBBx报道为正常肺或非特异性结果的患者中,9例手术肺活检诊断为特发性肺纤维化。9例TBBx认为存在特发性肺纤维化的患者,手术肺活检确认只有2例。TBBx没有诊断出有肺朗格汉斯细胞组织细胞增生症和结节病的9例患者。在另一项研究中,大多数TBBx诊断为非特异性慢性间质性炎症和纤维化的患者,表现出疾病发展或消退的过程与活检提示的疾病自然进程相反[177]。总之,TBBx不能被用来诊断普通型间质性肺炎,或是将它从特发性肺纤维化的其他组织学亚型中区分出来,如非特异性间质性肺炎[178]。目前基于指南的证据不推荐特发性肺纤维化患者进行TBBx[179]。

经支气管活检偶尔可以诊断出肺出血-肾炎综合征(Goodpasture综合征)、韦格纳肉芽肿病和变应性肉芽肿性血管炎(Churg-Strauss综合征)[180,181]。但是,大多数患者不能通过经支气管活检明确这些诊断。比如在一项研究中,虽然19例患者中的17例能通过经支气管活检获得足够肺泡,但是只有2例患者能通过组织学结果明确诊断为韦格纳肉芽肿病[182]。大多数患者报道为非特异性结果。相应地,通常建议用手术肺活检来诊断肺血管炎。相似地,矽肺、石棉肺、胶原血管病和药物毒性肺病等职业性肺病导致的肺弥漫性浸润也要求必须在组织诊断的时候进行手术肺活检。

TBBx标本中体积小的和伪组织[183]会给分析的病理医师造成相当大的诊断问题。为了获取更大的组织标本,一些检查者近来用柔性冷刀获取TBBx标本。在一项研究中,41例弥漫性肺病患者经历了标准的TBBx,然后在同一处肺段进行了冷刀活检[184]。这项研究中所有进行手术的患者在支气管镜检查前都插入了气管导管。检查者用2.4 mm的柔性冷刀获取活检组织。冷刀通过纤维支气管镜的工作通道进入,并在透视引导下推进到感兴趣区域,离胸壁10 mm的距离。探头冷却大约4秒后,和冷冻的肺组织一起退出。冷刀标本在组织玻片上中央区域的大小是15.22 mm^2,而标准经支气管活检为5.82 mm^2。检查者在冷刀活检标本上没有发现伪组织。10例进行冷刀活检的患者能明确诊断为非特异性间质性肺炎。但是,这项研究中的任何患者都没有经手术肺活检确认。冷刀活检后没有明显出血。这个结果和另外一组对15例弥漫性肺病患者报道的结果相似[185]。这些研究提供了有用的柔性冷刀的初步数据,以及关于如何获取更大组织标本,且又不存在破碎组织的可行性问题。目前需要前瞻性研究来调查冷刀活检对弥漫性肺病诊断的准确性,可以用手术肺活检作为参考标准。

孤立肺结节的低诊断率

明确孤立肺结节的组织诊断是呼吸科最困难的挑战之一。传统纤维支气管镜下TBBx的方法对这些患者的诊断率比较低。比如直径<2 cm的肺结节,有10个研究的数据表明纤维支气管镜平均诊断率为11%~76%、平均值为34%[37]。最近一项研究根据多变量分析发现,纤维支气管镜从肺结节获取诊断组织标本的独立预测因子是恶性病因(比值比4.8)、直径>2 cm(比值比3.6)和阳性支气管体征(比值比2.4)。这个结果再次强调了肿块大小和支气管体征可作为传统支气管镜诊断率的重要决定因素[186]。孤立肺结节的良性病因很少能通过经支气管活检明确。孤立肺结节的恶性病因不能根据支气管镜和经支气管活检结果阴性排除。TBBx 在孤立肺结节中诊断率低主要由于两个原因：①透视下不能看见病灶[187]；②在肿瘤-支气管关系不理想的情况下，无法将活检钳送到靶位置。

最近几年做了许多尝试来减少传统支气管镜检查方法的局限性，设法从外周结节中获取组织样本。特别是一些先进的技术被设计用来解决从小的肺结节中活检取样时碰到的困难。比如说，CT 透视和径向支气管内超声检查已经被用来在获取活检标本前改善病灶成像的可能性。虚拟支气管镜定位和电磁导航支气管镜已经用来帮助支气管镜医师选择最合适的路径到达活检靶位置。超薄支气管镜使得支气管镜在操作者的直接控制下能到达第七到第九级支气管，再加上电磁导航支气管镜使用的可引导探头和径向支气管内超声使用的双关节刮匙都改善了检查的操作性。在许多情况下，联合使用前面提及的技术已经被用来最大化从直径小于2~3 cm 的外周病灶获取诊断组织的机会。

许多研究调查了使用 CT 透视引导从外周肺结节获取活检标本的可行性。它的主要优势是能在横轴面定位活检钳，并且能直观确认活检钳和病灶是否接触[188]。在一项研究中，CT 透视引导下 TBBx 能正确诊断 12 例患者中的 8 例（67%），他们的外周病灶平均直径为 2.2 cm[189]。在另一项研究中，因为病灶直径<15 mm，所以 CT 透视引导下 TBBx 能明确 45 例患者中 22 例（49%）的诊断。相比之下，传统透视引导只能诊断 26 例患者中的 3 例（12%）[190]。与之相反，在最近的一项随机研究中，没有发现 CT 透视引导下 TBBx 的诊断敏感性与传统透视引导有差异[191]。在这个研究中，只有 33% 大小≤3 cm 的病灶能够通过 CT 引导下或传统透视引导下的 TBBx 诊断出。

在 CT 透视下进行传统支气管镜检查还存在许多问题。能够对病灶进行成像并不确保检查者能够操作活检设备到达靶位置。同时，在 CT 室进行支气管镜检查会造成手术排程和后期供养的困难。支气管镜通常对患者和操作者都是一次不愉快的体验，并且 CT 室可能装备不良，无法治疗严重的支气管镜相关并发症。可能最重要的缺陷是患者和操作者会有辐射过多的风险。根据目前的估计，CT 透视造成的患者辐射量是传统透视方法的 2~5 倍[189,191]。随着经导向鞘引导的支气管内超声检查（EBUS-GS）和 VBN 这类中等辐射替代方法的出现，再为了定位而使用 CT 透视就和临床上辐射合理化和优化使用的指导原则直接冲突[192]。

近来许多研究明确了 EBUS-GS 能用于活检钳定位肺小结节（第四章）。在一项研究中，使用 EBUS-GS 从 150 例存在外周病灶的患者中获取了 116 例（77%）患者的诊断组织[193]。虽然病灶大小>3 cm 时的诊断率（92%）显著高于病灶大小≤3 cm 时（74%）的，但是检查者也能明确 81 例病灶大小≤2 cm 的患者中 59 例（73%）的诊断。另外，检查者能明确 54 例病灶大小≤2 cm、不能借助透视定位的患者中 40 例（74%）的诊断。在一个前瞻性随机研究中，在 221 例患者中对比了 EBUS-GS 引导下和传统透视方法引导下的 TBBx 诊断率的区别[194]。对于患肺癌的患者，EBUS-GS 组（79%）比标准 TBBx 组（55%）诊断敏感性显著升高。在一个亚组分析中，两种技术对>3 cm 病灶的诊断敏感性相似。但是，EBUS-GS 对直径<3 cm（75% vs. 31%）和直径<2 cm（71% vs. 23%）病灶的诊断敏感性显著高于标准 TBBx 技术。

EBUS-GS 的主要优势是对那些传统透视方法不可见病灶的活检。比如说在一项前瞻性研究中，检查者能获得 54 例患者中 38 例（70%）的组织诊断，这些患者病灶直径平均为 2.2 cm，并且在透视下不可见[187]。这项技术的另一个优势在于它能够使用穿入导向鞘的双关节刮匙，来增加活检设备到达靶病灶的定位能力[193]。这个技术通常被用在支气管内超声不能定位病灶的病例中。

这个技术的一些局限性也必须被提到。首先，不是所有研究都得出对直径<2 cm 孤立肺结节的高诊断率。比如在一项研究中，对 100

例肺结节直径<2 cm 的患者进行 EBUS-GS 引导下 TBBx[195]。检查者能够用支气管内超声定位其中 67 例患者（67%）的病灶，并获取 46 例患者（46%）的诊断组织。相似地，在另一项研究中，EBUS-GS 引导下 TBBx 对直径>2 cm 外周病灶的诊断率为 76%，但是对直径≤2 cm 病灶的诊断率只有 30%[196]。另外，最近一项包含 246 例患者的随机试验没有发现 EBUS-GS 组（36%）和传统支气管镜组（44%）的癌症检出率有任何差异[197]。实际上在这项研究中，对于直径<3 cm 的病灶，透视引导下传统 TBBx 的诊断率高于 EBUS-GS 引导的活检。这项技术在报道结果中的一些变异可能和手术操作者的经验和培训有关。

电磁导航支气管镜（ENB）是一个影像引导的定位系统，它能够在纤维支气管镜检查时实时引导活检设备到达小的外周病灶（第 6 章）。许多研究报道了使用这项技术从小的外周病灶中获取活检标本，结果鼓舞人心。在一项前瞻性研究中，来自诊所的检查者报道了对 54 例外周病灶平均直径为 2.28 cm 患者的诊断率为 74%[198]。这项研究中 31 例病灶直径≤2 cm 患者中的 23 例（74%）被明确诊断。在许多其他研究中，对所有大小病灶的整体检出率范围为 63%~84%，对直径≤2 cm 病灶的检出率为 50%~76%[199-203]。ENB 对伴有 CT 支气管征的病灶的诊断率高于不存在明显指征的[202]。该技术表现出一个陡峭的学习曲线[203]。这项技术的劣势在于无法实时确认活检标本是否从病灶获取。另一些劣势在于设备的高成本和手术时使用的一次性配件的高费用。

虚拟支气管镜定位作为一种重要的方法出现，它能帮助支气管镜精确定位，使活检设备到达小的外周病灶（第 7 章）。在这项技术中，支气管树的虚拟图像通过 CT 的数据进行重建，模仿真实的支气管镜检查。在虚拟支气管镜图像上展现出最合适的到达靶病灶的经支气管途径，帮助检查者操作支气管镜到达通往靶病灶的正确气道。除了定位的功能外，最新的放置支气管镜定位系统能使图像旋转，并且能向前向后模拟实际的支气管镜图像。在大多数的病例系列中，检查者结合虚拟支气管镜定位和超薄支气管镜，来达到尽可能靠近病灶的目的。在一些研究中，活检可以在 CT 透视下[204]和其他标准透视引导下进行[205]。联合超薄支气管镜使用虚拟支气管镜定位进行 TBBx 的整体检出率范围是 63%~82%，对直径≤2 cm 外周病灶的诊断率在不同研究中的范围是 62%~82%[206-209]。在支气管镜检查时应用这项技术不需要额外的辐射照射或昂贵的配件。但是，借助超薄支气管镜可以获取最好的结果，虽然它通常不常见。另外，大多数关于虚拟支气管镜定位应用的数据来自对这项技术高度熟悉的检查者。

为了进一步改善支气管镜检查对小的肺外周结节的诊断率，许多最新的研究将电磁导航支气管镜或虚拟支气管镜定位系统用来定位支气管镜、用配件将它们靠近靶位置，并且在获取活检标本前用径向支气管内超声确认到达靶位置。使用这种多模态方法报道的结果非常鼓舞人。Eberhardt 等在一项前瞻性随机试验中研究了 ENB 和 EBUS-GS 联合使用的有效性[210]。39 例患者只使用 EBUS-GS 进行活检。39 例患者只使用 ENB，40 例患者联合使用 EBUS-GS 和 ENB。ENB 合并 EBUS-GS 引导的检查诊断率为 88%，显著高于 EBUS-GS（69%）或 ENB（52%）引导的诊断率。在另一项研究中，Asano 等研究了虚拟支气管镜定位、超薄支气管镜（BF-P260F，外径 4.0 mm，工作通道 2.0 mm，Olympus）和 EBUS-GS 联合使用获取 32 例外周病灶标本的诊断率[211]。总共 32 例病灶中的 27 例（84%）可以获得诊断标本，24 例直径≤3 cm 病灶中 22 例（79%）可以获得。来自这项研究的初步结果被最近的一项随机试验证实，试验中 199 例外周病灶直径≤3 cm 的患者被随机分配进行虚拟支气管镜定位合并 EBUS-GS（n=102）或单独进行 EBUS-GS（n=97）[212]。虚拟支气管镜定位合并 EBUS-GS 组诊断率（80%）显著高于 EBUS-GS 组（67%）。

对于直径＜2 cm病灶的诊断率联合方法为76%，单独EBUS-GS为59%。毋庸置疑，对一些透视引导下传统TBBx无法诊断的病灶，应用多项先进技术能够增加获取活检标本的能力。不幸的是，这些技术当中许多是昂贵的，因此在将它们整合进常规临床实践前需要充分的性价比研究。

CT引导下细针抽吸术仍是诊断肺外周结节常用的方法。它的诊断敏感性是90%（范围65%~94%），但是它和15%~43%的气胸相关（中位数27%），其中4%~18%的病例（中位数5%）需要放置胸导管[213]。CT引导下细针抽吸术的诊断敏感性依赖于病灶大小。当病灶直径＜2 cm时，CT引导下细针抽吸术的诊断敏感性范围是74%~77%，术后气胸风险是22%~28%[214,215]。在这些患者中，上面讨论的先进支气管镜技术提供了一些更安全、气胸风险更低的替代方法，而它们的诊断率和CT引导下细针抽吸术相似或更高。

经支气管活检并发症

TBBx通常比较安全，但是偶尔也会出现严重的甚至危及生命的手术相关并发症。根据最近日本的一个全国调查，对肺外周病灶进行活检后并发症的发生率是1.79%[216]。相对地，来自一个大学附属医院的对173例手术的回顾得出TBBx的并发症发生率为6.8%[217]。TBBx最常见的两个并发症是出血和气胸。

经支气管活检后报道的出血发生率在不同病例系列中的范围是0~26%。1%~2%经过经支气管活检的患者出现严重出血[1,218]。在免疫抑制患者和潜在肾功能不全患者中，出血的风险明显更高[6,8,81]。TBBx后由于出血不受控制导致的死亡非常罕见，但是也有可能是没有报道。在之前提到的日本的调查中，57 199例患者中的0.85%在TBBx后出现显著出血，但是没有死亡病例[216]。

经支气管活检后的出血并发症会使人紧张，但是大多数情况下出血能够在支气管镜室得到控制，没有出现严重结果[219]。经支气管活检后出血的主要危险是血被吸入未出血肺段，而不是失血的风险。所以，最紧急的措施是防止大量血流入气道。一旦发现显著出血，立刻倾斜支气管镜台让流血侧受限制。控制出血最有效的办法是维持楔形位置，覆盖出血部位直到形成凝血块。有时候，当拉出活检钳时无法维持楔形位置。在这些情况下，支气管镜检查医师应该尽最大努力尽快将支气管镜放回支气管。一些情况下，由于血液会模糊支气管镜视野，所以可能需要透视引导。维持支气管镜楔形位置大概5分钟后轻轻退出。如果看到突然的大量出血，支气管镜医师应该随时准备好重新恢复楔形位置。由于血液的稀释效应和远端出血，TBBx后使用冷生理盐水灌洗液或局部应用稀释的肾上腺素通常不能成功控制出血。如果采取局部措施后仍然持续出血，或是支气管镜已经滑出了出血部位，最好的选择是通过气管插管来保证气道通畅，并且考虑进行球囊填塞或对侧肺选择性置管。硬质支气管镜设备应该准备好随时治疗纤维支气管镜无法控制的出血发作。咯血的治疗在第14章中进一步讨论。

经支气管活检后1%~6%的患者报道出现气胸[1,24,220]。经支气管活检时没有控制咳嗽会极大地增加气胸的风险。接受正压机械通气的患者在经支气管活检后发生气胸的可能性也会更大。存在大泡性肺气肿和肺孢子虫肺炎患者的风险也可能更高[102]。经支气管镜活检时合理的透视引导会减少气胸的风险。透视检查能在活检后立刻发现气胸，但是在一些情况下，在手术完成后会缓慢出现迟发性气胸[1]。经支气管活检后张力性气胸非常常见。但是由于潜在的肺部受限，一些经历纤维支气管镜检查的患者轻度到中度的气胸可能会引起不成比例的症状。如果在手术后4小时没有出现症状，就不大可能出现临床上显著的气胸。当临床上怀疑气胸时，即使活检后立刻进行的透视结果正常，也应该在活检完成后半小时到 1 小时进行胸部平片。症状的严重度和胸部平片的范围决定了支气管镜检查后气胸的治疗。吸氧和住院观察在大多数情况下是足够的。中等症状的显著气胸患者可以通过在支气管镜套件里放置 Heimlich 瓣膜治疗。这些患者在放置 Heimlich 瓣膜观察 4~6 小时后,如果重复胸片发现气胸没有加重就可以出院。出现严重症状的张力性气胸患者和那些放置 Heimlich 瓣膜后气胸没有缓解的患者,就需要放置胸导管。当机械通气患者出现气胸时,也应该尽快放置胸导管。

结 论

经支气管活检是每个支气管镜医师的基本技能。经支气管活检通常在门诊室内患者意志清醒镇静的状态下进行。一个成功的 TBBx 可以避免手术肺活检的需要,后者侵犯性更强,并且需要全麻。TBBx 最普遍的指征是为了从肺外周肿块中获取活检标本。TBBx 对周围型肺癌的诊断率依赖于肿瘤的大小和是否存在支气管体征。TBBx 也能用于评估疑似肺结核、真菌感染、免疫抑制宿主和肺移植后不明原因肺浸润的患者,对肺移植患者同时可以监测和评估排斥反应或条件性感染。在非感染性疾病中,TBBx 最常用于结节病、淋巴管癌病和肺郎格汉斯细胞组织细胞增生症与淋巴管平滑肌瘤病的诊断。经支气管活检不能用于特发性肺纤维化的组织学诊断和区分特发性间质肺炎的组织学亚型。它对直径小于 2~3 cm 肺结节的诊断率也不理想。许多最新的技术,像 EBUS-GS、ENB 和虚拟支气管镜定位技术已经被用来提高 TBBx 对孤立肺结节的诊断率。咯血和气胸是 TBBx 的两大并发症,发生率 < 2%。我们相信所有的支气管镜医师都必须提高 TBBx 的水平,并且能治疗手术引起的并发症。

参考文献

1. Ahmad M, Livingston DR, Golish JA, Mehta AC, Wiedemann HP. The safety of outpatient bronchoscopy. Chest. 1986;90:403–5.
2. Blasco LH, Hernandez IMS, Garrido VV, et al. Safety of the transbronchial biopsy in outpatients. Chest. 1991;99:562–5.
3. Herth FJF, Becker HD, Ernst A. Aspirin does not increase bleeding complications after transbronchial biopsy. Chest. 2002;12q2:1461–4.
4. Ernst A, Eberhardt R, Wahidi M, Becker HD, Herth FJF. Effect of routine clopidogrel use on bleeding complications after transbronchial biopsy in humans. Chest. 2006;129:734–7.
5. Wahidi MM, Rocha AT, Hollingsworth JW, Govert JA, Feller-Kopman D, Ernst A. Contraindications and safety of transbronchial biopsy via flexible bronchoscopy. Respiration. 2005;72:285–95.
6. Cunningham JH, Zavala DC, Corry RJ, Keim LW. Trephine air drill, bronchial brush, and fiberoptic transbronchial lung biopsies in immunosuppressed patients. Am Rev Respir Dis. 1977;115:213–20.
7. Mehta NL, Harkin TJ, Rom WN, Graap W, Addrizzo-Harris DJ. Should renal insufficiency be a relative contraindication to bronchoscopy biopsy? J Bronchol. 2005;12:81–3.
8. Jain P, Sandur S, Meli Y, Arroliga AC, Stoller JK, Mehta AC. Role of flexible bronchoscopy in immunocompromised patients with lung infiltrates. Chest. 2004;125:712–22.
9. Morris MJ, Peacock MD, Mego DM, Johnson JE, Anders GT. The risk of hemorrhage from bronchoscopic lung biopsy due to pulmonary hypertension in interstitial lung disease. J Bronchol. 1998;5:117–21.
10. Diaz-Guzman E, Vadi S, Minai OA, Gildea TR, Mehta AC. Safety of diagnostic bronchoscopy in patients with pulmonary hypertension. Respiration. 2009;77:292–7.
11. Naidich DP, Harkin TJ. Airway and lung: correlation of CT with fiberoptic bronchoscopy. Radiology. 1995;197:1–12.
12. Cadranel J, Gillet-Juvin K, Antoine M, et al. Site directed bronchoalveolar lavage and transbronchial biopsy in HIV-infected patients with pneumonia. Am J Respir Crit Care Med. 1995;152:1103–6.
13. Loube DI, Johnson JE, Weiner D, Andres GT, Blanton HM, Hayes JA. The effect of forceps size on the adequacy of specimens obtained by transbronchial biopsy. Am Rev Respir Dis. 1993;148:1411–3.
14. Wang KP, Wise RA, Terry PB, et al. Comparison of standard and large forceps for transbronchial lung biopsy in the diagnosis of lung infiltrates. Endoscopy. 1980;12:151–4.
15. Smith LS, Seaquist M, Schillaci RF. Comparison of forceps used for transbronchial lung biopsy. Bigger may not be better. Chest. 1985;87:574–6.
16. Milligan SA, Luce JM, Golden J, Stulbarg M, Hopewell PC. Transbronchial biopsy without fluoroscopy in patients with diffuse roentgenographic infiltrates and the acquired immunodeficiency syndrome. Am Rev Respir Dis. 1988;137:486–8.
17. Cox ID, Bagg LR, Russell NJ, et al. Relationship of radiologic position to the diagnostic yield of fiberoptic bronchoscopy in bronchial carcinoma. Chest. 1984;85:519–22.
18. Jain P, Fleming P, Mehta AC. Radiation safety for the health care workers in bronchoscopy suite. Clin Chest Med. 1999;20:33–8.
19. Ernst A, Smith L, Gryniuk L, et al. A simple teaching intervention

significantly decreases radiation exposure during transbronchial biopsy. J Bronchol. 2004;11:109–11.
20. Jain P, Mehta AC. Infection control and radiation safety in the bronchoscopy suite. In: Wang KP, Mehta AC, Turner JF editors. Flexible bronchoscopy. 3rd ed. Oxford: Wiley-Blackwell, 2012. p. 6–31.
21. Kvale PA. Bronchoscopic lung biopsy. How I do it. J Bronchol. 1994;1:321–6.
22. Zavala DC. Transbronchial biopsy in diffuse lung disease. Chest. 1978;73:727S–33.
23. Frazier WD, Pope TL, Findley LJ. Pneumothorax following transbronchial biopsy. Low diagnostic yield with routine chest roentgenograms. Chest. 1990;97:539–40.
24. Descombes E, Gardiol D, Leuenberger P. Transbronchial lung biopsy: an analysis of 530 cases with reference to the number of samples. Monaldi Arch Chest Dis. 1997;52:324–9.
25. Curley FJ, Johal JS, Burke ME, Fraire AE. Transbronchial lung biopsy. Can specimen quality be predicted at the time of biopsy? Chest. 1998; 113:1037–41.
26. Gilman MF, Wang KP. Transbronchial biopsy in sarcoidosis. An approach to determine the optimal number of biopsies. Am Rev Respir Dis. 1980;122:721–4.
27. Rothe RA, Fuller PB, Byrd RB, et al. Transbronchial lung biopsy in sarcoidosis. Optimal numbers and sites for biopsy. Chest. 1980;77:400–2.
28. Popovich Jr J, Kvale PA, Eichenhorn MS, Radke JR, Ohorodnik JM, Fine G. Diagnostic accuracy of multiple biopsies from flexible fiberoptic bronchoscopy. A comparison of central versus peripheral carcinoma. Am Rev Respir Dis. 1982;125:521–3.
29. Anders GT, Linville KC, Johnson JE, Blanton HM. Evaluation of float sign for determining adequacy of specimens obtained with transbronchial biopsy. Am Rev Respir Dis. 1991;144:1406–7.
30. Fraire AE, Cooper SP, Greenberg SD, Rowland LP, Langston C. Transbronchial lung biopsy. Histopathologic and morphometric assessment of diagnostic utility. Chest. 1992;102:748–52.
31. Wu CC, Maher MM, Shepard JA. Complications of CT-guided percutaneous needle biopsy of the chest: prevention and management. AJR Am J Roentgenol. 2011;196:678–82.
32. Andersen HA. Transbronchial lung biopsy for diffuse pulmonary disease. Results in 939 patients. Chest. 1978;73:734S–6.
33. Ellis JH. Transbronchial lung biopsy via the fiberoptic bronchoscope. Experience with 107 consecutive cases and comparison with bronchial brushing. Chest. 1975;68:524–32.
34. Hanson RR, Zavala DC, Rhodes ML, Keim LW, Smith JD. Transbronchial biopsy via flexible bronchoscope: results in 164 patients. Am Rev Respir Dis. 1976;114:67–72.
35. Mitchell DM, Emerson CJ, Collins JV, Stableforth DE. Transbronchial lung biopsy with the fiberoptic bronchoscope: analysis of results in 433 patients. Br J Dis Chest. 1981;75:258–62.
36. Zellweger JP, Leuenberger PJ. Cytologic and histologic examination of transbronchial lung biopsy. Eur J Respir Dis. 1982;63:94–101.
37. Rivera MP, Mehta AC. Initial diagnosis of lung cancer. ACCP evidence-based clinical practice guidelines. 2nd edition. Chest. 2007;132:131S–48.
38. Mazzone P, Jain P, Arroliga AC, Matthay RA. Bronchoscopic and needle biopsy techniques for diagnosis and staging of lung cancer. Clin Chest Med. 2002;23:137–58.
39. Maxfield RA, Aranda CP. The role of fiberoptic bronchoscopy and transbronchial biopsy in the diagnosis of Pancoast's tumor. NY State J Med. 1987; 87:326–9.
40. Miller JI, Mansour KA, Hatcher Jr CR. Carcinoma of the superior pulmonary sulcus. Ann Thorac Surg. 1979;28:44–7.
41. Torrington KG, Hooper RG. Diagnosis of lymphangitic carcinomatosis with transbronchial biopsy. South Med J. 1978;71:1487–8.
42. Aranda C, Sidhu G, Sasso LA, Adams FV. Transbronchial lung biopsy in the diagnosis of lymphangitic carcinomatosis. Cancer. 1978; 42:1995–8.
43. Mohsenifar Z, Chopra SK, Simmons DH. Diagnostic value of fiberoptic bronchoscopy in metastatic pulmonary tumors. Chest. 1978;74:369–71.
44. Baaklini WA, Reinoso MA, Gorin AB, Sharafkaneh A, Manian P. Diagnostic yield of fiberoptic bronchoscopy in evaluating solitary pulmonary nodules. Chest. 2000;117:1049–54.
45. Tsuboi E, Ikeda S, Tajima M, et al. Transbronchial biopsy smear for diagnosis of peripheral pulmonary carcinomas. Cancer. 1967;20:687–98.
46. Gaeta M, Barone M, Russi EG, et al. Carcinomatous solitary pulmonary nodule: evaluation of tumor bronchi relationship with thin-section CT. Radiology. 1993;187:535–9.
47. Naidich DP, Sussman R, Kutcher WL, Aranda CP, Garay SM, Ettenger NA. Solitary pulmonary nodules. CT-Bronchoscopic correlation. Chest. 1988;93:595–8.
48. Bilaceroglu S, Kumcuoglu Z, Alper H, et al. CT-bronchus sign guided bronchoscopic multiple diagnostic procedures in carcinomatous pulmonary nodules and masses. Respiration. 1998;65:49–55.
49. Gaeta M, Pandolfo I, Volta S, et al. Bronchus sign on CT in peripheral carcinoma of the lung. Value in predicting results of transbronchial biopsy. AJR Am J Roengenol. 1991;157: 1181–5.
50. Gaeta M, Russi EG, La Spada F, et al. Small bronchogenic carcinomas presenting as solitary pulmonary nodules. Bioptic approach guided by CT-positive bronchus sign. Chest. 1992; 102:1167–70.
51. Shure D, Fedullo PF. Transbronchial needle aspiration of peripheral masses. Am Rev Respir Dis. 1983;128:1090–3.
52. Feinsilver SH, Fein AM, Niederman MS, Schultz DE, Faegenburg DH. Utility of fiberoptic bronchoscopy in nonresolving pneumonia. Chest. 1990;98:1322–6.
53. Arancibia F, Ewig S, Martinez JA, et al. Antimicrobial treatment failures in patients with community acquired pneumonia: causes and prognostic implications. Am J Respir Crit Care Med. 2000;162:154–60.
54. Wallace JM, Deutsch AL, Harrell JH, Moser KM. Bronchoscopy and transbronchial biopsy in evaluation of patients with suspected active tuberculosis. Am J Med. 1981;70:1189–94.
55. Danek SJ, Bower JS. Diagnosis of pulmonary tuberculosis by flexible fiberoptic bronchoscopy. Am Rev Respir Dis. 1979;119:677–9.
56. Charoenratanakul S, Dejsomritrutai W, Chaiprasert A. Diagnostic role of fiberoptic bronchoscopy in suspected smear negative pulmonary tuberculosis. Respir Med. 1995;89:621–3.
57. Tamura A, Shimada M, Matsui Y, et al. The value of fiberoptic bronchoscopy in culture positive pulmonary tuberculosis patients whose pre-bronchoscopic sputum specimen were negative both for smear and PCR analyses. Intern Med. 2010;49:95–102.
58. Kennedy DJ, Lewis WP, Barnes PF. Yield of bronchoscopy for the diagnosis of tuberculosis in patients with human immunodeficiency virus infection. Chest. 1992;102:1040–4.
59. Chan CHS, Chan RCY, Arnold M, Cheung H, Cheung SW, Cheng AFB. Bronchoscopy and tuberculostearic acid assay in the diagnosis of sputum negative pulmonary tuberculosis: a retrospective study with the addition of transbronchial biopsy. Q J Med. 1992;82:15–23.
60. Salzman SH, Schindel ML, Aranda CP, Smith RL, Lewis ML. Role of bronchoscopy in the diagnosis of pulmonary tuberculosis in patients at risk for HIV infection. Chest. 1992;102:143–6.

61. Jett JR, Cortese DA, Dines DE. The value of bronchoscopy in the diagnosis of mycobacterial disease. A five-year experience. Chest. 1981;80:575–8.
62. Griffith DE, Aksamit T, Brown-Elliot BA, et al. An official ATS/IDSA statement: diagnosis, treatment and prevention of nontuberculous mycobacterial diseases. Am J Respir Crit Care Med. 2007;175:367–416.
63. Sabonya RE, Barber RA, Wiens J, et al. Detection of fungi and other pathogens in immunocompromised patients by bronchoalveolar lavage in an area endemic for coccidioidomycosis. Chest. 1990;97:1349–55.
64. Patel RG, Patel B, Petrini MF, Carter RR, Griffith J. Clinical presentation, radiographic findings, and diagnostic methods of pulmonary blastomycosis: a review of 100 consecutive cases. South Med J. 1999; 92:289–95.
65. Martynowicz MA, Prakash. Pulmonary blastomycosis: an appraisal of diagnostic techniques. Chest. 2002;121:768–73.
66. Malabonga VM, Basti J, Kamholz SL. Utility of bronchoscopic sampling techniques for cryptococcal disease in AIDS. Chest. 1991;99:370–2.
67. Wallace JM, Catanzaro A, Moser KM, Harrell JH. Flexible fiberoptic bronchoscopy for diagnosing pulmonary coccidioidomycosis. Am Rev Respir Dis. 1981;123:286–90.
68. Salzman SH, Smith RL, Aranda CP. Histoplasmosis in patients at risk for the acquired immunodeficiency syndrome in a nonendemic setting. Chest. 1988;93:916–21.
69. DiTomasso JP, Ampel NM, Sobonya RE, Bloom JW. Bronchoscopic diagnosis of pulmonary coccidioidomycosis. Comparison of cytology, culture, and transbronchial biopsy. Diagn Microbiol Infect Dis. 1994;18:83–7.
70. Stover DE, Zaman MB, Hajdu SI, et al. Bronchoalveolar lavage in the diagnosis of diffuse pulmonary infiltrates in the immunosuppressed host. Ann Intern Med. 1984;101:1–7.
71. Eriksson B-M, Dahl H, Wang F-Z, et al. Diagnosis of pulmonary infections in immunocompromised patients by fiberoptic bronchoscopy with bronchoalveolar lavage and serology. Scand J Infect Dis. 1996;28:479–85.
72. Cazzadori A, Di Perri G, Todeschini G, et al. Transbronchial biopsy in the diagnosis of pulmonary infiltrates in immunocompromised patients. Chest. 1995;107:101–6.
73. Matthay RA, Farmer WC, Odero D. Diagnostic fiberoptic bronchoscopy in the immunocompromised host with pulmonary infiltrates. Thorax. 1977; 32:539–45.
74. Puska S, Hutcheon MA, Hyland RH. Usefulness of transbronchial biopsy in immunosuppressed patients with pulmonary infiltrates. Thorax. 1983;38:146–50.
75. Springmeyer SC, Silvestri RC, Sale GE, et al. The role of transbronchial biopsy for the diagnosis of diffuse pneumonias in immunocompromised marrow transplant recipients. Am Rev Respir Dis. 1982;126:763–5.
76. Feldman NT, Pennington JE, Ehrie MG. Transbronchial lung biopsy in the compromised host. JAMA. 1977;238:1377–9.
77. Nishio JN, Lynch III JP. Fiberoptic bronchoscopy in the immunocompromised host: the significance of a nonspecific transbronchial biopsy. Am Rev Respir Dis. 1980;121:307–12.
78. Pennington JE, Feldman NT. Pulmonary infiltrates and fever in patients with hematologic malignancy. Assessment of transbronchial biopsy. Am J Med. 1977;62:581–7.
79. Shelhamer JH, Towes GB, Masur H, et al. Respiratory disease in the immunosuppressed patient. Ann Intern Med. 1992;117:415–31.
80. Mulabecirovic A, Gaulhofer P, Auner HW, et al. Pulmonary infiltrates in patients with hematological malignancies: transbronchial lung biopsy increases the diagnostic yield with respect to neoplastic and toxic pneumonitis. Ann Hematol. 2004; 83:420–2.
81. White P, Bonacum JT, Miller CB. Utility of fiberoptic bronchoscopy in bone marrow transplant patients. Bone Marrow Transplant. 1997;20:681–7.
82. Patel NR, Lee PS, Kim JH, Weinhouse GL, Koziel H. The influence of diagnostic bronchoscopy on clinical outcomes comparing adult autologous and allogenic bone marrow transplant patients. Chest. 2005;127:1388–96.
83. Peikert T, Rana S, Edell ES. Safety, diagnostic yield and therapeutic implications of flexible bronchoscopy in patients with febrile neutropenia and pulmonary infiltrates. Mayo Clin Proc. 2005;80:1414–20.
84. Shannon VR, Andersson BS, Lei X, Champlin RE, Kontoyiannis DP. Utility of early versus late fiberoptic bronchoscopy in the evaluation of new pulmonary infiltrates following hemopoietic stem cell transplantation. Bone Marrow Transplant. 2010; 45:647–55.
85. Dunagan DP, Baker AM, Hurd DD, Haponik EF. Bronchoscopic evaluation of pulmonary infiltrates following bone marrow transplantation. Chest. 1997; 111:135–41.
86. Poe RH, Utell MJ, Israel RH, Hall WJ, Eshleman JD. Sensitivity and specificity of non-specific transbronchial lung biopsy. Am Rev Respir Dis. 1979; 119:25–31.
87. Nisho JN, Lynch JP. Fiberoptic bronchoscopy in the immunocompromised host: the significance of a non-specific transbronchial biopsy. Am Rev Respir Dis. 1980;121:307–12.
88. Canham EM, Kennedy TC, Merrick TA. Unexplained pulmonary infiltrates in the compromised patient. An invasive investigation in a consecutive series. Cancer. 1983;52:325–9.
89. Kramer MR, Berkman N, Mintz B, et al. The role of open lung biopsy in the management and outcome of patients with diffuse lung disease. Ann Thorac Surg. 1998;65:198–202.
90. White DA, Wong PW, Downey R. The utility of open lung biopsy in patients with hematologic malignancies. Am J Respir Crit Care Med. 2000; 161:723–9.
91. Jaffe JP, Maki DG. Lung biopsy in immunocompromised patients: one institution's experience and an approach to management of pulmonary disease in the compromised host. Cancer. 1981;48:1144–53.
92. Catterall JR, Mccabe RE, Brooks RG, et al. Open lung biopsy in patients with Hodgkin's disease and pulmonary infiltrates. Am Rev Respir Dis. 1989; 139:1274–9.
93. Cockerill III FR, Wilson WR, Carpenter HA, et al. Open lung biopsy in immunocompromised patients. Arch Intern Med. 1985;145:1398–404.
94. Leight Jr GS, Michaelis LL. Open lung biopsy for the diagnosis of acute, diffuse pulmonary infiltrates in the immunosuppressed patient. Chest. 1978;73:477–82.
95. Ellis ME, Spence D, Bouchama A, et al. Open lung biopsy provides a higher and more specific yield compared to bronchoalveolar lavage in immunocompromised patients. Scand J Infect Dis. 1995;27:157–62.
96. oledo-pereyra LH, DeMeester TR, Kinealey A, et al. The benefits of open lung biopsy in patients with previous non-diagnostic transbronchial lung biopsy. A guide to appropriate therapy. Chest. 1980;77:647–50.
97. Santamauro JT, Mangino DA, Stover DE. The lung in immunocompromised host: diagnostic methods. Respiration. 1999;66:481–90.
98. Miller RF, Leigh TR, Collins JV, Mitchell DM. Tess giving an etiological diagnosis in pulmonary disease in patients infected with the human immunodeficiency virus. Thorax. 1990;45:62–5.
99. Murray JF, Felton CP, Garay SM, et al. Pulmonary complications of the acquired immunodeficiency syndrome. N Engl J Med. 1984;310:1682–8.

100. Stover DE, White DA, Romano PA, Gellene RA. Diagnosis of pulmonary disease in acquired immune deficiency syndrome (AIDS). Role of bronchoscopy and bronchoalveolar lavage. Am Rev Respir Dis. 1984;130:659–62.
101. Harcup C, Baier HJ, Pitchenik AE. Evaluation of patients with the acquired immunodeficiency syndrome (AIDS) by flexible bronchoscopy. Endoscopy. 1985;17:217–20.
102. Broddus C, Dake MD, Stulbarg MS, et al. Bronchoalveolar lavage and transbronchial biopsy for diagnosis of pulmonary infections in the acquired immunodeficiency syndrome. Ann Intern Med. 1985;102:747–52.
103. Batungwanayo J, Taelman H, Lucas S, et al. Pulmonary disease associated with the human immunodeficiency virus in Kigali, Rawanda. A fiberoptic bronchoscopy study of 111 cases of undetermined etiology. Am J Respir Crit Care Med. 1994;149:1591–6.
104. Rosen MJ, Tow TW, Teirstein AS, Chuang MT, Marchevsky A, Bottone EJ. Diagnosis of pulmonary complications of acquired immunodeficiency syndrome. Thorax. 1985;40:571–5.
105. Eisner MD, Kaplan LD, Herndier B, Stulbarg MS. The pulmonary manifestations of AIDS related non-Hodgkin's lymphoma. Chest. 1996;110:729–36.
106. Ognibene FP, Steis RG, Macher AM, et al. Kaposi's sarcoma causing pulmonary infiltrates and respiratory failure in the acquired immunode fi ciency syndrome. Ann Intern Med. 1985;102:471–5.
107. Meduri GU, Stover DE, Lee M, Myskowski PL, Caravelli JF, Zaman MB. Pulmonary Kaposi's sarcoma in the acquired immunodeficiency syndrome. Clinical, radiological, and pathological manifestations. Am J Med. 1986;81:11–8.
108. Suffredini AF, Ognibene FP, Lack EE, et al. Nonspecific interstitial pneumonitis: a common cause of pulmonary disease in the acquired immunodeficiency syndrome. Ann Intern Med. 1987;107:7–13.
109. Sattiler F, Nichols L, Hirano L, et al. Non-specific interstitial pneumonitis mimicking Pneumocystis carinii pneumonia. Am J Respir Crit Care Med. 1997;156:912–7.
110. Golden JA, Hollander H, Stulbarg MS, Gamsu G. Bronchoalveolar lavage as the exclusive diagnostic modality for pneumocystis carinii pneumonia. A prospective study among patients with acquired immunodeficiency syndrome. Chest. 1986;90:18–22.
111. Menon L, Patel R, Varadarajalu L, Sy E, Fuentes GD. Role of transbronchioal lung biopsy in HIV positive patients suspected to have Pneumocystis jirovecii pneumonia. J Bronchol. 2007;14:165–8.
112. Jules-Elysee KM, Stover DE, Zaman MB, Bernard EM, White DA. Aerosolized pentamidine: effect on diagnosis and presentation of Pneumocystis carinii pneumonia. Ann Intern Med. 1990;112:750–7.
113. Bonfils-Roberts EA, Nickodem A, Nealon TF. Retrospective analysis of the efficacy of open lung biopsy in acquired immunodeficiency syndrome. Ann Thorac Surg. 1990;49:115–7.
114. Trachiotis GD, Hafner GH, Hix WR, Aaron BL. Role of open lung biopsy in diagnosing pulmonary complications of AIDS. Ann Thorac Surg. 1992;54:898–902.
115. Miller RF, Pugsley WB, Griffith MH. Open lung biopsy for investigation of acute respiratory episodes in patients with HIV infection and AIDS. Genitourin Med. 1995;71:280–5.
116. Fitzgerald W, Bevelaqua FA, Garay SM, Aranda CP. The role of open lung biopsy in patients with the acquired immunodeficiency syndrome. Chest. 1987;91:659–61.
117. Chhajed PN, Tamm M, Granville A. Role of flexible bronchoscopy in lung transplantation. Semin Respir Crit Care Med. 2004;25:413–23.
118. Glanville AR. Bronchoscopic monitoring after lung transplantation. Semin Respir Crit Care Med. 2010; 31:208–21.
119. Trulock EP, Ettinger NA, Brunt EM, Pasque MK, Kaiser LR, Cooper JD. The role of transbronchial biopsy in the treatment of lung transplant recipients. An analysis of 200 consecutive procedures. Chest. 1992;102:1049–54.
120. Hopkins PM, Aboyoun CL, Chhajed PN, et al. Prospective analysis of 1235 transbronchial lung biopsies in lung transplant recipients. J Heart Lung Transplant. 2002;21:1062–7.
121. McWilliams TJ, Williams TJ, Whitford HM, Snell GI. Surveillance bronchoscopy in lung transplant recipients: risk versus benefit. J Heart Lung Transplant. 2008;27:1203–9.
122. Valentine VG, Taylor DE, Dhillon GS, et al. Success of lung transplantation without surveillance bronchoscopy. J Heart Lung Transplant. 2002;21:319–26.
123. Kesten S, Chamberlain D, Maurer J. Yield of surveillance transbronchial biopsies performed beyond two years after lung transplantation. J Heart Lung Transplant. 1996;15:384–8.
124. Tamm M, Sharples LD, Higenbottom TW, Stewart S, Wallwork J. Bronchiolitis obliterans syndrome in heart-lung transplantation: surveillance bronchoscopies. Am J Respir Crit Care Med. 1997;155:1705–10.
125. Valentine VG, Gupta MR, Weill D, et al. Singleinstitution study evaluating the utility of surveillance bronchoscopy after lung transplantation. J Heart Lung Transplant. 2009;28:14–20.
126. Higenbottom T, Stewart S, Penketh A, Wallwork J. Transbronchial lung biopsy for the diagnosis of rejection in heart-lung transplant patients. Transplantation. 1988;46:532–9.
127. Scott JP, Fradet G, Smyth RL, et al. Prospective study of transbronchial biopsies in the management of heart-lung and single lung transplant patients. J Heart Lung Transplant. 1991;10:626–37.
128. Kukafka DS, O'Brien GM, Furukawa S, Criner GJ. Surveillance bronchoscopy in lung transplant recipients. Chest. 1997;111: 377–81.
129. Chan CC, Abi-Saleh WJ, Arroliga AC, et al. Diagnostic yield and therapeutic impact of flexible bronchoscopy in lung transplant recipients. J Heart Lung Transplant. 1996;15:196–205.
130. Lehto JT, Koskinen PK, Anttila VJ, et al. Bronchoscopy in the diagnosis and surveillance of respiratory infections in lung and heart-lung transplant recipients. Transpl Int. 2005;18:562–71.
131. Sibley RK, Berry GJ, Tazelaar HD, et al. The role of transbronchial biopsies in the management of lung transplant recipients. J Heart Lung Transplant. 1993;12:308–14.
132. Aboyoun CL, Tamm M, Chhajed PN, et al. Diagnostic value of follow-up transbronchial lung biopsy after lung rejection. Am J Respir Crit Care Med. 2001;164:460–3.
133. Lee P, Minai O, Mehta AC, et al. Lung nodules in lung transplant recipients etiology and outcome. Chest. 2004;125:165–72.
134. Yousem SA, Paradis IL, Dauber JH, Griffith BP. Efficacy of transbronchial biopsy in the diagnosis of bronchiolitis obliterans in heart lung transplant recipients. Transplantation. 1989;47:893–5.
135. Kramer MR, Stoehr C, Whang JL, et al. The diagnosis of obliterative bronchiolitis after heart lung and lung transplantation: low yield of transbronchial biopsy. J Heart Lung Transplant. 1993;12:676–81.
136. Heng D, Sharples L, McNeil K, Stewart S, Wrenghitt T, Wallwork J. Bronchiolitis obliterans syndrome: incidence, natural history, prognosis and risk factors. J Heart Lung Transplant. 1998;17:1255–63.
137. Hopkins PM, Aboyoun CL, Chhajed PN, et al. Association of minimal rejection in lung transplant recipients with obliterative bronchiolitis. Am J Respir Crit Care Med. 2004;170:1022–6.
138. Glanville AR, Aboyoun CL, Havryk A, Plit M, Rainer S, Malouf M. Severity of lymphocytic bronchiolitis predicts long-term

outcome after lung transplantation. Am J Respir Crit Care Med. 2008; 177:1033–40.
139. Burton CM, Iversen M, Scheike T, Carlsen J, Andersen CB. Is lymphocytic bronchiolitis a marker of acute rejection? An analysis of 2697 transbronchial biopsies after lung transplantation. J Heart Lung Transplant. 2008;27:1128–34.
140. Turner JS, Wilcox PA, Hayhurst MD, Potgieter PD. Fiberoptic bronchoscopy in the intensive care unit-a prospective study of 147 procedures in 107 patients. Crit Care Med. 1994;22:259–64.
141. Papin TA, Grum CM, Weg JG. Transbronchial biopsy during mechanical ventilation. Chest. 1986; 89:168–70.
142. Pincus PS, Kallenbach JM, Hurwitz MD, et al. Transbronchial biopsies during mechanical ventilation. Crit Care Med. 1987;15:1136–9.
143. Bulpa PA, Dive AM, Mertens L, et al. Combined bronchoalveolar lavage and transbronchial lung biopsy: safety and yield in ventilated patients. Eur Respir J. 2003;21:489–94.
144. O'Brien JD, Ettinger NA, Shevlin D, Kollef MH. Safety and yield of transbronchial biopsy in mechanically ventilated patients. Crit Care Med. 1997; 25:440–6.
145. Flabouris A, Myburgh J. The utility of open lung biopsy in patients requiring mechanical ventilation. Chest. 1999;115:811–7.
146. Warner DO, Warner MA, Divertie MB. Open lung biopsy in patients with diffuse pulmonary infiltrates and acute respiratory failure. Am Rev Respir Dis. 1988;137:90–4.
147. Koerner SK, Sakowitz AJ, Appelman RI, Becker NH, Schoenbaum SW. Transbronchial lung biopsies for the diagnosis of sarcoidosis. N Engl J Med. 1975;293:268–70.
148. Bilaceroglu S, Perim K, Gunel O, Cagirici U, Buyuksirin M. Combining transbronchial aspiration with endobronchial and transbronchial biopsy in sarcoidosis. Monaldi Arch Chest Dis. 1999;54:217–23.
149. Koontz CH. Lung biopsy in sarcoidosis. Chest. 1978;74:120–1.
150. Trisolini R, Lazzari AL, Cancellieri A, et al. Transbronchial needle aspiration improves the diagnostic yield of bronchoscopy in sarcoidosis. Sarcoidosis Vasc Diffuse Lung Dis. 2004;21:147–51.
151. Shorr AF, Torrington KG, Hnatiuk OW. Endobronchial biopsy for sarcoidosis. A prospective study. Chest. 2001;120:109–14.
152. Leonard C, Tormey VJ, O'Keane C, Burke CM. Bronchoscopic diagnosis of sarcoidosis. Eur Respir J. 1997;10:2722–4.
153. Navani N, Booth HL, Kocjan G, et al. Combination of endobronchial ultrasound-guided transbronchial needle aspiration with standard bronchoscopic techniques for the diagnosis of stage I and stage II pulmonary sarcoidosis. Respirology. 2011;16:467–72.
154. Travis WD, Borok Z, Roum JH, et al. Pulmonary Langerhans cell granulomatosis (histiocytosis-X). A clinicopathological study of 48 cases. Am J Surg Pathol. 1993;17:971–86.
155. Housini I, Tomashefski JF, Cohen A, Crass A, Kleinerman J. Transbronchial biopsy in patients with pulmonary eosinophilic granuloma. Comparison with findings on open lung biopsy. Arch Pathol Lab Med. 1994;118:523–30.
156. Leslie KO, Gruden JF, Parish JM, Scholand MB. Transbronchial biopsy interpretation in the patient with diffuse parenchymal lung disease. Arch Pathol Lab Med. 2007;131:407–23.
157. Auerswald U, Barth J, Magnussen H. Value of CD-1 positive cells in bronchoalveolar lavage fluid for the diagnosis of pulmonary histiocytosis-X. Lung. 1991; 169:305–9.
158. Urban T, Lazor R, Lacronique J, et al. Pulmonary lymphangioleiomyomatosis. A study of 69 patients. Medicine. 1999;78: 321–37.
159. Bonetti F, Chiodera PL, Pea M, et al. Transbronchial biopsy in lymphangiomyomatosis of the lung. HMB 45 for diagnosis. Am J Surg Pathol. 1993;17:1092–102.
160. Torre O, Harari S. The diagnosis of cystic lung disease: a role for bronchoalveolar lavage and transbronchial biopsy? Respir Med. 2010;104: S81–5.
161. Epler GR, Colby TV, McLoud TC, Carrington CB, Gaensler EA. Bronchiolitis obliterans organizing pneumonia. N Engl J Med. 1985;312:152–8.
162. Cordier J-F. Cryptogenic organizing pneumonia. Clin Chest Med. 1993;14:677–92.
163. Bartter T, Irwin RS, Nash G, Balikian JP, Hollingsworth HH. Idiopathic bronchiolitis obliterans organizing pneumonia with peripheral infiltrates on chest roentgenogram. Arch Intern Med. 1989;149:273–9.
164. Azzam ZS, Bentur L, Rubin AH, Ben-Izhak O, Alroy G. Bronchiolitis obliterans organizing pneumonia. Diagnosis by transbronchial biopsy. Chest. 1993 ;104:1899–901.
165. Polpetti V, Cazzato S, Minicuci N, Zompatori M, Burzi M, Schiattone ML. The diagnostic value of bronchoalveolar lavage and transbronchial biopsy in cryptogenic organizing pneumonia. Eur Respir J. 1996;9:2513–6.
166. Cordier JF. Cryptogenic organizing pneumonia. Eur Respir J. 2006;28:422–46.
167. Coleman A, Colby TV. Histologic diagnosis of extrinsic allergic alveolitis. Am J Surg Pathol. 1988; 12:514–8.
168. Lacasse Y, Fraser RS, Fournier M, Cormier Y. Diagnostic accuracy of transbronchial biopsy in acute farmer's lung disease. Chest. 1997;112:1459–65.
169. Gruden JF, Webb WR, Naidich DP, McGuinness G. Multinofdular disease: anatomic localization at thin section CT-multireader evaluation of a simple algorithm. Radiology. 1999;210:711–20.
170. Munk PL, Muller NL, Miller RR, Ostrow DN. Pulmonary lymphangitic carcinomatosis: CT and pathologic findings. Radiology. 1988;166:705–9.
171. Goldstein LS, Kavuru MS, Curtis-McCarthy P, Christie HA, Farver C, Stoller JK. Pulmonary alveolar proteinosis: clinical features and outcomes. Chest. 1998;114:1357–62.
172. Kim CH, Kim S, Kwon OJ, Han SK, Lee JS, Kim KY. Pulmonary diffuse alveolar septal amyloidosis–diagnosed by transbronchial lung biopsy. Korean J Intern Med. 1990;5:63–8.
173. Cale WF, Petsonk EL, Boyd CB. Transbronchial biopsy of pulmonary alveolar microlithiasis. Arch Intern Med. 1983;143:358–9.
174. Churg A. Transbronchial biopsy. Nothing to fear. Am J Surg Pathol. 2001;25:820–2.
175. Berbescue EA, Katzenstein AL, Snow JL, Zisman DA. Transbronchial biopsy in usual interstitial pneumonia. Chest. 2006;129:1126–31.
176. Wall CP, Gaensler EA, Carrington CB, Hayes JA. Comparison of transbronchial and open biopsies in chronic infiltrative lung diseases. Am Rev Respir Dis. 1981;123:280–5.
177. Wilson RK, Fechner RE, Greenberg SD, et al. Clinical implications of a non-specific transbronchial biopsy. Am J Med. 1978;65:252–6.
178. Churg A, Schwarz M. Transbronchial biopsy and usual interstitial pneumonia. A new paradigm? Chest. 2006;129:1117–8.
179. Raghu G, Collard HR, Egan JJ, et al. An official ATS/ERS/JRS/ALAT statement: idiopathic pulmonary fi brosis: evidence-based guidelines for diagnosis and management. Am J Respir Crit Care Med. 2011;183:788–824.
180. Lombard CM, Duncan SR, Rizk NW, Colby TV. The diagnosis of Wegener's granulomatosis from transbronchial biopsy specimens. Hum Pathol. 1990;21:838–42.
181. Givens CD, Newman JH, McCurley TL. Diagnosis of Wegener's granulomatosis by trsnbronchial biopsy. Chest. 1985;88:794–6.
182. Schnabel A, Holl-Ulrich K, Dalhoff K, Reuter M, Gross WL. Efficacy of transbronchial biopsy in pulmonary vasculitides. Eur

Respir J. 1997;10:2738–43.
183. Kendell DM, Gal AA. Interpretation of tissue artifacts in transbronchial lung biopsy specimen. Ann Diagn Pathol. 2003;7:20–4.
184. Babiak A, Hetzel J, Krishna G, et al. Transbronchial cryobiopsy: a new tool for lung biopsies. Respiration. 2009;78:203–8.
185. Griff S, Ammenwerth W, Schonfeld N, et al. Morphometrical analysis of transbronchial cryobiopsies. Diagn Pathol. 2011;6:53.
186. Rial MB, Delgado MN, Sanmartin AP, et al. Multivariate study of predictive factors for clearly defined lesions without visible endobronchial lesions in transbronchial biopsies. Surg Endosc. 2010;24:3031–6.
187. Herth FJH, Eberhardt R, Brcker HD, Ernst A. Endoscopic ultrasound guided transbronchial lung biopsy in fluoroscopically invisible solitary pulmonary nodules. A prospective study. Chest. 2006;129:147–50.
188. Wagner U, Walthers EM, Gelmetti W, Klose KJ, von Wichert P. Computer-tomograpghically guided fiberbronchoscopic transbronchial biopsy of small pulmonary lesions: a feasibility study. Respiration. 1996;63:181–6.
189. White CS, Weiner EA, Patel P, Britt J. Transbronchial needle aspiration. Guidance with CT fluoroscopy. Chest. 2000;118:1630–8.
190. Tsushima K, Sone S, Hanaoka T, Takayama F, Honda T, Kubo K. Comparison of bronchoscopic diagnosis for peripheral pulmonary nodule under fluoroscopic guidance with CT guidance. Respir Med. 2006; 100:737–45.
191. Ost D, Shah R, Anasco E, et al. A randomized trial of CT-fluoroscopic guided bronchoscopy vs conventional bronchoscopy in patients with suspected lung cancer. Chest. 2008;134:507–13.
192. Wrixon AD. New ICRP recommendations. J Radiol Prot. 2008;28:161–8.
193. Kurimoto N, Miyazawa T, Okimasa S, et al. Endobronchial ultrasound using a guide sheath increases the ability to diagnose peripheral lesions endoscopically. Chest. 2004;126:959–65.
194. Paone G, Nicastri E, Lucantoni G, et al. Endobronchial ultrasound-driven biopsy in the diagnosis of peripheral lung lesions. Chest. 2005;128:3551–7.
195. Eberhardt R, Ernst A, Herth FJF. Ultrasound-guided transbronchial biopsy of solitary pulmonary nodules less than 20 mm. Eur Respir J. 2009;34:1284–7.
196. Yoshikawa M, Sukoh N, Yamazaki K, et al. Diagnostic value of endobronchial ultrasonography with a guide sheath for peripheral pulmonary lesions without x-ray fluoroscopy. Chest. 2007;131:1788–93.
197. Roth K, Eagan TM, Andreassen AH, Leh F, Hardie JA. A randomized trial of endobronchial ultrasound guided sampling in peripheral lung lesions. Lung Cancer. 2011;74:219–25.
198. Gildea TR, Mazzone PJ, Karnak D, Meziane M, Mehta AC. Electromagnetic navigation bronchoscopy. A prospective study. Am J Respir Crit Care Med. 2006;174:982–9.
199. Eberhardt R, Anantham D, Herth F, Feller-Kopman D, Ernst A. Electromagnetic navigation diagnostic bronchoscopy in peripheral lung lesions. Chest. 2007;131:1800–5.
200. Makris D, Scherpereel A, Leroy S, et al. Electromagnetic navigation diagnostic bronchoscopy for small peripheral lung lesions. Eur Respir J. 2007;29:1187–92.
201. Mahajan AK, Patel S, Hogarth DK, Wightman R. Electromagnetic navigational bronchoscopy. An effective and safe approach to diagnose peripheral lung lesions unreachable by conventional bronchoscopy in high-risk patients. J Bronchology Interv Pulmonol. 2011;18:133–7.
202. Seijo LM, de Torres J, Lozano MD, et al. Diagnostic yield of electromagnetic navigation bronchoscopy is highly dependent on the presence of bronchus sign on CT imaging. Results from a prospective study. Chest. 2010;138:1316–21.
203. Lamprecht B, Porsch P, Wegleitner B, Strasser G, Kaiser B, Studnicka M. Electromagnetic navigation bronchoscopy (ENB): increasing diagnostic yield. Respir Med. 2012;106(5):710–5.
204. Shinagawa N, Yamazaki K, Onodera Y, et al. Virtual bronchoscopy navigation system shortens the examination time-feasibility study of virtual bronchoscopic navigation system. Lung Cancer. 2007;56:201–6.
205. Tachihara M, Ishida T, Kanazawa K, et al. A virtual bronchoscopic navigation system under x-ray fluoroscopy for transbronchial diagnosis of small peripheral pulmonary lesions. Lung Cancer. 2007;2007:322–7.
206. Shinagawa N, Yamazaki K, Onodera Y, et al. CT-guided transbronchial biopsy using an ultrathin bronchoscope with virtual bronchoscopic navigation. Chest. 2004;125:1138–43.
207. Asano F, Matsuno Y, Shinagawa N, et al. A virtual bronchoscopic navigation system for pulmonary peripheral lesions. Chest. 2006;130:559–66.
208. Iwano S, Imaizumi K, Okada T, Hasegawa Y, Naganawa S. Virtual bronchoscopy-guided transbronchial biopsy for aiding the diagnosis of peripheral lung cancer. Eur J Cancer. 2011;79:155–9.
209. Omiya H, Kikuyama A, Kubo A, et al. A feasibility and Efficacy study on bronchoscopy with a virtual navigation system. J Bronchology Interv Pulmonol. 2010;17:11–8.
210. Eberhardt R, Anantham D, Ernst A, Feller-Kopman D, Herth F. Multimodality bronchoscopic diagnosis of peripheral lung lesions. A randomized controlled trial. Am J Respir Crit Care Med. 2007;176:36–41.
211. Asano F, Matsuno Y, Tsuzuku A, et al. Diagnosis of peripheral pulmonary lesions using a bronchoscope insertion guidance system combined with endobronchial ultrasonography with a guide sheath. Lung Cancer. 2008;60:366–73.
212. Ishida T, Asano F, Yamazaki K, et al. Virtual bronchoscopic navigation combined with endobronchial ultrasound to diagnose small peripheral pulmonary lesions: a randomized trial. Thorax. 2011;66:1072–7.
213. Wahidi MM, Govert JA, Goudar RK, GouldMK MCDC. Evidence for the treatment of patients with pulmonary nodules: when is it lung cancer? ACCP evidence-based clinical practice guidelines (2nd edition). Chest. 2007;132:94S–107.
214. Huanqi L, Boiselle PM, Shepard JO, Trotman-Dickenson B, McCloud TC. Diagnostic accuracy and safety of CT-guided percutaneous needle aspiration biopsy of the lung: comparison of small and large pulmonary nodules. AJR Am J Roentgenol. 1996;167:105–9.
215. Ohano Y, Hatabu H, Takenaka D, et al. CT-guided transthoracic needle aspiration biopsy of small (≤20 mm) solitary pulmonary nodules. AJR Am J Roentgenol. 2003;180:1665–9.
216. Asano F, Aoe M, Ohsaki Y, et al. Deaths and complications associated with respiratory endoscopy: a survey by the Japan Society for respiratory endoscopy in 2010. Respirology. 2012; 17(3):478–85.
217. Pue CA, Pacht ER. Complications of fiberoptic bronchoscopy at a university hospital. Chest. 1995; 107:430–2.
218. Milman N, Fourschou P, Munch EP, Grode G. Trsnbronchial lung biopsy through fiberoptic bronchoscope. Results and complications in 452 examinations. Respir Med. 1994;88:749–53.
219. Cordasco EM, Mehta AC, Ahmad M. Bronchoscopically induced bleeding. A summary of nine years' Cleveland Clinic experience and review of literature. Chest. 1991;100:1141–7.
220. Pereira W, Kovnat DM, Snider GL. A prospective cooperative study of complications following flexible fiberoptic bronchoscopy. Chest. 1978;73:813–6.

第 3 章
经支气管针吸活检（TBNA）

Prasoon Jain, Edward F. Haponik, A. Lukas Loschner, and Atul C. Mehta

本章提要 经支气管针吸活检（TBNA）是一项通过纤维支气管镜技术跨越支气管树限制获取细胞学或组织学标本的技术。肺癌的纵隔分期是 TBNA 最常见的指征。这个检查也能用于诊断结节病和肺结核，它们会引起纵隔淋巴结肿大。检查在患者意识清醒镇静状态下进行，不需要昂贵的引导和追踪装置。这个检查性价比高、容易学习并且安全性优越。不幸的是，由于缺乏培训和关于它的效果和安全性的普遍误解，许多支气管镜医师从未在他们的临床实践中采用过这个技术。经支气管针吸活检是一个交叉技术，它是在支气管镜视野下使用 22 号穿刺针从病灶中获取细胞学标本。TBNA 提高了对黏膜下和支气管旁肺癌的诊断率。外周 TBNA 是一个在透视引导下从可疑的恶性周围型肺结节中获取细胞学标本的技术。在传统取样技术外再加上外周 TBNA 能改善支气管镜检查的诊断率，特别是对肿瘤-支气管关系 Tsuboi 类型 Ⅲ 型或 Ⅳ 型的患者。随着支气管内超声引导的经支气管针吸活检（EBUS-TBNA）的出现，传统 TBNA 的作用已经进一步成为热议话题。作者相信即便在 EBUS-TBNA 的时代，标准 TBNA 技术仍然在肺癌的诊断和分期中占有重要位置。

关键词 经支气管针吸活检，纵隔分期，肺癌分期，支气管镜下针吸活检，外周经支气管针吸活检。

引 言

TBNA 是一项通过纤维支气管镜技术跨越支气管树限制获取细胞学或组织学标本的技术，包括纵隔和肺门淋巴结[1]。肺癌纵隔分期是该检查最常见的指征[2,3]。在一些病例中，它也能用于肺癌、结节病和肺结核的诊断[4,5]。虽然纵隔镜检查还是肺癌纵隔分期的金标准，TBNA 分期比起侵犯性手术分期有许多显著优势。纵隔镜检查在全麻下进行，而 TBNA 可以在适度镇静下进行。比起纵隔镜 TBNA 检查费用更低、侵犯性更小、对患者来说更舒适[6]。TBNA 是一项容易学习的技术，不要求任何特殊的装备或引导装置。一份阳性 TBNA 报告可以避免纵隔镜检查或任何额外用于肺癌分期的侵犯性检测需要。

但是，许多先前的调查持续表明，由于缺乏对该技术的训练，对该技术的安全性和有效性也未经证实，许多人不愿意进行经支气管针吸活检[7,8]。近来 EBUS-TBNA 的出现，甚至使那些在这个领域有丰富知识的人也开始对这项技术的未来产生怀疑。

在本章中，我们讨论了标准 TBNA 的技术、临床应用以及局限性。我们的目标之一是要消除一些阻止这个技术在临床更好应用的恐惧和犹豫。我们讨论了目前关于经支气管针吸活检在肺癌纵隔分期中作用的证据，以及它在改善支气管镜对可见肺癌和外周肺结节和肿块诊断率中的作用。我们也通过这次机会来强调这样一个事实，即 EBUS-TBNA 的优势明显高于传统 TBNA 技术。

技　术

许多综述从技术层面对 TBNA 操作进行阐述[9,10]。在接下来的部分中，我们将从几个重要方面简单地介绍这项技术。

胸部 CT 检查

TBNA 涉及对操作者无法看见的管壁外淋巴结的采样。所以，在术前操作者必须研究 CT 图像上增大的淋巴结和气道以及周围血管的关系。一旦在 CT 上识别出增大的纵隔或肺门淋巴结，明确它对应的支气管解剖学标志，可以引导操作者选择合适部位进行气道穿刺。在这点上，气管隆突是最常见的用来选择穿刺部位的标志。虽然增强 CT 在这方面能提供更多信息，但是在不能注射造影剂的情况下可由普通 CT 代替。在一些研究中，PET/CT 已经被报道能够改善 TBNA 对肺癌纵隔分期的敏感性和阴性预测值[11,12]。但是从技术角度来看，PET/CT 相比胸部 CT 对引导操作者到达靶淋巴结并没有优势。

一般来说，临床医师已经使用 Moutain 和 Dressler 的 CT 图像系统来对增大的纵隔和肺门淋巴结进行分组[13]。最近，国际肺癌研究协会提议修正 CT 上淋巴结的定义，这个提议被第

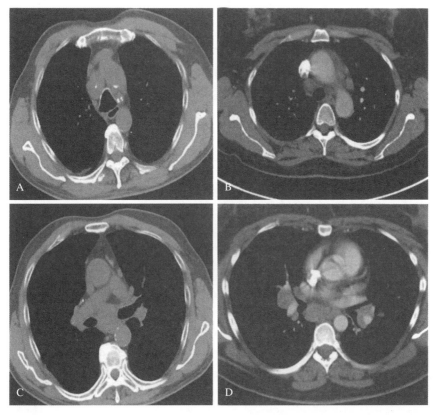

图 3.1　CT 图像显示增大的纵隔淋巴结。A. 右侧气管旁淋巴结（第 4R 组淋巴结）；B. 左侧气管旁淋巴结（第 4L 组淋巴结），主 - 肺动脉窗淋巴结也增大（第 5 组淋巴结），第 5 组不能通过经支气管针吸活检；C. 气管隆突下淋巴结（第 7 组淋巴结）；D. 右侧叶间淋巴结（第 11R 组淋巴结）和增大的左侧叶间淋巴结（第 11L 组淋巴结），气管隆突下淋巴结也增大

七版肺癌 TMN 分期所采纳[14]。临床医师现在应该按照国际肺癌研究协会的定义来识别肺癌患者增大淋巴结的分组（见后文图 5.1）。传统 TBNA 方法最适合对第 4R、4L 和 7 组淋巴结进行取样来定义 N2 或 N3 疾病，对第 10R、10L、11R 和 11L 组淋巴结取样定义 N1 疾病。常见的和 TBNA 相关的淋巴结分组在图 3.1 中已经注明。必须注意主肺动脉窗的淋巴结组（第 5 组）不能通过 TBNA 取样，因为它在动脉韧带外侧、左肺动脉第一级分支分叉处内侧。虽然增大的第 2R 和 2L 淋巴结可以通过 TBNA 取样，但是由于周围血管很近，最好使用支气管内超声活检从这些淋巴结组获取标本。另外，从这个位置异常组织的取样可能会由于对纵隔淋巴结的错误分析导致对肺癌病灶的分期过度。

TBNA 活检针

TBNA 可以使用的活检针有许多类型，对它的选择属于个人偏好。更重要的是对手术使用的活检针的熟悉。一根 22 号的 TBNA 活检针（MW-222）最常用来获取细胞学标本（图 3.2 A、B）。它的远端是可收缩的、带尖锐切边的 13 mm 针。当完全缩回时，活检针的尖锐段被包裹在一个金属外套中。活检针可以借助尖端的控制装置前进和缩回。透明塑料导管的外径为 1.9 mm。它可以通过 2.2 mm 或更大直径的工作通道穿入支气管镜。导管因为一根在内部穿行的金属针芯变硬。当活检针用力穿透气道壁的时候，导管的硬度能防止塑料导管扭转或弯曲。通过近端吸引侧孔，用一根 20 ml 或 50 ml 的注射管进行抽吸。

组织标本活检要求使用一根 19 号 TBNA 活检针[15]。MW-319 是活检常用的针（图 3.3 A~D）。它由 19 号可缩回的斜边针组成，针被包裹在金属外套中。当完全到位后，19 号针超过金属外套远端 15 mm。针的近端黏附在一个中空的弹簧上，弹簧穿过导管全段并且控制住 19 号针的运动。另一个 21 号斜边针被包裹在 19 号针中。安装完全后针头超过 19 号针远端 3 mm。21 号针近端被黏附在一个导丝上，导丝在中空弹簧壁的内侧。21 号针作为更大的 19 号针的套管针，能防止它被支气管组织和软骨塞住。为了获取组织标本，19 号和 21 号活检针都被推进到靶位置。21 号针穿透气道，并将导管固定到增大的淋巴结上。进行抽吸，确认导管没有在主要血管上。此时，21 号针被缩回，核心组织通过局部移动 19 号针进出淋巴结多次获取，同时维持注射器持续抽吸。然后将两根针都缩回，TBNA 导管从支气管镜中退出来收回标本。这个针的操作有些烦琐和复杂。最近的经验表明单腔 19 号 TBNA 活检针（MWF-319）在获取组织标本上同样成功，并且比起 MW-319 更容易使用。

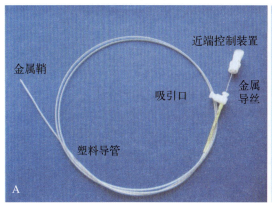
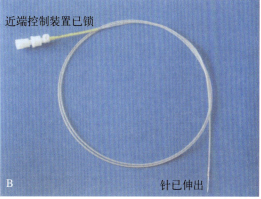

图 3.2　A. 远端带有 22 号穿刺针的 MW-222 活检针全部在金属外套内，当导管穿过工作通道时，确保穿刺针完全被金属外套包裹；B. 近端控制装置前进并锁定，用来弹出 TBNA 活检针

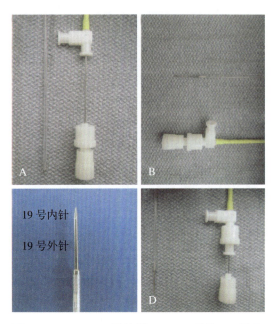

图 3.3 MW-319 活检针。A. 19 号和 21 号穿刺针都在导管内；B. 两种针都前进并锁定；C. 外侧 19 号穿刺针和内侧 21 号穿刺针的特写；D. 21 号穿刺针被缩回

计 划

所有 TBNA 操作前必须进行全面的临床评价。在进行最初的诊断性支气管镜检查时，从纵隔淋巴结获取组织标本进行分期通常先于对原发肿瘤组织进行标本的获取。在支气管镜检查前必须和助手先讨论好所有取样步骤和相应顺序，确保检查需要的所有附属设备都准备充分。为了对 TBNA 进行分期，最好在操作前把玻片标记好以避免对获取标本的淋巴结组出现任何困惑。与最高分期相关的淋巴结应该在对低分期的淋巴结组之前取样。所以，根据原发肿瘤的位置，N3 淋巴结应该在 N2 淋巴结前取样，N2 淋巴结在 N1 淋巴结之前。这种操作避免了在手术全程只使用 1 根活检针的情况下，来自低级淋巴结组的肿瘤细胞污染高级淋巴结组的细胞。

为了避免对工作通道无意的损害，操作者必须在 TBNA 导管进入到支气管镜工作通道前，确保活检针的斜边完全包裹在金属外套里面。必须在每一次 TBNA 前，都确认活检针的安装合适流畅。替换掉扭转或破坏的 TBNA 活检针。

操作过程

建议支气管镜检查尽可能使用鼻腔路径。相对口腔路径，支气管镜通过鼻腔时能握得更紧。TBNA 操作时运动更少可以增加操作的精确度，使得支气管镜医师能够穿刺支气管内目标部位。将 TBNA 导管插入工作通道时，操作者必须保持支气管镜的插入管和弯曲段尽可能直，防止对支气管镜造成任何无意损害。避免在 TBNA 分期前通过支气管镜工作通道进行抽吸，以减少呼吸道分泌物污染引起的假阳性结果风险。可以通过灭菌生理盐水冲洗掉覆盖在穿刺部位表面的分泌物。为了避免支气管内分泌物中恶性肿瘤细胞对工作通道的污染，TBNA 应在行进一步支气管检查或任何其他取样操作前进行。TBNA 导管应该被推进到支气管树，同时维持支气管镜尖端处于中间向前的观察位置。

大多数淋巴结组的穿刺部位在图 3.4 A~E 中注明。一旦识别穿刺的靶位置，TBNA 导管就被推进至超过支气管镜远端。在 TBNA 活检针到位前，能够清楚地看见远端金属外套很重要。但是导管应该只超过支气管镜尖端几毫米（图 3.5）。以这种方式，支气管镜的工作通道被用来夹住 TBNA 导管。如果看见导管超过支气管镜远端太长，那么必须缩回导管。不这样做的话操作时会扭转导管。一旦 TBNA 导管远端在操作时被扭转，那么将针穿刺到靶区域和从淋巴结抽吸组织都是不可能的。穿刺针应该穿插到软骨间隙。许多用来把针插入到气道壁的技术在表 3.1 中描述，在图 3.6 中注明。在缺乏任何对比研究的情况下，选择何种技术完全是个人的问题。一些情况下可能需要联合技术。不管怎样，必须保持 TBNA 活检针与气道壁垂直，至少和气道壁成 45°角来最大化活检针到达目标淋巴结核心部位的机会（图 3.7）。

第 1 篇 概　述

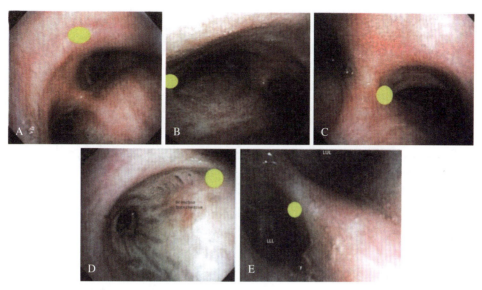

图 3.4　A. 第 4R 组淋巴结经支气管针吸活检位点在隆凸上第二或第三软骨间隙或其上 2 cm，相当于时钟的 1、2 点钟方向，不要在 3 点钟方向穿刺，避免损伤奇静脉；B. 第 4L 组淋巴结经支气管针吸活检位点在气道侧壁和隆凸水平的左主支气管，相当于 9 点钟方向；C. 第 7 组淋巴结经支气管针吸活检位点在第一隆凸下 3~5 mm 两侧，穿刺针指向内下侧；D. 第 11R 组淋巴结经支气管针吸活检位点在右上肺叶支气管分叉处、中间支气管侧壁 3 点钟方向；E. 第 11L 组淋巴结经支气管针吸活检位点在第二隆凸，位于左上和左下肺叶间的支气管，相当于 12 点钟至 2 点钟方向

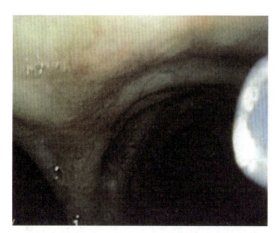

图 3.5　向前送 TBNA 活检针之前，应该能看见远端的金属外套

确认整段 TBNA 活检针都穿透气道壁，并且金属外套紧贴气道黏膜很重要（图 3.8）。一旦确认完毕，助手就会被要求使用注射器进行抽吸。在一些情况下，可以看见粉红色液体进入透明的塑料导管。这通常代表来自淋巴结的组织。在抽吸的时候，操作者频繁地将 TBNA 导管在淋巴结中前后移动，但是要确保活检针不会被拉出淋巴结和气道壁。几秒钟后助手会被指示停止抽吸，并且将活检针缩回到导管中。在活检针退出淋巴结前停止抽吸很重要。不这样做会让气道分泌物污染 TBNA 标本，因此增加假阳性的风险。当 TBNA 导管退出支气管树时，支气管镜远端应该伸直。

如果开始进行抽吸后马上看见血液充满导管，则提示穿刺到血管了。在这种情况下，支气管镜医师助手应该停止抽吸，并将活检针缩回到导管中。

穿刺次数

TBNA 的诊断率和每个淋巴结组的穿刺次数有关。在一项前瞻性研究中，Chin 等

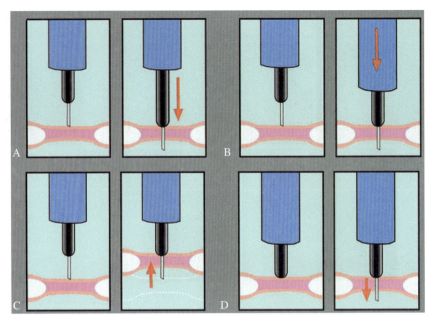

图 3.6 TBNA 活检针穿透气道壁的不同技术。A. 突刺法；B. 推进法；C. 咳嗽法；D. 鞘管贴近气道壁法

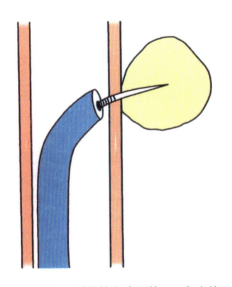

图 3.7 TBNA 活检针应该以约 90° 角来接近气道壁

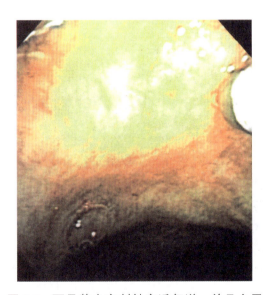

图 3.8 可见整个穿刺针穿透气道，并且金属外套紧靠气道壁

研究了获取 TBNA 最佳结果时每个淋巴结组的穿刺次数[16]。作者发现第一次采样能诊断 42% 的患者。在第七次 TBNA 后没有做出更多诊断。总之，93% 的诊断抽吸物可以在对单个淋巴组进行 4 次穿刺后得到。对于短轴 > 2 cm 的淋巴结，可以通过前两次的抽吸物

表 3.1 TBNA 活检针穿透气道壁的不同技术

突刺法
- 一旦看见 TBNA 导管，推进穿刺针完全进入中央气道
- 将大部分导管和部分穿刺针缩回到工作通道。针尖应该清晰可见
- 朝目标穿刺部位推进支气管镜和穿刺针
- 将穿刺针垂直气道壁放置
- 在鼻或嘴处握住支气管镜不动
- 导管向前刺向目标

鞘管贴近气道壁法
- TBNA 活检针完全缩回时，推进金属外套穿过支气管镜远端
- 将金属外套以 90° 角紧靠目标穿刺区域
- 在鼻或嘴处握住支气管镜不动
- 指导助手向前送 TBNA 活检针

推进法
- 将支气管镜靠近目标穿刺部位
- 推进导管直到金属外套远端可见
- 向前送穿刺针，并将它锁定在相应位置
- 使用小拇指在工作通道的活检孔稳定 TBNA 活检针导管
- 推进支气管镜，TBNA 活检针以 90° 角全部进入目标区域

咳嗽法
- 将支气管镜靠近目标穿刺部位
- 向前送 TBNA 活检针
- 在活检孔处稳定 TBNA 活检针导管
- 指导患者咳嗽。气道壁向穿刺针内侧移动以便于穿刺

明确 92% 病例恶性肿瘤的诊断。作者建议对单个淋巴结组进行 4~7 次的穿刺，这样能最大化对肺癌纵隔分期的诊断率。在另一项研究中，第 1、2、3 和 4 次穿刺的诊断率分别为 64%、85%、95% 和 98%[17]。作者建议用 3 次 TBNA 穿刺明确组织诊断，用 4~5 次进行纵隔肺癌分期。我们通常对每个淋巴结组进行 3~4 次穿刺来优化诊断率。

标本采集和分析

借助培训过的助手正确处理标本是操作的关键步骤，并且能改善 TBNA 的诊断率。直接制备细胞学标本是推荐的方法。这种方法是在支气管镜室将 TBNA 抽吸物制备成细胞学标本玻片。用抽吸样本的注射器中的空气将 TBNA 抽吸物置于载玻片上，用另一玻片覆盖，给予适当压力，然后分开玻片。用一张薄涂片盖在两张玻片上，立刻用 95% 乙醇溶液或商用喷雾固定剂进行固定。这一过程中任何的延迟都会由于干燥假象造成分析困难。

一些支气管镜医师使用液体法，该方法不使用玻片，将 TBNA 抽吸物打入 95% 乙醇中提交到细胞学实验室，然后通过标准方法进行处理。在一项前瞻性研究中，这种方法处理 TBNA 抽吸物的诊断率显著低于直接法[18]。基于这些结果，几乎没有理由选择使用液体法而非直接法。组织针获取的标本应该用福尔马林固定。任何可见的细胞学针获取的组织片也应该轻轻地移到福尔马林溶液中。TBNA 活检针和导管内残余标本应该用普通盐水冲刷到一个容器中，用于实验室的细胞封闭制备。

对标本仔细的分析是 TBNA 技术最优应用所必需的。一个合格的由淋巴结获得的标本应该主要是淋巴细胞，如果存在支气管上皮细胞，也应该是很少量的。

哪怕存在淋巴细胞，以最谨慎的态度分析阳性和阴性的 TBNA 结果是很重要的。TBNA 对肺癌分期的阴性预测值比较低。所以，如果来自纵隔淋巴结的 TBNA 抽吸物没有恶性肿瘤细胞，通常提示进行手术分期。反之，若 TBNA 抽吸物伴有一整块恶性肿瘤细胞，则可

以诊断淋巴结转移，避免了进一步的分期检查。但是，TBNA 标本中存在零散的恶性肿瘤细胞，不能充分证明淋巴结转移。任何类似的疑似情况都需要其他检查来进一步证实。假阳性的 TBNA 结果导致的错误分期存在严重的后果，因为它会导致错误的否定肺癌手术。虽然大多数研究发现 TBNA 检测淋巴结转移的敏感性达到 100%，但是也有一些假阳性的报道。支气管镜医师必须非常谨慎地去最小化 TBNA 出现假阳性的可能性（表 3.2）。

阳性结果的相关因素

持续研究报道，TBNA 对肺癌的诊断率比对良性疾病（如结节病）的更高[2]。在恶性诊断中，TBNA 对小细胞肺癌的诊断率高于非小细胞肺癌[19]。TBNA 的诊断率随着淋巴结大小的增加而增加。其他与 TBNA 高诊断率相关的因素在表 3.3 中列出[20,21]。

并发症

TBNA 是一个安全的技术，并发症发生率为 0.3%[22]。TBNA 术后出血通常很少，并且不明显。手术出现气胸[23]、纵隔气肿和纵隔积血[24]的报道也很少。TBNA 后只报道过 1 例化脓性心包炎[25]。没有关于手术相关死亡的报道。

临床应用

肺癌分期

TBNA 主要用于肺癌的纵隔分期。通过 TBNA 容易获取常见的淋巴结组（如第 4R、4L 和 7 组），这些淋巴结经常存在恶性细胞，可以用来定义 N2 或 N3 型疾病。从这些淋巴结获取的标本中识别肿瘤细胞能避免进一步侵犯性检查的需要，有助于立刻开始非手术性治疗。从肺门淋巴结（第 10、11 组）取样如前所述也是可行的，但是在这个位置出现肿瘤细胞只能定义为 N1 型疾病，不影响是否进行治疗性切除手术的决定。

在一项荟萃分析中，TBNA 对 34% 的纵隔转移患者进行纵隔分期，敏感性为 39%、特异性为 99%。但是在纵隔转移率为 81% 的研究中，它的敏感性为 78%[22]。在另一项系统性综述中，对于纵隔转移率为 70% 的患者，TBNA 的敏感性和特异性分别为 76% 和 96%[26]。TBNA 是一个便利的、性价比高、侵犯性低的方法，可以替代纵隔镜检查用于肺癌分期[3,27]。但是，当 TBNA 标本没有发现恶性细胞，或者获取的标

表 3.2　减少假阳性结果的方法

- 在气道检查或其他取样方法前进行经支气管针吸活检
- 在取得经支气管针吸活检标本前不进行抽吸
- 用生理盐水冲洗目标区域
- 先从更高级别的淋巴结组获取标本。所以，抽吸顺序为 N3>N2>N1
- 从淋巴结撤回穿刺针前停止抽吸
- 获取尽可能多的组织标本

表 3.3　经支气管针吸活检出现阳性结果的相关因素

- 恶性疾病
- 小细胞肺癌
- 右侧支气管旁和气管隆突下位置
- 淋巴结大小
- 使用组织活检针
- 直接法制备玻片
- PET 扫描上高 SUV 值
- 操作者和助手的技术和经验

本不足时，我们必须谨慎地分析它的结果。虽然 TBNA 的平均阴性预测值是 71%[26]，但是它依赖于肿瘤转移至淋巴结的发生率。在一个病例系列中，TBNA 对纵隔淋巴转移的阴性预测值只有 40%[28]。所以，作为一个普遍的原则，TBNA 阴性不能排除肿瘤的纵隔扩散，在给这些患者提供治疗性肺癌手术前还需要进一步检查。虽然纵隔镜检查是下一步检查的传统方法，但是最近的研究提示 EBUS-TBNA 是一个可行的替代治疗。

肺癌的重分期

关于 TBNA 对放化疗治疗后非小细胞肺癌ⅢA 期患者纵隔淋巴结分期的数据有限。在一项小型研究中，14 例非小细胞肺癌ⅢA 期患者在化疗或放化疗后通过 TBNA 对纵隔淋巴结进行重分期。TBNA 的准确性是 71%，5 例患者（36%）避免了纵隔镜检查[29]。最近的经验提示 EBUS-TBNA 相对标准的 TBNA 更适合这一指征。比如说在一项研究中，EBUS-TBNA 在化疗治疗后纵隔重分期的敏感性、特异性和精确性分别是 76%、100% 和 77%。但是，由于它的低阴性预测值，当 EBUS-TBNA 对纵隔淋巴结进行取样未发现恶性细胞时，还是提示进行手术分期[30]。

肺癌诊断

在许多情况下，虽然从原发肺肿块或结节进行组织取样无法得出诊断，但是从纵隔或肺门淋巴结获取的 TBNA 样本能提供组织诊断。在一些报道中，TBNA 是 18%~25% 存在肺实质病灶患者通过支气管镜进行组织诊断的唯一方法[3,19,27,31]。TBNA 避免了这些患者进一步诊断和分期的需要。

除了肺癌诊断之外，TBNA 也适合诊断上腔静脉综合征的患者。在一个前瞻性研究中，27 例上腔静脉综合征患者做了支气管镜检查，使用 22 号细胞学活检针对右淋巴结和其他淋巴结进行 TBNA[32]。96% 的患者能够通过 TBNA 标本明确组织诊断。在 82% 非小细胞肺癌和 47% 小细胞肺癌的患者中，TBNA 是唯一的诊断标本来源。没有发现手术相关并发症。

结节病

TBNA 对结节病的整体检出率在不同研究中的范围是 53%~94%[33,34]。对于这个疾病，应该获取多处 EBB、TBBx 和 TBNA 的标本来最大化支气管镜检查的诊断率。借助这个方法，能够明确 >90% 的结节病患者的诊断，其中 TBNA 能对 20%~60% 的患者进行排除诊断[33,35]。对两个分开的淋巴结组进行 TBNA 取样，能更加明确诊断[34]。在部分[33]而非全部[34]研究中，发现 TBNA 对Ⅰ期结节病的诊断率高于Ⅱ期结节病。虽然一些作者使用王氏 22 号细胞学活检针取得了不错的结果[36]，但是大多数作者为了获得一个更确信的诊断，更喜欢用 19 号的 TBNA 活检针来获取核心组织标本。

EBUS-TBNA 作为一个重要的结节病诊断工具，最近的研究报道它对Ⅰ期和Ⅱ期结节病的诊断敏感性为 85%[37]。在一项随机研究中，EBUS-TBNA 对结节病的整体检出率为 83.3%，而传统 TBNA 只有 53.8%[38]。虽然在这项研究中 EBB 和 TBBx 只在不到 50% 的患者中进行，但是支气管镜的整体检出率和 TBNA 对结节病的排除诊断率在两组中相似。基于这些数据，我们能够总结：在不进行 EBB 和 TBBx 的情况下，EBUS-TBNA 要优于传统 TBNA。

肺结核

TBNA 在诊断胸内结核性淋巴结炎中的作用已经被证实。在一项研究中，84 例纵隔淋巴结增大的 HIV 阴性患者使用 19 号组织学针进行 TBNA[39]。所有患者在支气管镜检查前痰标本抗酸杆菌染色阴性。诊断肺结节的敏感性、特异性、阳性和阴性预测值和准确性分别为 83%、100%、100%、38% 和 85%。TBNA 能提供 78% 的患者即刻诊断，并且是 68% 患者的唯一诊断来源。另外，27% 患者的 TBNA 标本培养分离出抗酸杆菌。在另一项研究中，在20例结核性纵隔淋巴结炎患者中通过22号TBNA活检针能明确65%患者的肺结核诊断[36]。

TBNA也能用于诊断HIV感染患者的纵隔淋巴结结核。在41例伴纵隔和肺门淋巴结病的HIV感染患者中研究了19号组织针进行TBNA的功效[40]。TBNA的整体检出率和排除诊断率分别是52%和32%。通过TBNA诊断出23例患者中20例（87%）的分枝杆菌病。74%的患者能够立刻得出诊断，61%的患者细胞培养阳性，并且48%的患者能够通过TBNA排除诊断淋巴结结核病。

最近的研究也报道了EBUS-TBNA对孤立结核性纵隔淋巴结炎的诊断率[41,42]。对于这部分患者TBNA与EBUS-TBNA诊断率的对比未曾有文献报道。

局限性和争议

"盲穿技术"

标准TBNA最主要的局限性是在操作过程中无法实时对纵隔淋巴结进行成像。由于这个原因，一些作者把传统TBNA称为盲穿技术。实际上，操作者和操作都不是盲目的。穿刺部位是在对胸部CT仔细评估后选择的，操作者清楚地知道淋巴结的位置及其与气道的关系。确实，一次成功的淋巴结穿刺要求对CT解剖全面的评估，以及操作技巧和自信。然而由于气道支气管树被全身和肺部的血管围绕，许多支气管镜医师还是对检查的安全性存在怀疑，哪怕出血和纵隔积血的报道只限于少数几个案例。然而，关于它的安全性的错误看法对这项技术的使用不足起到关键的作用。

血管和气道的关系比较固定。已经明确对许多淋巴结组进行TBNA的安全标志[43]。第7淋巴结组是最安全的淋巴结组，它的周围没有血管。相似地，对第4R淋巴结组进行的TBNA有非常良好的安全记录，特别是存在体积大的淋巴结时。然而我们必须承认，无法对靶部位进行成像确实使对较小的淋巴结（位于第2R和2L组）和一些肺门淋巴结组的定位变得困难。

在过去的20年已经探索了许多方法来克服标准TBNA技术的局限性。一些操作者在TBNA操作时使用CT透视来实时引导。虽然接近80%的患者能够成功[44,45]，但是由于在辐射安全方面存在的问题，以及更好的替代技术的出现，这种方法从未被主流支气管镜实践采用。另一个方法是通过电磁导管支气管镜来定位用于TBNA取样的淋巴结。这个技术主要被用来获取小的肺外周结节的活检组织[46-48]。但是它也能引导操作者更准确地到达淋巴结。Gildea等报道了在对31个淋巴结采样时，100%的合格标本获取成功率。这项研究的平均淋巴结大小为2.8 cm。在另一项研究中，通过这项技术获取了94.3%的纵隔淋巴结（平均大小1.8 cm）的合格标本[49]。然而，在缺乏对照组的情况下，这些数据只能明确电磁导航支气管镜的可行性，却不能说明电磁导航支气管镜引导下的TBNA比传统TBNA技术更好。这项技术是否比传统TBNA在获取小的纵隔淋巴结标本上更好，这个问题非常重要却又没有答案。仪器设备的高昂费用是这项技术相关的另一个问题[50]。

另一个方法是在TBNA检查前，通过多探头CT获得相关影像数据，生成虚拟支气管镜图像，从而引导TBNA。在这项技术中，进行实际支气管镜检查时，在屏幕上显示虚拟支气管镜图像。在TBNA时，通过半透明壁显示靶部位来引导支气管镜医师。在一项研究中，TBNA对支气管旁和肺门淋巴结的诊断率在使用虚拟支气管镜引导技术后，可从原来的69%上升到100%。两种方法对气管隆突下淋巴结的诊断率相似[51]。另外开发了一个CT支气管镜模拟软件，它不仅展示了位于透明气管壁后的靶病灶，还显示了虚拟针通向靶部位的最合适通道，避免损伤血管和其他脆弱结构。在一项前瞻性研究中，伴或不伴这款软件协助的情况下连续对28例患者的50个目标淋巴结进行TBNA[52]。淋巴结的平均大小是14 mm。伴CT支气管镜模拟的 TBNA 成功率为 58%，而传统技术的成功率为 30%。虽然 CT 支气管镜模拟不是一个实时引导的系统，但由于它不需要额外的感应和追踪装置或昂贵的附件，也不会有额外的辐射照射，所以它也有一些吸引力。从这些研究得到的初步结果需要其他独立研究的确认。

支气管内超声是目前最可靠、经临床验证的工具，可以为 TBNA 对壁外纵隔和肺门淋巴结进行成像[53]。EBUS-TBNA 在不同荟萃分析和系统性综述中的敏感性范围是 88%~100%[54-56]。这项技术是安全的，并且很快获得了全球范围支气管镜医师的认可。但是，这项技术要求专门的支气管镜，它不能用于其他取样操作，并且 EBUS-TBNA 活检针比标准技术使用的王氏针更笨重。另外，初始设备比较昂贵，并且由于费用的限制和专业知识缺乏，这项技术无法推广使用。然而，由于它能够对淋巴结进行成像，并实时追踪针道，在标准 TBNA 无法到达壁外结构这个问题上，EBUS-TBNA 提供了最有效的解决办法。

小的淋巴结的低诊断率

习惯上认为所有的纵隔淋巴结都是正常的，除非它的直径在 CT 上远远 > 1 cm。但是，将近 15%~20% 的肺癌患者手术切除大小 <1 cm 的纵隔淋巴结后，会意外地检测出肿瘤转移。如果要避免无意义的胸腔手术，在这些患者中检测出 N2 疾病很重要。累及 N1 淋巴结和中央部位的肿瘤是隐匿性 N2 疾病的高风险因素[59]。在未发现增大的纵隔淋巴结的情况下，推荐在开胸手术检测隐匿性 N2 疾病前，先对中央型肺癌和 N1 疾病患者进行纵隔分期[60,61]。标准 TBNA 不适用于这些患者的纵隔分期。一些研究报道 TBNA 对淋巴结短轴 < 1 cm 肺癌患者的诊断率很低，甚至可以忽略。比如在一个 TBNA 病例研究中，54 个从直径 <5 mm 的淋巴结获取的抽吸物中没有一个诊断出恶性，而从直径 5~9 mm 的淋巴结获取的抽吸物中有 15% 诊断出恶性[19]。在另一项研究中，从 75 例淋巴结大小 <10 mm 的患者中获取的 TBNA 标本，只有 1 例能得出诊断[31]。对于较小的纵隔淋巴结获得的 TBNA 标本的低诊断率有许多解释。使用标准 TBNA 方法对小淋巴结进行成功取样的首要障碍就是缺乏视觉引导。TBNA 操作时淋巴随着呼吸运动是另一个重要的原因。Piet 等在胸部 CT 四维成像中展示出纵隔淋巴结伴随呼吸在头尾向、内外向和腹背向有明显活动[62]。在这项研究中，淋巴结中心平均位移是（6.2±2.9）mm，气管的隆突运动是（6.5±2.5）mm，跟气管隆突相关的淋巴结在头尾向上的运动是（5.3±2.1）mm。另一个限制 TBNA 的因素是 CT/PET 上阴性的纵隔淋巴结转移病灶的大小。比如在一项研究中，在这类淋巴结中转移病灶的平均大小为（3.7±2.0）mm，68% 的病灶在组织学检查中 <4 mm[63]。总之，传统 TBNA 在这些患者中的低诊断率并非完全不可预计。

实时成像靶部位的能力是 EBUS-TBNA 在 <1 cm 的纵隔淋巴结取样方面明显优于标准 TBNA 的地方。许多研究报道，对于 CT 或 PET 扫描没有任何证据表明累及纵隔的患者，通过 EBUS-TBNA 检测 N2 疾病的敏感性、特异性和准确性都很高[64]。也有人报道 EBUS-TBNA 和超声内镜引导下细针穿刺活检术联合使用的高成功率[65]。现在看起来 EBUS-TBNA 作为比纵隔镜检查侵犯性更低的方法，在未来对肺癌患者的小的纵隔淋巴结分期指南中将更加强调。

其他误区

从 TBNA 的早期描述开始，就出现了许多没有充分理由的质疑。在之前的部分已经回答了未经证实的安全问题。有一个广泛传播的观念认为 TBNA 是一项复杂的技术，因此有很长的学习曲线。这是完全错误的。许多充满激情的操作者报道，他们只通过简单的自学入门工具，如书、教程和视频，没有经过任何正规的训练就得到与文献所报道的相似的结果[66,67]。另外，最近一个对 TBNA 的研究没有发现任何学习该技术周期长的证据，这项研究跟踪调查5位精通基础支气管镜技术的操作者在32个月时间里TBNA的诊断率[68]。学习开始时的诊断率为77%，32个月后为82%。

虽然许多研究证实这项技术的学习并不难，但是这并不表示正规教育和技术的提高不重要。实际上，持续有研究表明，教育干预和经验能改善TBNA的诊断结果。比如在一项为期3年的研究中，面向支气管镜医师、技术支持员工和病理分析医师的全面的、多角度的教育干预，能够将TBNA的诊断率从21.4%提高到47.6%[69]。许多其他研究得出相似的结论[70,71]。这些研究提出了一个普遍的主题，就是在TBNA操作中教育和培训支气管镜医师助手和正确处理标本的重要性。合理的患者选择、TBNA技术的一致性、熟悉活检针以及和细胞病理学医师的直接沟通对此也有帮助。以上这些问题也许可以解释为什么一些支气管镜医师从来不能达到和文献报道的相似的诊断率，因此放弃这一方法[8]。

另外也有人担心在TBNA的操作中，很有可能会损伤支气管镜。不正确的TBNA技术确实可能会损伤支气管镜的工作通道，因而需要昂贵的修理费用[72]。但是，这种情况比较罕见，如果能按照以下简单的原则进行，几乎就能完全避免。第一，在每次TBNA导管插入到支气管镜前，确保活检针的斜边全部都在远端的金属外套里面。如果它的前端超过金属外套，就会在插管时损伤工作通道。同时要确保活检针在前刺时，不要拉回靠近金属外套，因为它也可能穿透覆盖的塑料管并损伤工作通道。第二，当TBNA导管穿过支气管镜的时候，支气管镜的近端和远端应该尽量保持笔直。如果感受到阻力，不要用力让TBNA导管通过支气管镜远端。正确的操作是保持支气管镜远端为中立、前向位。第三，除非TBNA导管的远端确实超过支气管镜，并且能在气道内看见，否则不要进针。如果活检针就位的时候，TBNA导管仍在工作通道内，那么损伤导管的风险就很高。最后，一旦获得标本，支气管镜应该尽可能保持笔直，便于活检针平滑收回。

每次经支气管针吸活检后必须行急性泄漏测试，确保操作过程中没有损伤工作通道。

组织样本对比细胞样本

许多研究已经明确了通过TBNA技术从纵隔淋巴结获取组织标本的可行性[73,74]。因为诊断良性疾病组织标本优于细胞学标本，所以常规使用19号穿刺针进行TBNA可能是明智的。结节病或肺结核在鉴别诊断中特点鲜明。在肺癌的纵隔分期中，组织标本相比细胞学标本也有一些优势。比如说，TBNA组织标本中肿瘤的存在排除了肺癌分析假阳性的风险。一些研究也发现，TBNA组织标本在检测淋巴结转移时比细胞学标本更敏感。在一项Schenk等人的研究中，组织标本对肺癌纵隔分期的敏感性是89.1%，而细胞学标本只有52.7%[75]。一项多中心前瞻性研究也报道了相似结果，其中组织标本检测出57%的恶性肿瘤，而细胞学标本只有41%[19]。总之，如果在细胞学标本外同时获取组织标本，预计TBNA的诊断率将会上升14%~35%[76,77]。最后常规TBNA时从细胞学活检针转换为组织活检针，也会减少对肺癌纵隔分期手术操作的需要[2]。然而，关于这点的文献有冲突。在一项研究中，在22号穿刺针外又使用19号穿刺针后，淋巴结转移检测诊断率的上升无显著统计学差异[78]。

使用19号穿刺针的TBNA有良好的安全记录。没有证据表明19号TBNA活检针比起22号穿刺针，出现并发症的风险更高或更容易损伤支气管镜。但是，使用19号组织针穿透气管壁比22号穿刺针更困难。因此，不可能每个患者都能通过19号TBNA活检针获取合格的组织标本[73,79]。因为用19号穿刺针进行TBNA在技术上更有挑战性，所以只有在使用22号TBNA活检针上有足够的经验和熟练度时，才可以考虑转换使用19号穿刺针[2,71]。

快速原位评估

快速原位评估是一种类似术中冰冻切片检查的策略。在支气管镜检查时，细胞学病理医师和技师也在场，并且将TBNA标本的质量和初步结果立刻反馈给支气管镜医师。对支气管镜医师来说，快速原位评估的诉求是直观的和明显的[80]。如果使用快速原位评估确认恶性肿瘤细胞的存在，那么TBNA的进一步尝试可以被终止。如果通过快速原位评估做出明确的诊断，那么支气管镜医师可以选择放弃进一步的取样步骤，比如刷检和TBBx。相反，如果通过最初尝试无法获得合格的标本，那么支气管镜医师可以选择继续进一步尝试、重新查看解剖标记、选择另一个活检区域和改变经支气管针吸活检针。对那些努力想要改善自己的技术和诊断率的人，立即的反馈是非常有用的。快速原位评估也给了病理医师和顾问机会，以最适合他们偏好和实验室技术的方式来制备标本。快速原位评估最明显的障碍是由于细胞学病理医师在支气管镜室所花的额外时间所造成的费用的增加。由于时间限制和补偿问题，对于细胞学病理医师来说拒绝快速原位评估的要求是很常见的。然而，成本分析表明，当与TBNA操作一起使用时，快速原位评估是一个经济有效的策略[81,82]。

早期关于快速原位评估的研究表明，这项技术的整体检出率增加，有更高的机会在TBNA标本中检测出癌症，并且不合格标本的比例降低[83,84]。但是，与预期相反的是，在许多这类研究中快速原位评估并不影响每个淋巴结部位的穿刺次数[81,84]。

但是，最近关于快速原位评估的前瞻性随机研究与先前研究的结论恰恰相反，而先前的研究设计要么是回顾性的，要么是观察性的。在一项这样的研究中，快速原位评估对TBNA的诊断率、癌症诊断、合格标本的比例、活检针穿刺次数、操作时间和操作时镇静药使用的数量没有影响[85]。然而，作者注意到快速原位评估组TBBx数量的减少趋势。在另一项随机研究中报道了相似的结果，但是在这项研究中，被分配到快速原位评估组的患者的并发症发生率比进行传统TBNA组显著降低（6% vs. 20%，$P=0.01$）。一旦通过快速原位评估明确诊断，就避免了经支气管活检，导致快速原位评估组的并发症发生率减少[86]。在这些数据的启发下，现在常规快速原位评估显得没有必要，特别是当一位有经验的操作者进行TBNA时。当感觉有需要用一个比TBBx侵犯性更低的TBNA技术来确保诊断时，尤其是在高风险的患者中，快速原位评估可能还扮演重要的角色。

支气管内针吸活检

支气管内针吸活检（EBNA）是一项使用经支气管活检针从支气管内可见病灶获取细胞学标本的技术。许多研究表明，在传统诊断方法（如支气管内活检和刷检）外使用EBNA时，支气管镜的诊断率显著改善。EBNA在黏膜下和支气管旁疾病患者（图3.9A）中应用增加的收益要高于外生性肿块病灶的患者（图3.9B）。更重要的优势在于，对怀疑是小细胞肺癌的患者，活检钳取标本时会破坏组织学结构，影响正确的诊断。而EBNA获取细胞学标本不存在破坏组织学结构的问题，所以EBNA在这些病例中相比传统方法有更明显的优势[87]。

技术

EBNA的技术比较简单，还需根据取样的支气管内肿瘤类型。操作通常借助王氏经支气管22号细胞学活检针进行。为了从黏膜下和支气管旁疾病患者获取标本，活检针需要以30°~45°的倾斜角进入黏膜下肿瘤（图3.10A）。在病灶为外生性肿块的病例中，活检针需要以90°角进入肿瘤，来确保最大的穿刺深度，因为在这些病例中穿刺的目标是尽可能从肿瘤中心

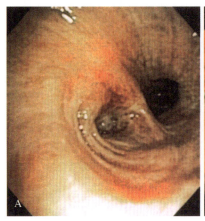 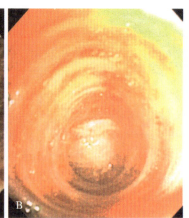

图 3.9　A. 黏膜下和支气管旁肿瘤；B. 外生性肿块

获取细胞学标本（图 3.10B）。虽然最佳的穿刺次数没有明确定义，但是大多数情况下 2~3 次穿刺应该是足够的。

临床应用

为了从内镜下可见的肺癌中获取细胞学标本，EBNA 伴随其他取样技术一起进行。根据 2012 年的综述，在 7 项报道的研究中，EBNA 的联合平均诊断率为 80%，范围在 68%~91%[88]。从那以后，许多其他的研究报道了相似的结果[89,90]。在大多数研究中，EBNA 的单独诊断率超过了传统取样技术（如支气管内活检和刷检）的单独诊断率[89,91]。

在传统取样步骤外加上 EBNA，能增加支气管镜对内镜下可见肺癌的诊断率[89-92]。比如在一项前瞻性研究中，我们组报道了纤维支气管镜下传统取样方法的诊断率为 76%，而联合 EBNA 和传统方法的诊断率增加到 96%[91]。Govert 等报道了相似的结果，即在传统取样方法外进行 EBNA 时，支气管镜的诊断率从 82% 增加到 95%[92]。

EBNA 特别适用于获取黏膜下和气管旁的病灶标本，这种肿瘤主要累及黏膜下层面。活检钳取样和刷检等传统方法倾向于对黏膜表面取样，可能会错过黏膜下肿瘤，更不用说位于支气管壁外肿瘤。从这些患者获取活检钳标本的另一个困难在于活检钳容易在支气管壁上

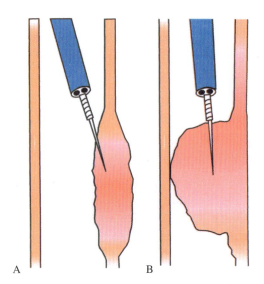

图 3.10　A. TBNA 活检针以 30°~45° 角进入黏膜下肿瘤；B. TBNA 活检针以 90° 角进入外生性肿瘤

打滑，因为在一些情况下覆盖的黏膜由于黏膜下浸润而变硬变厚。当活检钳斜向靠近被肿瘤累及的支气管壁时，获取好的活检标本同样有挑战性。在这些情况下，将支气管内活检针插入支气管壁的深层时，从黏膜下和支气管旁肿瘤获取标本更加容易。实际上，持续有研究表明 EBNA 对黏膜下和气管旁疾病患者的诊断作用优于外生性肿块病灶。比如，在一项研究中黏膜下和气管旁疾病的诊断率从传统诊

断方法的 65% 增加到 EBNA 合并传统诊断方法的 96%[91]，在另一项研究中从 64% 升高到 94%[89]。基于这些结果，EBNA 应该考虑和传统方法一起作为获取黏膜下和气管旁疾病标本的标准方法。

EBNA 在病灶为外生性肿块的患者中诊断效果的增加没那么显著。虽然有人报道诊断率有增加的趋势，但是在大多数研究中没有统计学上的差异[89,91]。所以，不推荐对这些患者在传统诊断方法外常规附加 EBNA。根据我们的经验，EBNA 能够提高支气管镜检查对镜下淡白色、体积大的外生性肿块病灶患者的诊断率。在这些患者中，表面活检和刷检可能只能获取坏死组织，不能得出可信的组织诊断。经支气管活检针穿透组织表面增加了它从肿瘤核心获取存活细胞的可能性，因此改善了支气管镜的诊断率。获取出血性肿瘤标本时，EBNA 也被认为比传统方法更好，因为 EBNA 的出血风险比活检钳方法更低。如果第一次支气管镜检查只使用传统取样技术无法获取标本，也提示可以对外生性肿块病灶的患者进行 EBNA。

局限性

EBNA 增加了操作的总持续时间和前期费用。但是，根据一项成本最小化分析，当 EBNA 的费用低于 250 欧元而诊断率增加超过 5.2% 时[93]，联合使用活检、刷检和 EBNA 比只进行活检和刷检更经济。常规进行 EBNA 至少对黏膜下和气管旁疾病患者是一个经济合理的决定，它对这类患者诊断率的增加更显著。EBNA 另一个潜在的缺点是它损伤支气管镜的风险比传统方法更高。显然从这方面来说，再怎样强调培训和经验的重要性也不过分。最后，来自 EBNA 的细胞学标本相比组织标本不太适合免疫组化和分子学研究，以进一步明确肿瘤的特征。

外周经支气管针吸活检

外周经支气管针吸活检（P-TBNA）是一个简单安全的技术，用于在透视引导下从孤立肺结节和肺肿块获取细胞学标本。尽管它对周围型肺癌诊断的作用被广泛接受，但是这个技术并未得到充分利用。

技术

外周经支气管针吸活检（P-TBNA）应该在其他取样方法前进行。操作时通常使用 22 号细胞学 TBNA 活检针。首先，通过透视成像识别病灶。然后将支气管镜插入到对应病灶的支气管。TBNA 活检针通过支气管镜的活检通道，确保活检针远端完全缩回到金属外套中。在一些情况下，支气管镜的远端需要伸直，并拉回到近端气道，帮助 TBNA 活检针进入气道。一旦看见金属外套，就开始在透视引导下向靶病灶的外边缘推进 TBNA 活检针。当金属外套接触病灶外周时就会感觉到阻力。不要在操作时使用过大的力，避免扭转 TBNA 导管，因为这样会导致操作基本上无效。通过旋转荧光镜 C 臂来确认活检针的位置。C 臂旋转时如果金属外套和肿块病灶维持一个持续的关系，那么 TBNA 活检针的位置就是合适的。

一旦确认金属外套的位置正确，助手就会被要求放置 22 号穿刺针并将其推向外周肿块（图 3.11A、B）。在透视下确认活检针位置后，助手就会被要求使用注射器进行抽吸，而操作者会轻轻地在病灶内前后移动活检针来切下细胞。在获取标本后，将活检针拉回到金属外套中，同时从偏转控制杆移开大拇指来伸直支气管镜的远端。通常需要向中央气道缩回支气管镜，来伸直支气管镜远端。尽可能在保持支气管镜笔直的同时移除活检针。使用标准方法收集细胞学标本。两次活检针穿刺足够从外周肿瘤获取细胞学标本。建议在检查的最后进行 X 线检查，来排除气胸的存在。

临床应用

P-TBNA 主要用于怀疑存在原发性肺癌的患者。P-TBNA 的诊断率范围是 36%~69%，平

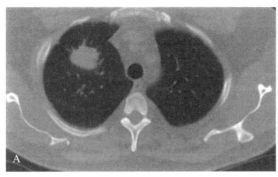
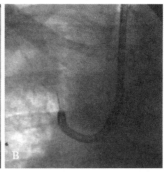

图 3.11　A. 胸部 CT 显示右上肺肿块；B. 可见 TBNA 活检针在肿块内，病理检查提示肺腺癌

均诊断率为 60%[88]。大多数关于这个话题的各项研究都表明，P-TBNA 的诊断率高于其他取样技术，如刷检和活检。作为 8%~35% 患者的唯一诊断来源，除了传统诊断方法外再使用 P-TBNA 能够增加纤维支气管镜对周围型肺癌的整体检出率。比如在一项研究中，在支气管冲洗术、刷检和经支气管活检外再使用 P-TBNA 能将纤维支气管镜的诊断率从 46% 增加到 70%[94]。

最近在意大利的一项大型前瞻性研究中，重新确认了 P-TBNA 在诊断周围型肺部肿瘤中的重要作用[95]。在这项研究中，218 例伴有外周结节或肺肿块的患者在一次检查中接受了支气管冲洗术、TBBx 和 P-TBNA。这个研究中将近 60% 的病灶 <3 cm。大多数病灶（88%）的病因是恶性的。P-TBNA 的诊断率是 65%，TBBx 的诊断率是 45%，支气管冲洗术的诊断率是 22%。P-TBNA 是 21% 患者的唯一诊断来源。8 例患者（3.7%）出现主要并发症，包括 4 例患者出现气胸，另外 4 例出现严重出血。不确定研究中的哪个步骤引发主要并发症。

病灶大小是影响 P-TBNA 诊断率的重要因素。在一项研究中，P-TBNA 对 <3 cm 恶性肿瘤的诊断率为 27.5%，对 >3 cm 恶性肿瘤的诊断率为 65.5%[96]。相似地，在另一项 Wang 等的研究中[97]，P-TBNA 对 <3 cm 病灶的诊断率为 46.7%，对 >3 cm 病灶的诊断率为 80%。在 Trisolini 等人的研究中[95]，P-TBNA 对 <2 cm 病灶的诊断准确率低于 >2 cm 的病灶，比值比是 0.25（95% 可信区间，0.12~0.7）。实际上，没有证据表明对于直径 <2 cm 的外周肿瘤，P-TBNA 的诊断率优于传统诊断方法[95,97,98]。

肿瘤-支气管关系是另一个影响不同取样方法对周围型肺部肿瘤诊断率的重要因素。比如在一项研究中，高分辨率胸部 CT 下肿瘤-支气管关系为 3 型或 4 型的外周肿瘤患者共 26 例，P-TBNA 能诊断出其中 20 例（77%），而 TBBx 诊断出 5 例（19%）[99]。P-TBNA 在 3 型和 4 型病灶中的高成功率是由于 TBNA 活检针能穿透支气管扭曲或狭窄的节段，到达肿瘤的深部。而活检钳要么被推开（3 型中），要么不能到达目标位置（4 型中）。所以在支气管镜检查前行胸部 CT 检测为 3 型或 4 型肿瘤-支气管关系时，应该考虑进行 P-TBNA。

外周经支气管针吸活检的局限性

应该注意 P-TBNA 存在着许多局限性。第一，P-TBNA 获取的是细胞学标本，比起组织标本不太适合进行免疫组化研究或分子学研究。第二，P-TBNA 的诊断价值或多或少限制于识别恶性病灶[95]。诊断良性病变时，TBBx 获取的组织标本相比 P-TBNA 获取的细胞学标本有明显优势。可能 P-TBNA 最重要的局限是它不能改善对 <2 cm 的外周病灶的诊断率。CT 的广泛应用使得意义不明的小病灶的检出率明显增加，同时也伴随着支气管镜活检的增加。对于

这些患者，包括 P-TBNA 在内的传统方法的诊断率低，而在径向探头支气管内超声、虚拟支气管镜定位和电磁导航支气管镜引导下获取标本会有很大帮助。在其中任一技术帮助下，外周病灶标本均可通过标准支气管镜技术（如经支气管活检和刷检）获取。在一个随机前瞻性试验中，Chao 等对比了 202 例存在外周病灶的患者，探讨分别使用径向探头支气管内超声引导下的传统诊断方法，以及伴或不伴径向探头支气管内超声引导下的 P-TBNA 的诊断率[100]。接受支气管内超声引导下 P-TBNA 的患者外周病灶平均大小为 3.5 cm，并且操作者在操作过程中没有使用导向鞘。同时进行 P-TBNA 和传统检查患者的诊断率显著高于只进行传统诊断方法的患者（78.4% vs. 60.6%）。支气管内超声引导下 P-TBNA 的诊断率为 62.5%，而支气管内超声引导下 TBBx 为 48.9%。虽然支气管内超声探头位于病灶内（78.3%）比在病灶附近（47.2%）能达到的诊断率更高，但是支气管内超声引导下 P-TBNA 不受支气管内超声探头和病灶相对位置的影响。支气管内超声引导下 P-TBNA 没有出现手术相关并发症。

虽然从这项研究中获得的初步结果是鼓舞人心的，但是需要更多的工作来对这些结果进行独立验证。同样，对支气管内超声引导下 P-TBNA 在改善 <3 cm 肺部病灶的诊断率中可能的作用的研究也是值得的。

经支气管针吸活检术的现状

支气管内超声引导下经支气管针吸活检（EBUS-TBNA）的日益普及引发了关于标准经支气管针吸活检（TBNA）在支气管镜实践中现有价值的讨论[101]。我们认为一个简单安全又不昂贵、临床价值可靠的技术，不应该毫无根据地被放弃。有许多理由支持学习标准的经支气管针吸活检技术，并将它有效地应用在每天的支气管镜检查实践中。

没有研究直接地对比凸面探头 EBUS-TBNA 和传统 TBNA 技术对肺癌纵隔分期诊断率的区别。我们也必须指出在大量的研究中，EBUS-TBNA 通常通过气道导管或喉罩气道在全麻下进行，而传统 TBNA 通常在最初支气管镜检查的适度镇静下进行。EBUS-TBNA 比标准 TBNA 费用更高，并且当地是否具备检查的装备和专业人员都是限制该技术广泛应用的重要问题。如果要在单次操作中完成诊断和分期，那么操作者必须在经支气管针吸活检后退出支气管内超声，并使用标准纤维支气管镜获取其他标本，而这会增加支气管镜检查的费用和持续时间。

包括支气管源性癌在内的肺部疾病在第三世界国家更加流行。对来自这部分地区的呼吸内科医师来说，进行 EBUS-TBNA 的费用和所要求的培训仍然是很大的阻力。另外，还必须掌握凸面探头超声支气管镜的技术、熟悉 EBUS-TBNA 的复杂设计、收集超声系统的使用指导，并且学会怎样读超声图像。想要对这项技术建立信心大概要求经过 50 次操作。一个社区支气管镜医师可能需要长达 1 年的时间来克服学习曲线。另外，每年至少还要进行 25 次操作来维持这一检查技术。后者在三级护理中心和所谓的卓越中心比较有可能完成。在这方面，对于传统呼吸内科医师，传统 TBNA 仍然是检查方法之一。

我们坚定地相信传统经支气管针吸活检无论是在当前还是未来的临床实践中，均会是纵隔分期的主要力量。对于位于经支气管针吸活检能够到达的淋巴结组（第 4R 组和第 7 组）中的大淋巴结，EBUS-TBNA 相比标准技术没有优势。通过传统经支气管针吸活检进行分期在绝大多数患者中都足够了。让这些患者习惯性接受 EBUS-TBNA 是错误的建议，只会增加检查的持续时间和费用。然而，如果传统 TBNA 不能明确这些患者的 N2 或 N3 病诊断，那么 EBUS-TBNA 将会是合理的下一步检查。

另外，CT 或 PET/CT 上提示正常或轻微增大的淋巴结，传统 TBNA 不太可能提供分期信息。在这种情况下，谨慎的办法是放弃传统

TBNA，并在早期支气管镜检查时进行 EBUS-TBNA。诊断位于第 2R 和 2L 组的小淋巴结时，EBUS-TBNA 也优先于传统 TBNA。借助 19 号穿刺针进行经支气管针吸活检、支气管内活检和经支气管活检，是对怀疑 I 期和 II 期结节病患者合理的诊断方法。但是，当支气管镜下肺活检不能进行的时候，EBUS-TBNA 优先于传统 TBNA。怀疑结核性纵隔淋巴炎的患者，也建议进行经支气管针吸活检。EBUS-TBNA 也能用于这些患者，但是不清楚是否优于标准 TBNA。TBNA 对淋巴瘤的独立检测作用还未验证。

TBNA 能够改善支气管镜对黏膜下和支气管旁肿瘤的诊断率已经证实。在外生性肿块病灶中，TBNA 在支气管镜显示存在表面广泛坏死的情况下是有用的。不推荐在外生性肿块病灶中常规应用 TBNA。

P-TBNA 改善了支气管镜对周围型肺部肿瘤患者的诊断率。推荐所有周围型肺部肿瘤患者都接受诊断性支气管镜。当支气管镜检查前 CT 结果表明肿瘤 - 支气管关系为 3 型或 4 型时，这项技术是最有用的。

参考文献

1. Dasgupta A, Mehta AC. Transbronchial needle aspiration. An underused diagnostic technique. Clin Chest Med. 1999;20:39–51.
2. Patel NM, Pohlman A, Husain A, Noth I, Hall JB, Kress JP. Conventional transbronchial needle aspiration decreases the rate of surgical sampling of intrathoracic lymphadenopathy. Chest. 2007;131:773–8.
3. Shah PL, Singh S, Bower M, Livni N, Padley S, Nicholson AG. The role of transbronchial fine needle aspiration in an integrated care pathway for the assessment of patients with suspected lung cancer. J Thorac Oncol. 2006;1:324–7.
4. Cetinkaya E, Yildiz P, Kadakal F, et al. Transbronchial needle aspiration in the diagnosis of intrathoracic lymphadenopathy. Respiration. 2002;69:335–8.
5. Khoo KL, Chua GSW, Mukhopadhyay A, Lim TK. Transbronchial needle aspiration: initial experience in routine diagnostic bronchoscopy. Respir Med. 2003;97:1200–4.
6. Jeune IL, Baldwin D. Measuring the success of transbronchial needle aspiration in everyday clinical practice. Respir Med. 2007;101:670–5.
7. Prakash UBS, Offord KP, Stubbs SE. Bronchoscopy in North America: the ACCP survey. Chest. 1991; 100:1668–75.
8. Haponik EF, Shure D. Underutilization of transbronchial needle aspiration. Experience of current pulmonary fellows. Chest. 1997;112:251–3.
9. Rajamani S, Mehta AC. Transbronchial needle aspiration of central and peripheral nodules. Monaldi Arch Chest Dis. 2001;56:436–45.
10. Wang KP. Transbronchial needle aspiration. J Bronchol. 1994;1:63–8.
11. Bernasconi M, Chhajed PN, Gambazzi F, et al. Combined transbronchial needle aspiration and positron emission tomography for mediastinal staging of NSCLC. Eur Respir J. 2006;27:889–94.
12. Hsu LH, Ko JS, You DL, Liu CC, Chu NM. Transbronchial needle aspiration accurately diagnoses subcentimeter mediastinal and hilar lymph nodes detected by integrated positron emission tomography and computed tomography. Respirology. 2007;12:848–55.
13. Mountain CF, Dressler CM. Regional lymph node classification for lung cancer staging. Chest. 1997; 111:1718–23.
14. Rusch VW, Asamura H, Watanabe H, et al. The IASCL lung cancer staging project. A proposal for a new international lymph node map in the forthcoming seventh edition of the TMN classification for lung cancer. J Thorac Oncol. 2009;4:568–77.
15. Wang KP. Transbronchial needle aspiration to obtain histology specimen. J Bronchol. 1994;1:116–22.
16. Chin R, McCain TW, Lucia MA, et al. Transbronchial needle aspiration in diagnosing and staging lung cancer. How many aspirates are needed? Am J Respir Crit Care Med. 2002;166: 377–81.
17. Diacon AH, Schuurmans MM, Theron J, et al. Transbronchial needle aspirates: how many passes per target site? Eur Respir J. 2007;29:112–6.
18. Diacon AH, Shuurmans MM, Theron J, et al. Transbronchial needle aspirates. Comparison of two preparation methods. Chest. 2005;127:2015–8.
19. Harrow EM, Abi-Saleh W, Blum J, et al. The utility of transbronchial needle aspiration in the staging of bronchogenic carcinoma. Am J Respir Crit Care Med. 2000;161:601–7.
20. Seijo LM, Campo A, de Torres JP, et al. FDG uptake and the diagnostic yield of transbronchial needle aspiration. J Bronchology Interv Pulmonol. 2011;18:7–14.
21. Horrow E, Halber M, Hardy S, Halterman W. Bronchoscopic and roentgenographic correlates of a positive transbronchial needle aspiration in the staging of lung cancer. Chest. 1991;100:1592–6.
22. Holty JC, Kuschner WG, Gould MK. Accuracy of transbronchial needle aspiration for mediastinal staging of non-small cell lung cancer: a meta-analysis. Thorax. 2005;60:949–55.
23. Wang KP, Brower R, Haponik EF, Siegelman S. Flexible transbronchial needle aspiration for staging of bronchogenic carcinoma. Chest. 1983;84:571–6.
24. Kuchera RF, Wolfe GK, Perry ME. Hemomedidiastinum after transbronchial needle aspiration. Chest. 1986;90:466.
25. Epstein SK, Winslow CJ, Brecher SM, Faling LJ. Polymicrobial bacterial pericarditis after transbronchial needle aspiration. Case report with an investigation on the risk of bacterial contamination during fiberoptic bronchoscopy. Am Rev Respir Dis. 1992;146:523–5.
26. Toloza EM, Harpole L, Detterbeck F, McCrory DC. Invasive staging of non-small cell lung cancer. A review of current

evidence. Chest. 2003;123:157S–66S.
27. Medford ARL, Agrawal S, Free CN, Bennett JA. A prospective study of conventional transbronchial needle aspiration: performance and cost utility. Respiration. 2010;79:482–9.
28. Bilaceroglu S, Cagirici U, Gunel O, Bayol U, Perim K. Comparison of rigid and flexible transbronchial needle aspiration in the staging of bronchogenic carcinoma. Respiration. 1998;65:441–9.
29. Kunst PWA, Lee P, Paul MA, Senam S, Smit EF. Restaging of mediastinal nodes with transbronchial needle aspiration after induction chemoradiation for locally advanced non-small cell lung cancer. J Thorac Oncol. 2007;2:912–5.
30. Herth FJF, Annema JT, Eberhardt R, et al. Endobronchial ultrasound with transbronchial needle aspiration for restaging the mediastinum in lung cancer. J Clin Oncol. 2008;26:3346–50.
31. Oki M, Saka H, Kamazava A, Sako C, Ando M, Watanabe A. The role of transcranial needle aspiration in the diagnosis and staging of lung cancer:computed tomographic correlates of a positive result. Respiration. 2004;71:523–7.
32. Selcuk ZT, Firat P. The diagnostic yield of transbronchial needle aspiration in superior vena cava syndrome. Lung Cancer. 2003;42:183–8.
33. Bilacerglu S, Perin K, Gunel O, Cagirici U, Buyuksirin M. Combining transbronchial aspiration with endobronchial and transbronchial biopsy in sarcoidosis. Monaldi Arch Chest Dis. 1999;54:217–23.
34. Trisolini R, Tinelli C, Cancellieri A, et al. Transbronchial needle aspiration in sarcoidosis: yield and predictors of a positive aspirate. J Thorac Cardiovasc Surg. 2008;135:837–42.
35. Trisolini R, Lazzari L, Cancellieri A, et al. The value of flexible transbronchial needle aspiration in the diagnosis of stage I sarcoidosis. Chest. 2003;124:2126–30.
36. Cetinkaya E, Yildiz P, Altin S, Yilmaz V. Diagnostic value of transbronchial needle aspiration by Wang 22-gauge cytology needle in intrathoracic lymphadenopathy. Chest. 2004;125:527–31.
37. Navani N, Booth HL, Kocjan G, et al. Combination of endobronchial ultrasound-guided transbronchial needle aspiration with standard bronchoscopic techniques for the diagnosis of stage I and stage II pulmonary sarcoidosis. Respirology. 2011;16:467–72.
38. Trembley A, Stather DR, MacEachern P, Khalil M, Field SK. A randomized controlled trial of standard vs endobronchial ultrasonography guided transbronchial needle aspiration in patients with suspected sarcoidosis. Chest. 2009;136:340–6.
39. Bilaceroglu S, Gunel O, Eris N, Cagirici U, Mehta AC. Transbronchial needle aspiration in diagnosing intrathoracic tuberculous lymphadenitis. Chest. 2004;126:259–67.
40. Harkin TJ, Ciotoli C, Addrizzo-Harris DJ, Naidich DP, Jagirdar J, Rom WN. Transbronchial needle aspiration (TBNA) in patients infected with HIV. Am J Respir Crit Care Med. 1998;157:1913–8.
41. Hassan T, McLaughlin AM, O'Connell F, Gibson N, Nicholson S, Keane J. EBUS-TBNA performs well in the diagnosis of isolated thoracic tuberculous lymphadenopathy. Am J Respir Crit Care Med. 2011;183:136–7.
42. Navani N, Molyneaux PL, Breen RA, et al. Utility of endobronchial ultrasound-guided transbronchial needle aspiration in patients with tuberculous intrathoracic lymphadenopathy: a multicenter study. Thorax. 2011;66:889–93.
43. Wang K-P. Staging of bronchogenic carcinoma by bronchoscopy. Chest. 1994;106:588–93.
44. Garpestad E, Goldberg SN, Herth F, et al. CT fluoroscopy guidance for tracheobronchial needle aspiration. An experience in 35 patients. Chest. 2001;119:329–32.
45. White CS, Weiner EA, Patel P, Britt EJ. Transbronchial needle aspiration. Guidance with CT fluoroscopy. Chest. 2000;118:1630–8.
46. Gildea TR, Mazzone PJ, Karnak D, Meziane M, Mehta AC. Electromagnetic navigation diagnostic bronchoscopy. A prospective study. Am J Respir Crit Care Med. 2006;174:982–9.
47. Makris D, Scherpereel A, Leroy S, et al. Electromagnetic navigation diagnostic bronchoscopy for small peripheral lung lesions. Eur Respir J. 2007;29:1187–92.
48. Mahajan AK, Patel S, Hogarth DK, Wightman R. Electromagnetic navigational bronchoscopy. An effective and safe approach to diagnose peripheral lung lesions unreachable by conventional bronchoscopy in high risk patients. J Bronchology Interv Pulmonol. 2011;18:133–7.
49. Wilson DS, Bartlett RJ. Improved diagnostic yield of bronchoscopy in a community practice: combination of electromagnetic navigation system and rapid on-site evaluation. J Bronchol. 2007;14:227–32.
50. Gildea TR. Electromagnetic navigation: a rosy picture. J Bronchol. 2007;14:221–2.
51. McLennan G, Ferguson JS, Thomas K, Delsing AS, Cook-Granroth J, Hoffman EA. The use of MDCTbased computer aided pathway finding for mediastinal and perihilar lymph node biopsy: a randomized controlled prospective trial. Respiration. 2007;74:423–31.
52. Weiner GM, Schulze K, Geiger B, Ebhardt H, Wolfe KJ, Albrecht T. CT bronchoscopic simulation for guiding transbronchial needle aspiration of extramural mediastinal and hilar lesions. Initial clinical results. Radiology. 2009;250:923–31.
53. Cameron SHE, Andrade RS, Pambuccian SE. Endobronchial ultrasound guided transbronchial needle aspiration cytology: a state of the art review. Cytopathology. 2010;21:6–26.
54. Gu P, Zhao YZ, Jiang LY, et al. Endobronchial ultrasound guided transbronchial needle aspiration for staging of lung cancer. Eur J Cancer. 2009;45:1389–96.
55. Adams K, Shah P, Edmonds L, et al. Test performance of endobronchial ultrasound and transbronchial needle aspiration biopsy for mediastinal staging in patients with lung cancer: systemic review and meta-analysis. Thorax. 2009;64:757–62.
56. Varela-Lema L, Fernandez-Villar A, Ruano-Ravina A. Effectiveness and safety of endobronchial ultrasound transbronchial needle aspiration: a systemic review. Eur Respir J. 2009;33:1156–64.
57. Kerr KM, Lamb D, Wathen CG, Walker WS, Douglas NJ. Pathological assessment of mediastinal lymph nodes in lung cancer: implications for non-invasive mediastinal staging. Thorax. 1992;47:337–41.
58. Gomez-Caro A, Garcia S, Reguart N, et al. Incidence of occult mediastinal nodal involvement in cN0 nonsmall cell lung cancer patients after negative uptake of positron emission tomography/computer tomography scan. Eur J Cardiothorac Surg. 2010;37:1168–74.
59. Verhagen AFT, Bootsma GP, Tjan-Heijnen VCG, et al. FDG-PET in staging lung cancer. How does it change the algorithm? Lung Cancer. 2004;44:175–81.
60. Detterbeck FC, Jantz MA, Wallace M, Vansteenkiste J, Silvestri GA. Invasive mediastinal staging of lung cancer. ACCP evidence-based clinical practice guidelines. Chest. 2007;132:202S–20S.
61. Leyn PD, Lardinois D, Van Schil PE, et al. ESTS guidelines for preoperative lymph node staging for non-small cell lung cancer. Eur J Cardiothorac Surg. 2007;32:1–8.
62. Piet AHM, Lagerwaard FJ, Kunst PWA, Van de Sornsen Koste JR, Slotman BJ, Senam S. Can mediastinal nodal mobility explain the low yield rates for transbronchial needle aspiration without real time imaging. Chest. 2007;131:1783–7.
63. Kanzaki R, Higashiyama M, Fugiwara A, et al. Occult mediastinal lymph node metastasis in NSCLC patients diagnosed as clinical N0-1by preoperative integrated FDG-PET/CT and CT:

64. Herth FJF, Eberhardt R, Krasnik M, Ernst A. Endobronchial ultrasound guided transbronchial needle aspiration of lymph nodes in the radiologically and positron emission tomography-normal mediastinum in patients with lung cancer. Chest. 2008;133:887–91.
65. Szlubowski A, Zielinski M, Soja J, et al. A combined approach of endobronchial and endoscopic ultrasound guided needle aspiration in the radiologically normal mediastinum in non-small cell lung cancer staging—a prospective trial. Eur J Cardiothorac Surg. 2010;37:1175–9.
66. Boonsarngsuk V, Pongtippan A. Self learning experience in transbronchial needle aspiration in diagnosis of intrathoracic lymphadenopathy. J Med Assoc Thai. 2009;92:175–89.
67. Kupeli E, Memis L, Ozdemirel TS, Ulubay G, Akcay S, Eyuboglu FO. Transbronchial needle aspiration by the book. Ann Thorac Med. 2011;6:85–90.
68. Herman FHW, Limonard GJM, Termeer R, et al. Learning curve of conventional transbronchial needle aspiration in pulmonologists experienced in bronchoscopy. Respiration. 2008;75:189–92.
69. Haponik EF, Cappellari JO, Chin R, et al. Education and experience improve transbronchial needle aspiration performance. Am J Respir Crit Care Med. 1995;151:1998–2002.
70. Hsu LH, Liu CC, Ko JS. Education and experience improve the performance of transbronchial needle aspiration. A learning curve at a cancer center. Chest. 2004;125:532–40.
71. Phua GC, Rhee KJ, Koh M, Loo CM, Lee P. A strategy to improve the yield of transbronchial needle aspiration. Surg Endosc. 2010;24:2105–9.
72. Mehta AC, Curtis PS, Scalzitti ML, et al. The high price of bronchoscopy. Maintenance and repair of the flexible fiberoptic bronchoscope. Chest. 1990;98:448–54.
73. Mehta AC, Kavuru MS, Meeker DP, Gephardt GN, Nunez C. Transbronchial needle aspiration for histology specimens. Chest. 1989;96:1228–32.
74. Schenk DA, Strollo PJ, Pickard JS, et al. Utility of Wang 18-gauge transbronchial histology needle in the staging of lung cancer. Chest. 1989;96:272–4.
75. Schenk DA, Chambers SL, Derdak S, et al. Comparison of Wang 19-gauge and 22-gauge needles in the mediastinal staging of lung cancer. Am Rev Respir Dis. 1993;147:1251–8.
76. Hermens FHW, Limonard GJM, Hoevenaars BM, de Kievit I, Janssen JP. Diagnostic value of histology compared with cytology in transbronchial aspiration samples obtained by histology needle. J Bronchol. 2010;17:19–21.
77. Stratakos G, Porfyridis I, Papas V, et al. Exclusive diagnostic contribution of the histology specimens obtained by 19-gauge transbronchial aspiration needle in suspected malignant intrathoracic lymphadenopathy. Chest. 2008;133:131–6.
78. Patelli M, Agli LL, Poletti V, et al. Role of fiberoptic transbronchial needle aspiration in the staging of N2 disease due to non-small cell lung cancer. Ann Thorac Surg. 2002;73:407–11.
79. Herman FHW, van Engelenburg TCA, Visser FJ, Thunnissen FBMJ, Termeer R, Janssen JP. Diagnostic yield of transbronchial histology needle aspiration in patients with mediastinal lymph node enlargement. Respiration. 2003;70:631–5.
80. Gasparino S. It is time for this ROSE to flower. Respiration. 2005;72:129–31.
81. Baram D, Garcia RB, Richman PS. Impact of rapid onsite cytologic evaluation during transbronchial needle aspiration. Chest. 2005;128:869–75.
82. Diacon AH, Schuurmans MM, Theron J, et al. Utility of on-site evaluation of transbronchial needle aspirates. Respiration. 2005;72:182–8.
83. Davenport RD. Rapid on-site evaluation of transbronchial aspirates. Chest. 1990;98:59–61.
84. Diette GB, White P, Terry P, Jenckes M, Rosenthal D, Runin HR. Utility of onsite cytopathology assessment for the bronchoscopic evaluation of lung masses and adenopathy. Chest. 2000;117:1186–90.
85. Yarmus L, van der Kloot T, Lechtzin N, Napier M, Dressel D, Feller-Kopman D. A randomized prospective trial of the utility of rapid on-site evaluation of transbronchial needle aspirate specimen. J Bronchology Interv Pulmonol. 2011;18:121–7.
86. Trisolini R, Cancellieri A, Tinelli C, et al. Rapid onsite evaluation of transbronchial aspirates in the diagnosis of hilar and mediastinal adenopathy: a randomized trial. Chest. 2011;139:395–401.
87. Jones DF, Chin R, Cappellari JO, Haponik EF. Endobronchial needle aspiration in the diagnosis of small cell carcinoma. Chest. 1994;105:1151–4.
88. Mazzone P, Jain P, Arroliga AC, Matthay RA. Bronchoscopy and needle biopsy techniques for diagnosis and staging of lung cancer. Clin Chest Med. 2002;23:137–58.
89. Kacar N, Tuksavul F, Edipoglu O, Sulun E, Guclu SZ. Effectiveness of transbronchial needle aspiration in the diagnosis of exophytic endobronchial lesions and submucosal/peribronchial disease of the lung. Respir Med. 2005;50:221–6.
90. Caglayan B, Akturk UA, Fidan A, et al. Transbronchial needle aspiration in the diagnosis of endobronchial malignant lesions. A 3-year experience. Chest. 2005;128:704–8.
91. Dasgupta A, Jain P, Minai OA, et al. Utility of transbronchial needle aspiration in the diagnosis of endobronchial lesions. Chest. 1999;115:1237–41.
92. Govert JA, Dodd LG, Kussin PS, Samuelson WM. A prospective comparison of fiberoptic transbronchial needle aspiration and bronchial biopsy for bronchoscopically visible lung tumors. Cancer. 1999;87:129–34.
93. Roth K, Hardie JA, Andreassen AH, Leh F, Eagan TML. Cost-minimization analysis for combination of sampling techniques in bronchoscopy of endobronchial lesions. Respir Med. 2009;103:888–94.
94. Katis K, Inglesos E, Zachariadis E, et al. The role of transbronchial needle aspiration in the diadnosis of peripheral lung masses or nodules. Eur Respir J. 1995;8:963–6.
95. Trisolini R, Cancellieri A, Tinelli C, et al. Performance characteristics and predictors of yield from transbronchial needle aspiration in the diagnosis of peripheral pulmonary lesions. Respirology. 2011;16:1144–9.
96. Reichenberger F, Weber J, Tamm M, et al. The value of transbronchial needle aspiration in the diagnosis of peripheral pulmonary lesions. Chest. 1999;116:704–8.
97. Wang KP, Haponik EF, Britt JB, Khouri N, Erozan Y. Transbronchial needle aspiration of peripheral pulmonary nodules. Chest. 1984;86:819–23.
98. Shure D, Fedullo PF. Transbronchial needle aspiration of peripheral masses. Am Rev Respir Dis. 1983;128:1090–2.
99. Bilaceroglu S, Kumcuoglu Z, Alper H, et al. CT bronchus sign guided bronchoscopic multiple diagnostic procedures in carcinomatous solitary pulmonary nodules and masses. Respiration. 1889;65:49–55.
100. Chao TY, Chien MT, Lie CH, Chung YH, Wang JL, Lin MC. Endobronchial ultrasonography-guided transbronchial needle aspiration increases the diagnostic yield of peripheral pulmonary lesions. A randomized trial. Chest. 2009;136:229–36.
101. Yarmus L, Feller-Kopman D, Browning R, Wang K-P. TBNA: should EBUS be used on all lymph node aspirations? J Bronchology Interv Pulmonol. 2011;18:115–6.

第 2 篇

诊断性介入支气管镜

Diagnostic Interventional Bronchoscopy

第 4 章
径向探头支气管内超声
Noriaki Kurimoto

本章提要 径向探头支气管内超声是一种利用一个小超声探头进入支气管腔内而获得支气管周围组织超声图像的技术。利用探头周围的水囊，可以明确气管支气管壁的五层结构。在中央气道中，这种技术用于明确支气管内肿瘤浸润管壁的深度是最有用的。导向鞘引导的支气管内超声是一种改良的支气管内超声技术，这个技术通过导向鞘引入径向超声探头，并深入周围型的肺部病灶。据报道，对 < 3 cm 的周围型的肺部病灶，这种技术的诊断率为74%。近年来，利用电磁导航或虚拟支气管镜定位，使超声探头和导向鞘更准确定位肿瘤位置，进一步提高周围型肺结节的诊断率。

关键词 支气管内超声，径向探头支气管内超声，周围型肺部病灶。

引 言

支气管内超声（EBUS）是利用微型超声探头导入气管支气管管腔从而得到支气管周围组织超声图像的一种诊断方式。

径向探头支气管内超声检查最常用于支气管镜活检前的周围型肺结节定位。本小组于1994 年 8 月开始使用径向探头 EBUS。最初，我们使用不带导向鞘的径向探头 EBUS 来诊断周围型肺部病灶，从 1996 年开始使用导向鞘准确定位周围型肺部病灶进行活检。EBUS 的另一个应用是用带水囊的探头对支气管壁结构进行观察[1]。

科学依据

超声学

人类耳朵可接受一定频率范围的声波。通常，人类耳朵接受的声音频率为 20~20 000 Hz。一般情况下，超声波指频率 > 20 000 Hz 的声波，这是人耳不能听见的频率范围。因此，我们经常用它们的用途来定义声音。超声不能被人类听见。音频告诉我们声波频率的高低。音频的单位是赫兹（Hz），就是它每秒振荡的次数。例如，一个声音的频率为 20 kHz，就是指每秒有 20 000 次振荡。一种声音频率为 1 兆赫（MHz），就是每秒有 1 000 000 次的振荡。医用超声设备产生的声音频率为 2~50 MHz。波长是声波的任何连续的相同部分间的距离，并与频率成反比，所以频率越高，波长越短。声音可以通过各种介质传播，如空气、水，声波在每个介质中传播的速度不同，通常认为，声音通过人体的速度为 1 530 m/s，然而通过不同器官和组织的实际速度是不同的。例如声音在脂肪中的传播速度是 1 450 m/s。

超声图像的形成

医学超声诊断应用的超声探头使用换能器，可以将电信号变成超声信号，超声信号变成电信号。当一个电信号作用于超声换能器的电极

(也是振荡器/变压器),从设备的表面会发射超声波,当设备表面接收到返回的超声时,会产生一个电信号。传导是指超声换能器产生的超声波通过介质进行传播。随着声波的传播,其振荡的能量被吸收和分散,并逐渐变弱,这种现象称为衰减。在一般情况下,超声频率越高,则衰减率越大。

与光一样,超声波在不同的介质边缘时一部分会发生反射,另一部分则穿透边缘继续向前传播。超声波换能器能发射超声波脉冲,并能接收来自于不同媒介边缘反射的超声波脉冲,超声波处理器通过分析这些反射来构造图像,超声波处理器通过计算发射超声波和接收介质边缘反射超声波脉冲的时间,来计算介质边缘距离探针的距离,并将反射的脉冲强度转换为图像亮度。

穿透深度

如上所述,超声波在介质内的传播是逐渐衰减的。也就是说,超声波只能从声源起传播有限的距离。因此,超声图像也能从超声探头延伸至一定距离。这个距离称为穿透深度。对于既定的一种介质,穿透深度取决于频率和换能器的大小(孔径面积)。超声波的衰减率随着频率的增加而增加,穿透深度随着频率的减少而增加。由于超声换能器的孔径面积增大后,它能发出更强的脉冲,并且可以将较弱的接收脉冲转换为电信号。所以随着换能器尺寸的增加,穿透深度增加。

临床应用

基于各种研究,目前的径向探头EBUS的应用如下:①测定肿瘤浸润气管/支气管壁的深度。②分析气道疾病(如气管支气管软化症)支气管壁的结构。③在支气管镜检查时确定周围型肺部病灶的位置。径向探头EBUS比荧光镜更能准确地确定病变与支气管的关系。因此,它缩短了确定活检部位和荧光透视检查的时间。④鉴别周围型肺结节性质的良恶性。⑤引导经支气管针吸活检,在这个方面径向探头EBUS大部分被凸面探头EBUS代替。

步 骤

中央型肺部病灶的水囊探头术

空气可干扰超声成像。获得中央病灶(如位于气管、主支气管、段支气管和亚段支气管)的超声图像需要用盐水囊包绕的EBUS探头。在亚段支气管以下,超声波探头可紧贴着支气管表面,故无须盐水囊包绕的EBUS探头,即可探测获得支气管壁和支气管周围结构的图像。

设备

我们曾经采用了20 MHz 机械径向超声探头(微型探头,Tokyo,Japan,Olympus)与水囊外鞘管(mh-246r,Olympus)。该外鞘管的直径为3.6 mm,只适合具备大工作通道的支气管镜(bf-st40,支气管镜工作通道直径3.7 mm)。近年来,我们使用一种更薄的20 MHz 机械径向超声探头(um-bs-20-26r,Olympus)与一个水囊外鞘管(mh-676r,Olympus),可以通过纤维支气管镜直径2.8 mm 的工作通道进入(bf-1t260,Olympus)(图4.1)。这些探头与超声内

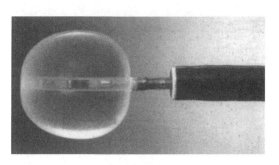

图4.1 EBUS的径向超声探头。中央病灶水囊法:我们使用一个更小的20 MHz 机械径向超声探头(um-bs-20-26r,Olympus)与水囊外鞘管(mh-676r,Olympus)通过2.8 mm 直径的纤维支气管镜的工作通道(bf-1t260,Olympus)

镜系统（eumel 和 eu-m 2000，Olympus）相连可获得 EBUS 图像。

水囊探头的准备

将超声探头插入水囊外鞘管中，探头和外鞘管由连接单元固定到位，连接单元的注射口接一 20 ml 的注射器，内含约 15 ml 的生理盐水。外鞘管内表面与探头外表面之间的大部分空气可通过抽吸此注射器 2~3 次排出。将注射器里的生理盐水注射到外鞘管中和顶端的水囊，注射 15 ml 的生理盐水后球囊的直径约为 15 mm。水囊顶部少量的空气可以经水囊的开放末端排出，水囊的开放末端可向后推入超声探头的中空部分。

使用水囊探头下进行 EBUS

我们使用工作通道直径为 2.8 mm 的纤维支气管镜（1T-40，1T-240R，Olympus），此通道适于所有水囊探头进行 EBUS。通过操作"图像方向"按钮，可翻转显示器的图像（图 4.2）。超声图像翻转后，术者使患者的从头端看到的左右成像与内镜所见图像是相同的。通常的胃肠超声内镜（EUS）中，正常超声图像是从足端方向看的，以便于与 CT 比较，但 EBUS 的超声图像需要与支气管镜图像重合，从而在气管支气管管腔中得到中央病灶的图像。不翻转图像的模式仅用于特殊情况下，比如与 CT 图像的对比。

为了避免剧烈的咳嗽，手术中水囊探针接触到的支气管部分要进行充分的局部麻醉。水囊探头通过支气管镜的工作通道到达病灶部位，然后注入生理盐水，获得支气管壁的四周 EBUS 图像后立即停止注入。缓慢退出探头进行扫描。避免从近端向远端推进探头，因为这可能导致探头受损。

在 EBUS 图像 12 点钟位置没有对应的支气管镜下 12 点钟位置时，参照支气管镜图像，旋转调整 EBUS 图像。当向上转动支气管镜时，应检查探头移动的角度。通常我们转动 EBUS 图像，与支气管镜图像保持一致。水囊探头应逐渐收回，以采集病灶短轴和支气管壁的 EBUS 图像。

我们提供以下使用水囊探头 EBUS 的两点建议：①保持探头在水囊的中心。②应于病灶第一层较厚处，且高回声处测量肿瘤深度。

20 MHz 的探头可通过超声图像，对肺外、肺内支气管的软骨部的 5 层结构进行识别（图 4.3）[1]。软骨部的第 1 层（高回声）是边缘层，第 2 层（低回声）代表的是黏膜组织，第 3 层（高回声）是支气管软骨内的边缘组织，第 4 层（低回声）代表的是支气管软骨，第 5 层（高回声）是支气管软骨外的边缘组织。在膜部，第 1 层（高回声）是一个边缘回声，第 2 层（低回声）是黏膜下组织，第 3 层（高回声）是外膜。

采用 EBUS 对气管肿瘤的浸润深度进行测定时，必须仔细检查与支气管软骨相对应的第 3 层和第 4 层。术前 EBUS 检查肿瘤浸润深度的一个重要局限在于，对肿瘤侵犯与淋巴细胞浸润的鉴别困难。因为超声对人体组织的可视化是基于超声波速度，而从 20 MHz 探头发出的超声波，穿过浸润性癌与通过淋巴细胞液和增生的支气管淋巴结时的传播速度是相似的。同样，

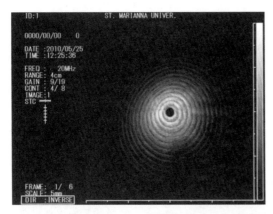

图 4.2 倒置图像。我们需要操作"图像方向"开关将显示的图像翻转。这使超声图像反转后左、右方向与从内镜方向看到的图像相同

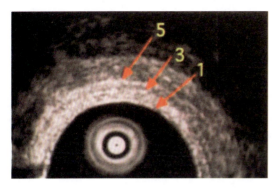

图4.3 支气管内超声检查显示支气管壁层。肺外支气管：气管的软骨部和肺外支气管有5层，膜部有3层。第1层（高回声）是一个边缘回声，第2层（低回声）代表黏膜下层，第3层（高回声）是内侧的支气管软骨边缘回声，第4层（低回声）代表支气管软骨，第5层（高回声）是在外侧的支气管软骨边缘回声。在肺外支气管的膜部，第1层（高回声）是一个边缘回声，第2层（低回声）代表黏膜下层，第3层（高回声）是外膜

在对食管癌患者的内镜超声检查（EUS）报道中，鉴别纤维组织增生与肿瘤侵袭的淋巴结同样是困难的[2,3]。例如，Arima等指出，一些组织中的变化如食管癌附近增生的淋巴滤泡细胞，纤维化滤泡细胞等经常被误认为肿瘤[2]。同样，Kikuchi等把EUS误诊大肠癌浸润深度的原因归结于超声波因肿瘤厚度而衰减，以及超声难以鉴别真正的肿瘤浸润和淋巴滤泡细胞浸润或黏膜下纤维化[4]。Menzel与Domschke[5]报道称，有可能由于超声诊断误诊把黏膜下炎症当作肿瘤，使食管癌分期更高。因此，操作者必须意识到EBUS探头在肿瘤气管壁受累程度的评估检查中具有局限性。

EBUS用于周围型病灶

近年来，径向探头EBUS成为诊断孤立性肺结节患者的一个重要技术。在对病灶组织标本活检诊断之前，径向探头EBUS有助于评估周围型肺结节的内部结构以及病灶定位。

周围型肺部病灶内部结构分析

一些研究者已经使用微型超声探头对周围型肺部病变进行评估，Hürter等报道了在20例患者中有19例成功地显示了周围型肺部病灶[6]，Goldberg等报道了25例患者中有18例，EBUS为其他诊断方法补充提供了独立的信息，此25例患者中6例为周围型病变，19例为肺门部肿瘤[7]。

为区分良性和恶性病变，确定肺癌的类型和分化程度，我们提出了一个分类系统[8]。对于周围型肺结节的超声成像，病灶的分类基于内部回声模式（同类或异类）、血管通畅度和强回声区（反映空气的存在和支气管的状态）的形态学。Ⅰ型病变为均质型，其中92%是良性；Ⅱ型病变为强回声点和弧线模式，其中99%是恶性的；Ⅲ型病变为多形性模式，其中99%为恶性。

Hosokawa等报道称，一个典型肿瘤性疾病的EBUS超声检查有以下几个特征：①连续边缘回声。②粗糙内部回声。③无代表支气管的强回声斑，或者即使存在也没有纵向的连续性[9]。Kuo等评估EBUS在区分良性和恶性病变可行性时，以下超声特征指示恶性：①连续边缘。②线性空气支气管充气征缺失。③异形回声结构[10]。没有这3种回声特征，恶性病变的阴性预测值是93.7%，有这3种里面的任何2种特征，恶性肿瘤的阳性预测值为89.2%。尽管CT和MRI扫描已经用于定性诊断周围型肺病，支气管镜下EBUS评价仍有多种优势：①可见病灶内通畅的血管。②可见病灶内气泡点（呈现为小白点）的分布。③可见病灶内坏死组织（无回声区）。④可见病灶的回声强度。

特别注意的是，20 MHz高频超声显示的病灶回声强度的变化与肿瘤细胞的分布和密度、黏液的存在、病变组织的间质增生有关。回声

强度取决于超声波在组织类型之间反射的程度。细支气管肺泡癌（黏液型）用CT扫描很难与肺炎区分，但在20 MHz高频超声中比肺炎有更强的回声，其产生的原因不明，但怀疑是由于黏液使肺泡间隔内肿瘤组织反射增加。

综上所述，EBUS对周围型肺部病灶的内部结构的可视化是令人兴奋的。尽管如此，仍需要更多的研究，去发现EBUS超声成像潜在的病理学和组织学意义。

导向鞘引导的支气管内超声（EBUS-GS）用于周围型病灶活检

自1996年以来，我们发明了一种带导向鞘的超声探头，探头可从顶端伸出，来确定病灶进行超声显像；移走超声探头，导向鞘保留在原来位置，然后用其他工具如活检刷和活检钳，通过导向鞘收集细胞或组织标本[11]（图4.4）。下面会对这一技术进行简单讨论。

仪器设备

我们分别使用了两个微型超声探头（UM-S20-20R，UM-S20-17R；20 MHz，机械径向，Olympus），外径分别为1.7 mm和1.4 mm。探头连接到超声内镜系统（EU-ME1EU-M2000，Olympus）。这个引导套装置（K-201-202，K-203-204，Olympus）包含一个导向鞘（外径分别为1.95 mm和2.55 mm），一次性活检刷（BC-204D-2010，BC-202D-2010：外径为1.4 mm和1.8 mm），一次性活检钳（FB-233D，BC-231D-2010：外径为1.5 mm和1.9 mm）。

EBUS-GS活检准备

首先，将用于纤维支气管镜活检（TBBx）的支气管刷（BC-202D-2010，BC-204D-2010，Olympus），或活检钳（FB-231D，FB-233D，Olympus），插入导向鞘中，使钳尖端到达鞘管的远端。同时，用固定装置将活检刷或钳固定在导向鞘的近末端。这将有利于在支气管镜下，将导向鞘内的刷子或活检钳插入适当的深度。

然后，在导向鞘中插入一个微型超声探头（SG-201C，SG-200C，Olympus）伸出导向鞘末端约2 mm。同时，用固定装置将探头和导向鞘固定在一起，并使探头的前端始终超出鞘的末端。

进行EBUS-GS活检

我们在所有手术中都使用一种纤维支气管镜（BF 1T-30，40，240R，260，或P260F）。在最

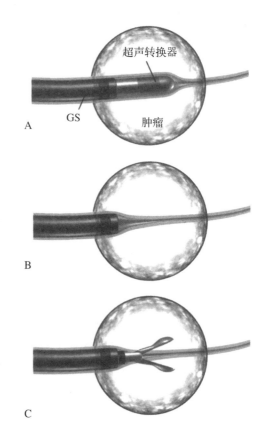

图4.4 EBUS-GS程序。A.探头向前推进，直到操作者感觉到阻力，然后拉回进行扫描；B.一旦EBUS明确病灶的位置，探头退出，导向鞘保留在原位置；C.将活检钳或支气管刷插入导向鞘中，到达标记的位置。在透视引导下用支气管刷来回刷动，采集样品；用活检钳通过导向鞘反复地抓取，获得肿瘤的活检组织

近几年中，我们偏好使用带有 2 mm 工作通道的 4 mm 支气管镜。在支气管镜进入声带后，可见所有支气管分支。根据影像学结果，将带有导向鞘的微型探头定位到需检查的支气管。对支气管的选择，需基于支气管检查前对 CT 图像仔细的研究。对于非常小的病灶，选择正确的支气管是非常困难的，预先列举 5~6 个支气管作为备选是非常有用的。

探头先向前推进，直到操作者感觉到阻力，然后边拉回边进行扫描（图 4.4A）。一旦获得病灶的 EBUS 图像并明确病灶的位置，便将探头退出，导向鞘留在原位置。

将活检钳或支气管刷插入导向鞘中，到达标记的位置。在透视引导下用支气管刷来回刷动，采集样品。

支气管刷退出后，将活检钳插入导向鞘中，直至活检钳到达的远端。打开钳尖，钳尖进入病变 2 mm 或 3 mm 时，在影像引导下闭合。获得足够多的活检标本后，将标本放入甲醛中保存，送实验室进行组织学检查。

导向鞘仍留在原处并按压活检部位约 2 分钟以控制出血。确认止血后，结束操作。

诊断率

我们以前报道过使用厚导向鞘的 EBUS（EBUS-thickGS）的总体诊断率为 77%（116/150），而 EBUS-GS 对良性和恶性病变的诊断率分别为 81%（82/101）和 73%（35/49）[11]。EBUS 成像时，探头进入病灶内的诊断率（105/121，87%）明显比探头在病灶附近进行 EBUS 成像的诊断率（8/19，42%）高。进行 TBBx 时，探头位于病灶内的诊断率（85/104，82%）比探头在病灶附近的诊断率（15/1，7%）高更多。

EBUS-GS 对肿块的诊断率（>30 mm，24/26，92%）比对结节的诊断率（<30 mm，92/124，74%）明显更高。但是，EBUS-GS 对 <10 mm 病灶的诊断率（16/21，76%）与 >10 mm 且 <15 mm（19/25，76%），>15 mm 且 <20 mm（24/35，69%），>20 mm 且 <30 mm（33/43，77%）病灶的诊断率相似。也就是说，对于 <30 mm 的病灶来说，病灶大小不影响 EBUS-GS 的诊断率，即使病灶 <10 mm 诊断率也不会降低。对于 <20 mm 的病灶，如果能用 X 线透视确认活检钳到达病灶的位置，诊断率有可能达到 81 例中 54 例能确诊。然而，这些病灶的诊断率为 74%（40/54）与 X 线透视辅助的诊断率（18/27，64%）相似。150 例有 2 例患者（1%）出现中度出血。没有出现死亡、气胸等严重的并发症。

利用 EBUS-GS 技术，现在能取得在过去只能通过 CT 引导下穿刺活检获取的病灶组织样本。Fielding 等做了 EBUS-GS 与 CT 引导下穿刺活检的对比研究[12]，对于 <2 cm 的病灶，CT 引导下穿刺活检有更高的诊断率，但是 EBUS-GS 有着更好的耐受性和更少的并发症。

成功进行 EBUS-GS 的技巧

这些技巧是为了确保导向鞘在病灶的位置，并在活检之前将病灶附近的探头移动到病灶内。

用导向鞘导致信号衰减

如上所述，导向鞘以及超声探头在病灶内的诊断率高于其在病灶旁边时的诊断率[11]。信号衰减方法可用于确定导向鞘是否在周围型肺病灶中。一旦 EBUS 扫描到外周型肺病变，当病灶最大、最清晰时，助手需保持导向鞘稳定，同时解开超声探头与导向鞘之间的连接装置，退出探头 2 mm 直到探头进入导向鞘中。当探头完全进入导向鞘时，超声脉冲被导向鞘阻断，超声图像会突然变得黑暗。如果超声探头完全在导向鞘内时，还可以看到病变，则提示导向鞘尖端精确地放置在周围型病灶上。

将导向鞘从病灶附近移到病灶内

如果导向鞘位于病灶附近，应努力在活检之前将其移到病灶内。然而，把导向鞘从相邻的位置移动到肿瘤内是具有挑战性的。以下几种技术有助于实现这一目标：①在支气管镜引导下选择另一个支气管来插入导向鞘。4 mm 的支气管镜可以使这一技术得以实现，因为其比标准的纤维支气管镜能直接检查更远端的支气管分支。如果一开始选择的支气管镜仅使超声传感器和导向鞘到达病灶附近，此时可将导向鞘撤回，超声探头可在支气管镜视野下进入另一个亚段支气管，便可能到达病灶。②透视引导下选择不同的支气管也可协助导向鞘进入病灶。当EBUS图像中探头位于病灶周围时，应将探头拉回来，在透视下改变支气管镜角度，向靶病灶方向推动探头。③另一个简单的方法是通过改变支气管镜的上下角度，来选择不同的支气管。当EBUS图像中探头在病灶附近时，可通过支气管镜的上下角度改变，引导探头移动。例如，向上改变角度，如果在EBUS图像上看到探头进入病变，导套和探头应拉回来一些，并从上方重新进入病变。④也可利用叫双链刮匙的引导装置来选择不同的支气管。当病灶图像不能通过EBUS获取时，超声波探头应撤出，导向鞘不移动，铰接刮匙插入导向鞘，直至其尖端并从导向鞘末端突出，接着将铰接刮匙的顶端向病灶方向弯曲，然后引导装置缓慢退出，直到在透视下移动到病变部位。这一操作的目的是进入能直接到达靶病灶的支气管分支，如果刮匙尖端移动方向正确，导向鞘将跟随着到达病变部位。有时候在刮匙进入一个支气管开口时，这样的分支点会感觉轻度的"弯曲"。这使得导向鞘在外周型肺病病灶中能够精确定位。移除刮匙，重新安置超声探头，再使用如上所述的标准技术对病变部位进行活检。

EBUS-GS 的优势

使用EBUS-GS技术对周围型肺部病灶进行活检、获取活检标本的主要优点如下：①当在透视下进行小病灶活检不可行时，在活检之前可对病灶进行准确定位。②在同一个支气管段可以多次使用活检钳。③可分析病灶的内部结构。④经支气管肺活检后出血少见。

如何确认通向靶病灶的支气管

准确识别支气管，是EBUS-GS技术对靶病灶成功组织采样的一个重要决定因素。这可以通过回顾支气管镜检查前CT或在虚拟支气管镜导航或者电磁导航系统帮助下完成。

运用CT成像技术

在许多情况下，仔细观察CT，确定通向病灶的支气管，并沿着它追溯至肺门是可行的。有了这些信息，支气管分支，其支气管段、亚段和通向靶病灶随后的分支都可以确认。CT图像上显示的路径结构，有助于支气管镜检查时确定通向靶病灶的支气管路径。例如，如果候选支气管是右侧B6c支气管，B6c病变在CT上的显示是在B6b区域附近，在支气管镜检查时，我们会将超声探头插入接近B6b支气管的右侧B6c支气管分支。

使用导航系统

近年来，两种精确定位周围型肺部病灶的导航系统被开发出来。作为一种定位装置，电磁导航系统可协助支气管设备放置到支气管或肺的理想区域。此系统采用低频电磁波，由置于气管镜桌垫下的一个电磁板发出[13]。该系统允许操作员引导探头传感器及扩展的工作通道到达病灶区域。一旦到达目标，径向探头EBUS可以将扩展的工作通道定位到病灶内。据报道，电磁导航和径向探头EBUS联合应用，比单独应用有更高的诊断率[14]。Harms等[15]提出了晚期周围型肺部肿瘤新的治疗方法是结合电磁导航系统与EBUS下3D支气管镜腔内治疗技术，Asano等[16-18]发明了支气管镜插入导引系统，这一系统通过自动调节，获取支气管产生的虚拟图像，并寻找通向目标支气管的路径。他们将该系统与细支气管镜和EBUS-GS结合。该系统可自动生成至平均第五级支气管的虚拟图像。93.8%的病例EBUS可视化成功，84.4%可提供组织诊断。使用该气管镜插入导引系统，可以很容易地产生虚拟图像，并成功地引导支气管镜到达目标。这种方法有望成为精确定位引导穿刺活检的常规技术。

未来方向

目前，我们使用的 4 mm 气管镜的工作通道直径为 2 mm，利用这个管道我们可通过 1.4~1.7 mm 外径的超声探头，在未来，我们希望通过更细的支气管镜进入更多的外周支气管，采用厚度较薄的导向鞘和超声探头检测早期病变。

目前的细胞学检查和组织活检是在透视下进行的，但当我们采用带有凸面探头的细支气管镜获得标本时，实时观察 EBUS 图像是非常有用的。

总　结

EUBS 使用的高频超声探头可以对气管支气管肿瘤的浸润深度进行测定，这对于其他诊断成像方法是不可能实现的。当外膜受到侵犯时，术前 EBUS 使用的 20 MHz 探头可清晰显现肿瘤组织内支气管软骨。虽然这种技术已经显示出了巨大的潜力，但使用 EBUS 探头用于肿瘤浸润深度测定，仍存在一些问题。主要的问题是无法可视化原位癌，以及肿瘤浸润与淋巴细胞浸润或支气管腺体增生之间鉴别困难。EBUS-GS 从周围型肺部病灶采集样品的定位比其他方法更精确。这种方法有利于在同一部位进行多次活检，防止活检部位出血进入临近的支气管，并能描绘周围型肺部病灶的内部结构。

参考文献

1. Kurimoto N, Murayama M, Yoshioka S, et al. Assessment of usefulness of endobronchial ultrasonography in determination of depth of tracheobronchial tumor invasion. Chest. 1999;115: 1500–6.
2. Arima M, Tada M. Endosonographic assessment of the depth of tumor invasion by superficial esophageal cancer, using a high-frequency miniature US probe: difficulties in interpretation and misleading factors. Stomach Intest. 2004;39:901–13.
3. Kawano T, Nagai Y, Inoue H, et al. Endoscopic ultrasonography for patients with esophageal cancer. Stomach Intest. 2001;36: 307–14.
4. Kikuchi Y, Tsuda S, Yurioka M, et al. Diagnosis of the depth infiltration in colorectal cancer-diagnosis and issues of the depth of infiltration investigated by endoscopic ultrasonography (EUS). Stomach Intest. 2001; 36:392–402.
5. Menzel J, Domschke W. Gastrointestinal miniprobe sonography: the current status. Am J Gastroenterol. 2000;95:605–16.
6. Hürter T, Hanarath P. Endobronchiale sonographie zur diagnostik pulmonaler und mediastinaler tumoren. Dtsch Med Wochenschr. 1990;115:1899–905.
7. Goldberg B, Steiner R, Liu J, et al. US-assisted bronchoscopy with use of miniature transducer-containing catheters. Radiology. 1994;190:233–7.
8. Kurimoto N, Murayama M, Yoshioka S, Nishisaka T. Analysis of the internal structure of peripheral pulmonary lesions using endobronchial ultrasonography. Chest 2002;122:1887–94.
9. Hosokawa S, Matsuo K, Watanabe Y, et al. Two cases of nodular lesions in the peripheral lung field, successfully diagnosed by endobronchial ultrasonography (EBUS). Kokyuu. 2004;23:57–60.
10. Kuo C, Lin S, Chen H, et al. Diagnosis of peripheral lung cancer with three echoic features via endobronchial ultrasound. Chest. 2007;132:922–9.
11. Kurimoto N, Miyazawa T, Okimasa S, et al. Endobronchial ultrasonography using a guide sheath increases the ability to diagnose peripheral pulmonary lesions endoscopically. Chest. 2004;126:959–65.
12. Fielding DI, Chia C, Nguyen P, et al. Prospective randomized trial of EBUS guide sheath versus CT guided percutaneous core biopsies for peripheral Lung Lesions. Intern Med J 2012;42:894–900.
13. Schwarz Y, Mehta AC, Ernst A, et al. Electromagnetic navigation during flexible bronchoscopy. Respiration. 2003;70:516–22.
14. Eberhardt R, Anantham D, Ernst A, Feller-Kopman D, Herth F. Multimodality bronchoscopic diagnosis of peripheral lung lesions. A randomized controlled trial. Am J Respir Crit Care Med. 2007;176:36–41.
15. Harms W, Krempien R, Grehn C, et al. Electromagetically navigated brachytherapy as a new treatment option for peripheral pulmonary tumors. Strahlenther Onkol. 2006;182:108–11.
16. Asano F, Matsuno Y, Matsushita T, et al. Transbronchial diagnosis of a pulmonary peripheral small lesion using an ultrathin bronchoscope with virtual bronchoscopic navigation. J Bronchol. 2002;9:108–11.
17. Asano F, Matsuno Y, Shinagawa N, et al. A virtual bronchoscopic navigation system for pulmonary peripheral lesions. Chest. 2006;130:559–66.
18. Asano F, Matsuno Y, Tsuzuku A, et al. Diagnosis of pulmonary peripheral lesions using a bronchoscope insertion guidance system combined with endobronchial ultrasonography with a guide sheath. Lung Cancer. 2008;60:366–73.

第 5 章
EBUS-TBNA 支气管镜检查
Sonali Sethi and Joseph Cicenia

本章提要 支气管内超声（EBUS）是一项不断发展的技术，该技术已成功用于在支气管镜检查过程中观察不能被观察到的中央气道毗邻结构。支气管内超声引导下经支气管针吸活检术（EBUS-TBNA）具有以下优点：耐受性好，创伤小，性价比高，对纵隔及肺门淋巴结能精确采样。其主要适应证包括肺癌诊断及分期，放化疗后再分期，胸腔外恶性肿瘤转移的诊断，结节病诊断，纵隔淋巴结结核以及其他病因导致的纵隔淋巴结肿大的诊断。本章主要探讨该检查的技巧、标本处理、麻醉等问题，以及 EBUS-TBNA 在各种疾病过程中的诊断率并与其他淋巴结采样方法的诊断率进行比较，同时探讨 EBUS-TBNA 的并发症及局限性。

关键词 支气管内超声，经支气管针吸活检术，支气管镜，纵隔淋巴结肿大，肺癌分期，EBUS-TBNA。

引 言

近 20 年来，支气管内超声（EBUS）技术已成为检查和评估肺部疾病的主要诊断方法，尤其是纵隔疾病。自 20 世纪 90 年代对其初次描述后，EBUS 的使用和普及在世界范围内呈指数增长。EBUS 最初的操作方法是将径向超声探头经标准支气管镜的工作通道与支气管壁接触[1]。径向探头 EBUS 仍然有多种用途：经支气管针吸操作之前确定纵隔淋巴结的位置[2]，评估肿瘤侵犯气管壁的深度[3]，以及指导支气管镜工具获取孤立性肺结节及周围病灶的组织标本[4]。尽管径向探头 EBUS 能使操作者观察到支气管壁以外的结构，但实际上对气道以外的病灶活检时进行引导是不可行的。为克服这个缺点，目前已开发出一种凸探头 EBUS，该探头直接置于支气管镜顶端，可实时观察并指导纵隔淋巴结活检[5]。该领域即"EBUS 穿刺领域"的发展，使肺科或胸外科医师在纵隔淋巴结或肿块取样方面能更广泛地应用该项技术[6]。由于使用方便且并发症发生率低，该技术已迅速应用于学术界以及社区卫生保健系统。本章节主要讨论 EBUS-TBNA 技术及其目前在肺癌分期中的临床地位，同时探讨 EBUS-TBNA 在诊断其他各种纵隔疾病中的作用。第 4 章讨论了径向探头 EBUS 在周围病变中的作用，并且在这些地方已做综述[7-11]。

纵隔取样的选择

纵隔镜检查历来是评估纵隔内疾病的金标准。然而，它是一种伴有一定并发症的侵入性过程（并发症尽管发生率较小但具有统计学意义）[12, 13]。此外，纵隔镜检查不能到达纵隔腔的所有区域，其最适合接近气管旁淋巴结（第 2、3、4 组）和隆突下区淋巴结（第 7 组）[14, 15]。纵隔镜很难到达隆突后部淋巴结。标准的经颈纵隔镜检查术亦不能到达主动脉弓下（第5组）、主动脉旁（第6组）、食管旁（第8组）、肺韧带（第9组）淋巴结等区域。事实上，在肺癌分期中，大部分纵隔镜检查的敏感性降低是由于未能检测到纵隔镜探测范围以外区域淋巴结[16]。此外，尽管该技术非常有用，在实际过程中，对于肺癌术前纵隔分期未必都会应用它，即使在临床诊断中也不一定应用[17]。依据适应证，纵隔镜的诊断率在不同研究中有差异[16-22]。对于肺癌分期，有报道指出经颈纵隔镜检查的平均敏感性为80%左右[16]，电视纵隔镜检查可提高敏感性，其平均敏感性接近90%。与常规纵隔镜相比，电视纵隔镜可探测到更多纵隔淋巴结并进行取样[23]。在过去的30年里，用于诊断肺癌分期的几项技术被开发出来，这些技术比纵隔镜创伤更小。传统的TBNA技术是针穿过支气管壁进行淋巴结穿刺（第3章）。Eduardo Schieppati于1949年首次对TBNA技术进行描述，他运用硬质支气管镜经支气管对纵隔淋巴结进行穿刺。该方法被认为对胸腔内恶性肿瘤分期、获取纵隔肿瘤组织样本以及诊断其他疾病引起的纵隔淋巴结肿大是安全有效的[25]。依据同样的原则，20世纪80年代初，Ko Pen Wang使用柔性纤维支气管镜开创了TBNA技术[26]。通过TBNA，第2、4、7、10、11组淋巴结很容易被采样。尽管该操作是安全的，但缺点在于不能直接观察到气道以外区域，因此该技术的诊断率具有不确定性[27]。TBNA的成功率依赖于以下几个因素：取样淋巴结大小，淋巴结短轴直径>20 mm 诊断率较高；淋巴结位置，位于第4组（右侧）和第7组区，诊断率极佳[27]；淋巴结恶性程度[16]；针吸操作次数[28, 29]；现场快速细胞学评估（ROSE）[29]。对于恶性疾病的诊断，TBNA具有高度特异性，但敏感性相对居中，为78%[16, 27]。TBNA对于良性疾病诊断率较低，因此，作为一种疾病诊断方法其使用受限。此外，由于缺乏专业培训以及对该技术安全性和临床实用性有误解，很多肺科专家从不使用该技术，这一点在第3章已讨论。

EBUS-TBNA作为一项新技术，将纵隔镜的高诊断率与TBNA的微创性两个优点结合起来。与传统TBNA技术相比，EBUS-TBNA的主要优点是在可视化条件下，定位淋巴结并采样。通过传统TBNA技术可到达的所有纵隔淋巴结同样EBUS-TBNA也可到达。此外，EBUS-TBNA在标准技术方面具有显著优势，能获取直径<1 cm的纵隔淋巴结样本，而传统TBNA技术很难做到。尽管目前没有精心设计的随机试验直接比较这两种技术在肺癌纵隔分期中的实用性，但有一些文献中的数据表明，EBUS-TBNA对纵隔分期比常规TBNA更敏感。

EBUS-TBNA 技术

EBUS技术用于观察纵隔内结构并获取标本，一旦观察到纵隔内淋巴结，通常需要描述其位置，依据IASLC（国际肺癌分期）示意图划分该淋巴结属于哪一组。图5.1显示IASLC示意图以及每组淋巴结的解剖学定义，包括淋巴结群所在的可能区域以及对预后判断的意义[30]。EBUS较一般支气管镜观察范围更广且稳定性更好（图5.2），Olympus EBUS 外部直径为6.2 mm，顶端直径6.9 mm，与此相对的标准支气管镜的平均直径为5~6 mm。EBUS上有一个直径2.0 mm的工作通道，引导22G或21G TBNA针进行穿刺，该技术能够同时显示两种图像：超声图像和气道图像。超声图像位于EBUS顶端轴向90°的位置，也包括该区域50°切线方向。探头频率为7.5 MHz，可获得深达9 cm的图像。利用超声显像特性，新一代EBUS技术具有多普勒成像能力，即从非血管结构中区分出血管结构。多普勒成像有两种模式：能量多普勒和彩色多普勒。能量多普勒对于探测淋巴结内血流十分敏感，但是不能探测血流方向（图5.3）。彩色多普勒对于探测血流敏感性相对较低，但能探测淋巴结内血流方向（图5.4）。运用能量多普勒和彩色多普勒

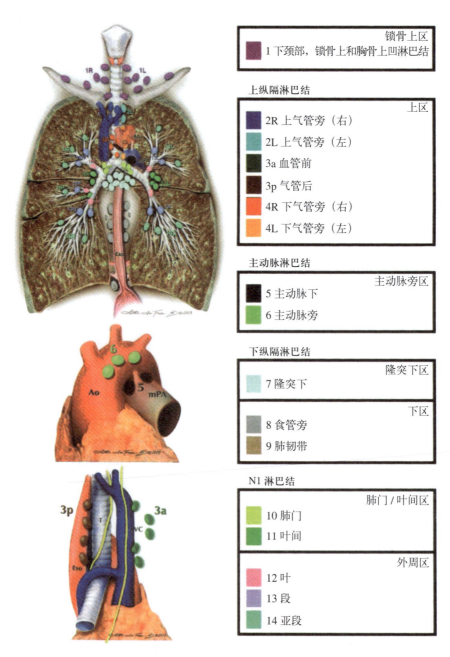

图 5.1 国际肺癌研究学会（IASLC）淋巴结图，包括淋巴结群位置分组以及对预后判断的意义（经 Aletta Frazier 博士允许，转载自国际肺癌研究学会）

成像对于评价淋巴结血管类型十分有用，而淋巴结血管类型对疾病具有诊断价值[31]。EBUS 的镜头角度为水平 30°，而非标准气管镜的为 0°。这一点具有实用意义，如果支气管镜在正中位置前进，为了获得正前方 0°视野，镜头必须弯曲到 -30°，否则操作者会不知不觉损伤声带和气管壁。气管镜大小以及可视范围可能使气道检查受限，只能到达段或亚段水平，因此对整个支气管内的检查必须运用标准支气管镜。EBUS-TBNA 内建立的活检针通道，将活检针置于整个气管镜并沿其轴线延伸 20°，直至其穿出末梢顶端。当活检针通过气道前进到达淋巴结时，必须保证通道的角度能实现实时超声可视化（图 5.5）。操作者进行 EBUS 时必须使用 TBNA 专用穿刺针，与标准 TBNA 穿刺针类似，EBUS-TBNA 穿刺针被置于鞘内。然而，EBUS-TBNA 穿刺针（40 mm）比标准 TBNA 活检针（13 mm）长，且末梢远端有沟槽（图 5.6），使之发出强回声，从而在超声显像上极易观察到更广泛的视野。EBUS-TBNA 穿刺针内有一根内芯，在穿刺淋巴结时可防止污染支气管细胞。EBUS 气管镜顶端安装有一个气囊，该气囊可充盈不等量生理盐水，从而使超声探头与气道壁接触良好（图 5.7）。因此，在某些情况下可更好地观察到气管腔以外的结构。气囊由乳胶材料制成，应避免使用在乳胶过敏患者身上。

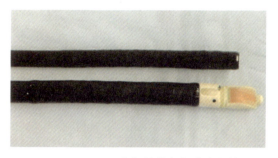

图 5.2　EBUS-TBNA 支气管镜与标准支气管镜的比较

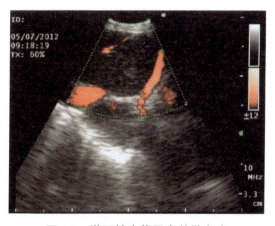

图 5.3　淋巴结内能量多普勒血流

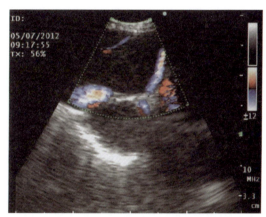

图 5.4　淋巴结内彩色多普勒血流

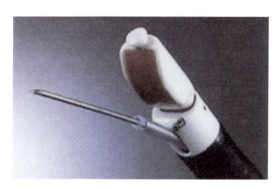

图 5.5　EBUS-TBNA 顶端以及插入式 TBNA 穿刺针

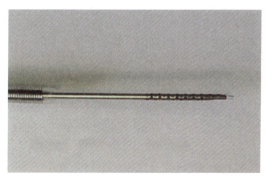

图 5.6　EBUS-TBNA 穿刺针上的沟槽使其出现高回声从而在超声图像上极易观察到更广泛的视野

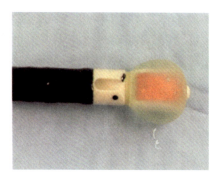

图 5.7　EBUS-TBNA 气管镜上充满生理盐水的膨胀球囊

操作技术

该气管镜可通过口腔，经声门上气道，如经过喉罩（LMA）或气管导管（ETT）进入气道。尽管一些操作者将该气管镜经鼻置入，但 EBUS 外围直径较大，使之较难通过且容易导致局部创伤，尤其是鼻道狭窄患者。因此，大部分情况下，最好使用经口腔导入 EBUS 的方法。尽管 EBUS-TBNA 的最佳方案已制定[32]，但因并无标准技术，故操作者和相关机构的操作方法略微存在差异。一般情况下，应遵循以下原则：运用超声成像识别结节，通过气管镜尖端所指位置直接观察或通过超声成像观察解剖结构以正确识别结节位置（图 5.8）。一旦识别结节，EBUS 穿刺针导管经工作通道前进并锁定该部位。在 EBUS 引导下进行 TBNA，为了更加娴熟地操作，操作者必须完全通晓 TBNA 专用穿刺针的每个方面（图 5.9）。表 5.1 总结了如何通过一步一步的操作获得靶淋巴结样本，当 EBUS 气管镜到达气道正中部位时，贯穿气管镜终端的穿刺针必须向前推进，由于穿刺针远端部分相对坚硬，如果操作者不慎对其施压使远端弯曲，将会造成 EBUS 气管镜损伤。一旦

表 5.1　EBUS-TBNA 操作步骤	
第 1 步	EBUS 活检穿刺针沿正中位置进入工作通道
第 2 步	滑动轮缘，锁定到位，固定穿刺针
第 3 步	松开保护套螺钉
第 4 步	显示器右上角可见时，固定保护套
第 5 步	松开穿刺针旋钮
第 6 步	运用超声成像定位需要活检的靶淋巴结
第 7 步	通过快速"穿刺"技术进针
第 8 步	观察穿刺针进入靶淋巴结
第 9 步	反复抽送内芯数次以去除穿刺针内残渣
第 10 步	撤出内芯
第 11 步	将注射器连接至活检穿刺针
第 12 步	抽吸
第 13 步	在超声可视化条件下，移动穿刺针进出 10~15 次
第 14 步	释放抽吸物
第 15 步	将穿刺针置入鞘内
第 16 步	打开并移除穿刺针和鞘，准备涂片

第 2 篇　诊断性介入支气管镜

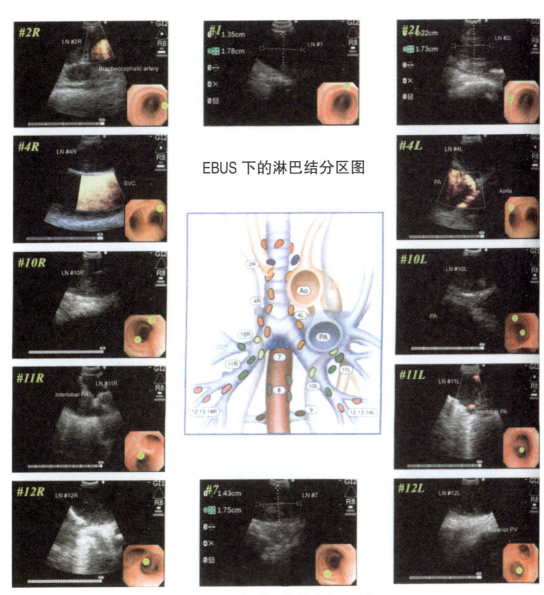

图 5.8　EBUS 成像以及相应支气管不同组淋巴结的分布 [引自 Yasufuku K. EBUS-TBNA Bronchoscopy. In：Ernst A, Herth FJX (eds.). Endobronchial Ultrasound：An Atlas and Practical Guide. New York：Springer Science + Business Media; 2009. With permission from Springer Science + Business Media]

穿刺针完全进入并锁定部位，针鞘继续进入直到气管镜末端突出可被看到为止。由于穿刺针有点硬，与没有穿刺针相比，气管镜最大弯曲程度会下降，淋巴结超声显像范围也会因此改变。因此，为了对可视淋巴结活检，EBUS 气管镜通常需要重新定位。一旦完成调整并准备对淋巴结活检，穿刺针需经气道壁刺入到达靶淋巴结（图 5.10）。穿刺针进入淋巴结在细胞学文献中定义为"偏移"，从进入淋巴结到撤出，穿刺针"穿刺"的过程是一系列"偏移"的集合。穿刺针一旦进入淋巴结，内芯应抽吸或反复稍微撤出和进入以弹出在插入过程中经气管壁携带的残渣。关于穿刺针的"偏移"次数，"偏移"速度，"偏移"部位（淋巴结皮质、髓质，还是

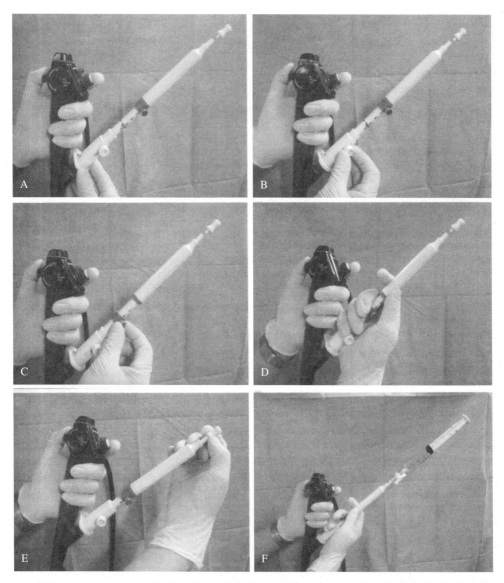

图 5.9 使用 EBUS-TBNA 专用针从淋巴结获得细胞学标本。A. 滑动轮缘将穿刺针连接到工作通道处并锁定位置；B. 鞘调节器旋钮旋松以调节长度；C. 旋开穿刺针调节器旋钮；D. 针头进入；E. 穿刺针进入淋巴结后，来回拉动内芯数次，去除碎片；F. 用注射器抽吸 [引自 Yasufuku K.EBUS-TBNA Bronchoscopy. In：Ernst A, Herth FJX(eds.). Endobrochial Ultrasound：An Atlas and Practical Guide. New York：Springer Science + Business Media; 2009. With permission from Springer Science + Business Media]

两部分都需要），"偏移"过程中是否进行抽吸，目前尚未达成共识。一旦完成活检，穿刺针必须再次沿中位线位置取下，以免损伤气管镜通道。不管什么穿刺技术，穿刺最理想的结果是获得淋巴组织或恶性肿瘤细胞，从而代替淋巴结取样。样本的处理和分析将在下一部分讲到。

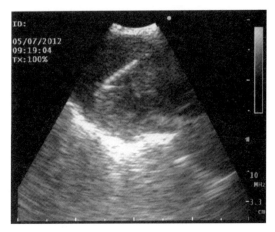

图 5.10 EBUS 成像显示肿大纵隔淋巴结以及其中清晰可见的活检穿刺针

样本处理

每次穿刺应该获得充足材料以制备涂片，并且有足够的剩余样本材料置于保存剂中制成细胞包埋。依据细胞病理学家的方法，涂片经空气干燥后以酒精固定，或者两者都可行。穿刺针自气管镜移出后，将内芯放回 TBNA 穿刺针，并将穿刺针的吸出物置于玻片进行涂片。涂片可置于 95% 乙醇或在空气中干燥。我们的惯例是，每次穿刺准备两张涂片，一张用酒精固定，另一张由空气干燥，用于 Diff-Quick 快速染色，剩余样本置于 Cytolyt®。内芯移出后，用大约 0.5 ml 生理盐水冲洗 TBNA 穿刺针，直到 TBNA 穿刺针内充满空气。这些生理盐水样本也置于 Cytolyt®。保存于 Cytolyt® 的样本材料用于液基薄层切片以及细胞块制备。有些研究中心更倾向于将初始样本置于防腐剂中对剩余样本进行涂片。此方法的目的是使外周血对涂片的污染程度降到最低。一旦获得样本，用湿纱布（生理盐水或乙醇）擦拭内芯，并放回 TBNA 穿刺针以备下次穿刺活检时使用。如果能进行快速细胞学检查（即 ROSE：快速当场评估），几种染色方法可迅速评估 EBUS-TBNA 所获样本的充足性以及分类。这些染色方法包括快速 H&E 染色（4 分钟），快速巴氏染色（6~8 分钟）以及 Diff-Quick 染色（约 1 分钟）。穿刺针吸出样本可分别进行流式细胞分析，微生物培养以及分子学检测等。ROSE 结果用于评估样本充足性以及分类，而不是最终诊断，这些结果类似于外科手术中快速冰冻切片。尽管有些研究发现，ROSE 对于传统 TBNA 有优势 [33-36]，目前并无文献表明 ROSE 可提高 EBUS-TBNA 的诊断率。从传统 TBNA 数据中可以十分直观地推断出，ROSE 可减少每站淋巴结穿刺的次数（基于样本充分性分析），与 EBUS-TBNA 联用时可减少操作时间 [37]。此外，通过对样本针对性分类，ROSE 也可能降低操作成本，因此减少不必要的检测，避免患者进行不必要的操作，以后的研究需要注重这些方面。

在不能进行 ROSE 的情况下，必须保证足够多的活检样本，以确保有能充分代表淋巴结的样本。在肺癌分期中，每个淋巴结有 3 个活检样本才足够，如果想要获得组织碎片，两次穿刺也是必要的 [38]。置于乙醇中的切片用巴氏染色进行处理，可更好地评价细胞形态。放置在防腐剂溶液中的样本被浓缩处理为液基薄层和细胞包埋。除肺癌之外，当怀疑为其他诊断时，应该将样本置于合适媒介中为其进行免疫分型或流式细胞仪检测。例如，若怀疑为恶性淋巴瘤，应运用 RPMI 培养基或与之相当的培养基，若怀疑感染，抽吸物应置于无菌生理盐水进行培养。

EBUS-TBNA 的麻醉方式

目前尚没有相关研究针对 EBUS-TBNA 最佳麻醉方式的选择。利用短效麻醉剂，比如丙泊酚和芬太尼以及短效肌松剂（罗库溴铵）进行全身麻醉或者深度镇静，能更好地固定患者，提供更好的操作条件，提高患者的舒适度，并最大限度地减少使用局部麻醉药。这种麻醉方式能使患者在体位固定时，通过优化内镜位置采集标本来缩短整个操作过程。另外，这些试剂的半衰期很短，因此这种麻醉方式能缩短患者复苏时间。然而，在绝大多数支气管镜检查中全身麻醉并不常用；即便真的需要使用这种麻醉方式，那也需要配备额外的医护人员与监护设备，这就增加了检查的整体费用。在临床实践过程中，EBUS-TBNA 通常在手术室内进行，这也带来了相关的安排困难及费用问题。在支气管镜检查时，清醒镇静更容易、更便捷，能够达到进行 EBUS-TBNA 检查时的镇静需求。在清醒镇静时不需要建立人工气道辅助呼吸，也不需要专门的麻醉人员。目前，尚不清楚在清醒镇静下 EBUS-TBNA 诊断的阳性率是否比全身麻醉下的低，尤其是在有经验的临床工作者操作时[39]。未来需要更多的研究来评估该检查过程中的其他变量，例如操作时间、患者舒适度以及获得确切诊断所需的操作环节的数量等，是否受到麻醉方式的影响。

如果使用全身麻醉，那么全身静脉麻醉（total intravenousanesthesia，TIVA）优于吸入麻醉，原因在于频繁地吸痰会导致患者吸入的挥发性麻醉气体量具有不均一性[40]。此外，挥发性麻醉剂具有污染手术室的可能，使操作人员暴露于麻醉剂气体中。为了达到 TIVA 效果，我们需要控制丙泊酚的静脉注射速度在 75~250 μg/（kg·min）[41]，可以间歇性联合使用短效麻醉剂芬太尼或者瑞芬太尼。这些麻醉剂的剂量需要因人而异，以确保在整个检查过程中患者处于足够深的麻醉状态下。为了保持患者肌肉松弛，我们可以使用短效肌松剂如罗库溴铵或者顺式阿曲库铵。在整个检查过程中，肌肉松弛有利于减少患者移动和咳嗽，这样就能观察到足够多的淋巴结，并准确地进行淋巴结穿刺取样。肌肉松弛不仅有利于 SGA，例如 LMA 和 ETT 的插入，也能松弛声带，消除绷紧的声带对气管镜的抵抗，最大限度地降低频繁插入导致的创伤。在松弛肌肉过程中，脑电双频指数监测（Bispectral indexmonitor，BIS Monitor®）（Covidien，都柏林，爱尔兰）能被用来监测麻醉深度，从而减少患者术中觉醒的可能性[42]。BIS 监测仪也能帮助麻醉医师调整麻醉剂用量，避免由于深度或者轻度麻醉而导致过度麻醉和血流动力学的紊乱，甚至可能因不理想剂量导致患者觉醒。

如果使用全身麻醉或者深度镇静，那么建议使用 LMA 或者 ETT。上述两种气道装置有利也有弊，需要根据不同患者分别选择，因此在进行相关检查之前，应先咨询麻醉医师，选择理想的气道装置。

SGA 是 EBUS-TBNA 的一个理想气道装置。4 号 LMA 具有足够宽的内径，能使相对较粗的 EBUS 支气管镜通过，并在与支气管镜的间隙中进行肺部通气（图 5.11）。另外，在 SGA 装置内，支气管镜能在气道内自由移动，调整其尖端紧邻支气管壁，而这一过程对于检查气道旁淋巴结尤为重要。但对于那些具有胃内容物误吸风险（严重胃食管反流或者食管裂孔疝）的患者，应谨慎使用 SGA。

如果使用 ETT，那么应该使用大规格的 ETT，以使其能容纳 EBUS 镜（常规 8.5，甚至更大）。ETT 应置入气管内偏上的位置，以免影响气道旁淋巴结的检查（图 5.12）。作为一个常规方法，ETT 能提供一个更安全的气道，对重度胃食管反流或者食管裂孔疝的患者大有裨益。值得注意的是，ETT 能保护声带，在支气管镜外部需要多次插入及抽回且时间较长的操作过程中，可避免反复摩擦导致的声带损伤。

如果使用清醒镇静这种麻醉方式，那么需要达到足够深的镇静效果，以便在检查过程中给予患者舒适，方便医师检查。最经典的镇静麻醉方式就是联用抗焦虑药（比如咪达唑仑）和麻醉剂（比如芬太尼）。一些随机研究证实，与单独使用苯二氮䓬类药物相比，联合使用苯二氮䓬类药物和阿片类药物能改善患者舒适度、耐受力，减少患者咳嗽[43]。但是这种麻醉方式最常见的问题是延长了检查时间，降低了患者对大直径 EBUS 支

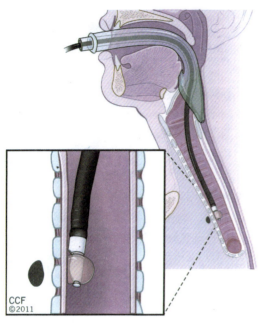

图 5.11　EBUS-TBNA 置于喉罩气道内（LMA）

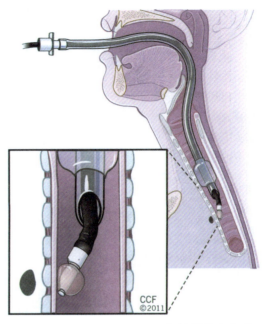

图 5.12　EBUS-TBNA 置于气管导管内表面

气管镜的耐受力。最终的结果是，为了获得患者较好的耐受力，镇静剂的使用剂量较常规支气管镜显著增加。另外，在这种检查过程中，局部麻醉剂常被用来最大限度地控制患者咳嗽。相比标准的支气管镜检查，该检查时间更长，使用局部麻醉剂来控制咳嗽的累计剂量更大，这会增加这些药物出现毒性副作用的风险[44]。在这些药物当中，利多卡因的总量必须严格限制在 7 mg/kg 及以下[45]。利多卡因中毒会导致患者出现不自主运动、精神状态异常、癫痫发作、呼吸抑制，甚至需要进行原本不必要的气管插管、住院，以及延长患者恢复时间。在检查过程中，如果遇到如下情况：不止一个淋巴结需要针吸穿刺采集标本；或者淋巴结相对来说很小；抑或是需要检查纵隔淋巴结进行疾病分期，那么整个检查过程将需要更长时间。

EBUS-TBNA 的适应证

EBUS-TBNA 主要的适应证包括纵隔和肺门的非小细胞肺癌（non-small-celllung cancer, NSCLC）的分期；无支气管病变，但有淋巴结肿大，且怀疑为肿瘤的鉴别诊断；NSCLC 患者化疗/放疗后的再分期或者复发。其他的适应证包括纵隔淋巴结病变的病因分析，比如可疑结节病、结核等感染，纵隔淋巴瘤、胸腺瘤以及纵隔囊肿。另外，EBUS-TBNA 能通过检测肿瘤侵犯气管壁的深度为选择治疗方案提供依据，也可以用来采集样本进行分子学检测，甚至组建组织样本库。更多的临床应用包括评估肺血管疾病和气道重塑。

EBUS-TBNA 的并发症和安全性

患者对 EBUS-TBNA 的耐受力较好，且后者与传统的 TBNA 有着同样的安全性[46,47]。与纵隔镜检查相比，EBUS-TBNA 侵袭性小，安全性高。但关于 EBUS-TBNA 后出现纵隔气肿、气胸、纵隔积血、纵隔炎以及菌血症等并发症仍然偶有报道[48-50]。与传统 TBNA 一样，出血并发症的发生率很低，即使在大血管被意外刺破时。

诊断价值

肺癌分期

本章节并不着重讨论 NSCLC 纵隔分期。EBUS-TBNA 能有效评估 NSCLC 患者发生肺门和纵隔淋巴结转移的情况[47,51]。纵隔镜可以系统地采集 NSCLC 患者的纵隔淋巴结样本。EBUS-TBNA 不具备这种作用[14,16,52],但是当遇到同样的指征时,我们要有从使用纵隔镜演变成使用 EBUS-TBNA 的直觉,未来需要更多的研究来证明 EBUS-TBNA 在肺癌的分期中更有效。另外,EBUS-TBNA 不具备传统纵隔镜采集 N1 淋巴结的功能,那么这个淋巴结数据是否需要被整合到 EBUS-TBNA 分期尚不清楚。此外,采集多大的淋巴结组织进行活检没有共识,确实在医学文献中淋巴结的采集大小比较宽泛,有的取短轴 10 mm 的组织块,有的取 5 mm。采集短轴 10 mm 组织块是依据 CT 扫描推断的[53-55];然而采集 5 mm 组织块进行活检不仅可行,也使 EBUS-TBNA 具备了对 NSCLC 患者进行分期的作用[37,56,57]。

有些推测认为 EBUS 影像上出现的淋巴结可以预示出现疾病的淋巴结转移[58],但是最近有研究报道对这一观念持怀疑态度[37]。一些研究表明,EBUS-TBNA 的多普勒影像图能预测恶性肿瘤的扩散[31,58,59],其机制正如超声内镜学(EUS)所描述的,是检测纵隔淋巴结内的血管图像[60,61]。

最初,在肿瘤分期上,我们将 EBUS 与放射影像学进行比较,特别是与正电子发射断层成像(positron emission tomography,PET)和计算机断层成像(computed tomography,CT)进行比较。对于纵隔肿瘤来说,PET 比传统 CT 更加灵敏,能评估淋巴结情况,但是其阴性预测值取决于组织中氟脱氧葡萄糖的亲和力和肿瘤位置[62]。多项研究[56,63-68]利用 CT 和 PET/CT 检查患者纵隔内正常或者是肿大的淋巴结,并依据 CT 和 PET/CT(表 5.2)的影像学诊断标准[53-55]对病变进行分期,并将其与 EBUS-TBNA 分期进行对比,发现在对 5~20 mm 淋巴结病变的检查上,尤其是高纵隔淋巴结转移、低 PET 活性的腺癌[64],EBUS-TBNA 分期优于放射影像学分期。另外,在诊断 CT 扫描上出现的亚厘米级结节时,联合使用 EBUS-TBNA 和 EUS-FNA 比单独使用更准确[68]。

EBUS-TBNA 与传统 TBNA 的对比

针对纵隔转移瘤,TBNA 阳性检出率差异大,文献报道为 20%~89%,这除了与病变的大小、位置有关,也与操作者的经验有关[26,69]。

表 5.2 EBUS-TBNA 分期与 CT/PET 分期的比较

研究	年份	患者数	敏感性(%)			特异性(%)			阴性预测值(%)			患病率(%)
			CT	PET	EBUS	CT	PET	EBUS	CT	PET	EBUS	
Yasufuku	2006	102	76.9	80	92.3	55.3	70.1	100	87.5	91.5	97.4	23.6
Herth	2008	97			89			100			98.9	82
Bauwens	2008	106		67	95			100		100	91	58
Wallace	2008	138	67	24	69			100			88	28
Hwangbo	2009	117		70	90		59.8	100		85.2	96.7	26
Rintoul	2009	109			91			100			60	71
Szlubowski	2010	120			68+EUS			98+EUS			91+EUS	22

几项临床实验针对肺癌分期将传统 TBNA 与 EBUS-TBNA 进行了比较。在一个包含 200 例（除了第 7 组淋巴结）可疑 NSCLC 患者的前瞻性对照实验中，EBUS-TBNA 的诊断率优于传统 TBNA（84% vs. 58%）。而第 7 组淋巴结的诊断率在统计学上是没有显著差异的，尽管作者指出 EBUS-TBNA 诊断率的趋势优于常规的 TBNA（86% vs. 74%）。然而，需要注意的是，在这个实验中是使用 EBUS 径向探头来定位淋巴结的，TBNA 用的是标准 TBNA 针和传统技术。换句话说，这项实验并不是 EBUS-TBNA 凸面探头与传统 TBNA 间的比较。事实上，EBUS 径向探头逐渐被 EBUS-TBNA 凸面探头取代。第二个前瞻性对照实验收集了 138 例已确诊或者 CT 显示可疑的肺癌患者的资料[67]。在该研究中，EBUS-TBNA 及 EUS-FNA 与传统 TBNA 对比，EBUS-TBNA 和 EUS-FNA 的敏感性为 69%，阴性预测值（NPV）为 88%。然而，传统 TBNA 的敏感性仅为 36%，NPV 为 78%。这项研究证实 EBUS-TBNA 在检查纵隔转移性疾病和肺门淋巴结上较传统 TBNA 敏感性更高。

EBUS-TBNA 与纵隔镜比较

多项研究已经证实了 EBUS-TBNA 在肺癌分期上的重要作用（表 5.3）。EBUS-TBNA 成功应用于肿瘤分期开始于对 EBUS-TBNA 能否取代纵隔镜作为纵隔分期方式的讨论[6,70]。大量研究证实其稳定的敏感性和阴性预测值[63,71-73]与胸腔镜类似[57,74-76]（表 5.4）。

早期应用 EBUS-TBNA 进行纵隔肿瘤分期能降低对胸腔镜检查的需求[77]。2007 年颁布的 ACCP 指南建议将 EBUS-TBNA 作为肺癌纵隔分期的一个检查方法。因为 EBUS-TBNA 没有 100% 的阴性预测值，因此当 EBUS-TBNA 取出的组织样本没有发现肿瘤转移时，建议做纵隔镜进一步确诊。例如，在来自 Mayo Clinic

表 5.3 EBUS-TBNA 评估肺癌分期的有用性研究

研究	年份	患者数量	研究设计	敏感性（%）(EBU)	特异性（%）(EBUS)	阴性（%）预测值	患病率（%）
Szlubowski	2009	206	前瞻性队列研究	89	100	84	61
Rintoul	2009	109	回顾性研究	91	100	60	71
Hwangbo	2010	150	前瞻性研究	84	100	93	
Andrade	2010	98	回顾性研究	88	97	84	

表 5.4 EBUS-TBNA 与 纵隔镜 (MED) 对肺癌分期的比较研究

研究	年份	患者数量	研究设计	敏感性（%）		特异性（%）	阴性预测值（%）		患病率（%）
				EBUS	MED		EBUS	MED	
Ernst	2008	66	前瞻交叉	87	68	100	78	59	89
Annema	2010	241	随机	94	79	100	93	86	49
Defranchi	2010	494	回顾性			100	72	81	
Yasufuku	2011	153	前瞻交叉	87	68	100	91	90	35

的一项研究中，29例确诊或者可疑N2期肺癌患者在EBUS-TBNA检查阴性的情况下进行纵隔镜检查，其中8例患者发现纵隔内转移性病灶（28%）[74]。为此，该学者得出结论：如果怀疑肿瘤患者已进入N2期，即便EBUS-TBNA检查结果阴性，也应该进一步进行纵隔镜检查。与此相反的是，其他研究建议这种验证性的纵隔镜检查在这些病例中没有必要[55,77]。显然，EBUS-TBNA的效果，特别是阴性预测值（NPV），是决定在其检查结果阴性后是否进一步应用验证性纵隔镜检查的重要影响因素。EBUS-TBNA的NPV受多种因素影响，包括操作者技巧、病理科能力、检查前恶性肿瘤的概率以及该人群中良性疾病（比如组织胞浆菌病）的发病率。因此，在临床实践过程中，除了有其他确切的检查结果，EBUS-TBNA检查结果阴性的患者一定要进行验证性纵隔镜检查。

需要强调的是EBUS-TBNA和纵隔镜应该是互补的检查方式，而不是多余的。为此，任何一个独立的医疗机构都应该在进行肿瘤纵隔分期前综合考虑操作者的经验、病理科的能力以及外科手术经验等因素。

EBUS-TBNA检查淋巴瘤

淋巴瘤的诊断需满足2008年WHO列出来的多个条件[78]。包括临床特征、形态学、免疫分型和基因型数据。既往，淋巴瘤的诊断和分型主要依据细胞形态分析，目前主要依据细胞免疫分析（特别是流式细胞仪分析）和基因型分析。形态特征分析所需要的组织块比FNA获得的组织样本要多得多，但FNA提供的组织样本足够进行细胞分型和基因型分析[79-81]。一些研究表明，EBUS-TBNA也可以用来诊断淋巴瘤[82-84]。其对淋巴瘤诊断的敏感性大致为76%；但由于采集的组织样本少，不足以进行淋巴瘤亚型分析，因此对淋巴瘤亚型（例如边缘细胞、滤泡状细胞和霍奇金淋巴瘤）的敏感性很低[85]。另外，在检测细胞学标本时，尽管细胞型分析和基因型检测有所进步，对一些淋巴瘤亚型，例如弥漫大B细胞淋巴瘤、套细胞淋巴瘤、伯基特淋巴瘤、滤泡状淋巴瘤以及霍奇金淋巴瘤的诊断仍很困难[86]。即便霍奇金淋巴瘤内一小部分缺少细胞标记物的Reed-Sternberg细胞，也能被流式细胞仪检测到[86]，但现在仍然在研发新的检测方法以使其能更容易地被流式细胞仪检测出来[87]。

EBUS-TBNA诊断良性疾病

结节病

由于结节病病理特征为非坏死性上皮样肉芽肿，该表现亦存在于其他很多疾病，因此结节病诊断较困难。其诊断依据临床症状、影像学改变以及病理活检辅助诊断。支气管镜检查及支气管镜活检对肺结节病诊断率极高。同样地，有几项研究表明运用传统TBNA从肿大的纵隔淋巴结获取样本来诊断结节病具有可行性。肺泡灌洗液淋巴细胞增多以及CD4/CD8＞3.5可能作为结节病诊断的依据，但不能直接诊断结节病[88]。有报道指出，依据操作者的经验以及是否使用19G病理穿刺针，传统TBNA对于结节病患者从纵隔淋巴结获取样本的诊断率存在差异[89,90]。EBUS-TBNA获取结节组织样本诊断结节病的诊断率为93%[91]，并且集中诊断率大约为80%[92]。在一些研究中，EBUS-TBNA可能优于传统TBNA[93]以及支气管镜活检[94]。基于这些研究，EBUS-TBNA作为诊断Ⅰ期和Ⅱ期结节病的初步检测方法十分合理，尤其是当支气管镜活检不可行或不能诊断时。

感染

几项研究显示，EBUS-TBNA有益于结核病的诊断，尤其是在涂片阴性时可结合肺泡灌洗液培养、核酸放大试验帮助诊断[95,96]。此外，EBUS-TBNA对诊断孤立性纵隔淋巴结结核（在所有病例中发生率高达9%）敏感性较高[97]。

其他

虽然数据有限,有研究指出 EBUS-TBNA 对不明原因的纵隔肿块诊断率较高[98],特别是良性病变。EBUS-TBNA 也可能在支气管囊肿的诊断和治疗中发挥作用[99, 100]。

EBUS-TBNA 的局限性

EBUS-TBNA 是一项令人振奋的新技术,虽然一直在改进,但为了进一步加强该技术在临床的应用,还需要克服很多挑战和局限性。EBUS 比标准支气管镜大,它不能进行全面的支气管内检查,除 TBNA 样本外它不能获取支气管镜范围内样本。因此,标准支气管镜需要与 EBUS-TBNA 伴随使用,这样不仅增加费用还花费更多时间。如果 EBUS-TBNA 外形设计合理,又具备标准支气管镜的检查能力,这将会增加其临床实用性。一些操作者通常在全麻下操作 EBUS-TBNA,这不仅增加了费用,易引起调度冲突,还增加了麻醉风险。更好的支气管镜设计可避免该过程全麻的需要,另一个主要问题是 TBNA 专用穿刺针的设计,其使用比传统 TBNA 穿刺针更为复杂烦琐。TBNA 穿刺针设计上的创新可以使其使用更加顺畅,在 TBNA 取样时使步骤有所减少。最后提到的是费用问题。在资源有限的条件下,EBUS 的初始费用是需要着重考虑的问题。而且,全麻下操作以及复苏等可能大大增加总体费用。另外还需指出的是,EBUS-TBNA 每个细节的维修费用显著高于标准纤维支气管镜[101]。最后,大部分肺科医师未接受超声成像方面的培训,在操作者会精准操作之前,需要对其进行教育和培训。

总　结

总之,EBUS-TBNA 是一项创新性技术,在世界范围内对良恶性疾病的诊断应用得越来越广泛。EBUS-TBNA 通过微创方式到达肺门和纵隔淋巴结,同时对淋巴结组织进行实时采样。与传统 TBNA 和纵隔镜相比,EBUS-TBNA 可能更适合应用于穿刺更小更远的肺门和纵隔淋巴结。EBUS-TBNA 对良恶性疾病的诊断率极高,与纵隔镜诊断率相近。虽然纵隔镜在纵隔疾病的诊断中发挥重要作用,但随着 EBUS-TBNA 专业知识和有效性的提升,EBUS-TBNA 将会继续广泛应用在这些疾病中。

参考文献

1. Hurter T, Hanrath P. Endobronchial sonography in the diagnosis of pulmonary and mediastinal tumors. Dtsch Med Wochenschr. 1990;115:1899–905.
2. Shannon JJ, Bude RO, Orens JB, et al. Endobronchial ultrasound-guided needle aspiration of mediastinal adenopathy. Am J Respir Crit Care Med. 1996;153:1424–30.
3. Kurimoto N, Murayama M, Yoshioka S, et al. Assessment of usefulness of endobronchial ultrasonography in determination of depth of tracheobronchial tumor invasion. Chest. 1999;115: 1500–6.
4. Herth FJ, Ernst A, Becker HD. Endobronchial ultrasound-guided transbronchial lung biopsy in solitary pulmonary nodules and peripheral lesions. Eur Respir J. 2002;20:972–4.
5. Yasufuku K, Chiyo M, Sekine Y, et al. Real-time endobronchial ultrasound-guided transbronchial needle aspiration of mediastinal and hilar lymph nodes. Chest. 2004;126:122–8.
6. Rusch VW. Mediastinoscopy: an obsolete procedure? J Thorac Cardiovasc Surg. 2011;142:1400–2.
7. Disayabutr S, Tscheikuna J, Nana A. The endobronchial ultrasound-guided transbronchial lung biopsy in peripheral pulmonary lesions. J Med Assoc Thai. 2010;93 Suppl 1:S94–101.
8. Wang Memoli JS, Nietert PJ, Silvestri GA. Metaanalysis of guided bronchoscopy for the evaluation of the pulmonary nodule. Chest. 2012;142(2):385–93.
9. Kurimoto N, Miyazawa T, Okimasa S, et al. Endobronchial ultrasonography using a guide sheath increases the ability to diagnose peripheral pulmonary lesions endoscopically. Chest. 2004; 126:959–65.
10. Yoshikawa M, Sukoh N, Yamazaki K, et al. Diagnostic value of endobronchial ultrasonography with a guide sheath for peripheral pulmonary lesions without X-ray fluoroscopy. Chest. 2007;131: 1788–93.
11. Chao TY, Chien MT, Lie CH, et al. Endobronchial ultrasonography-guided transbronchial needle aspiration increases the diagnostic yield of peripheral pulmonary lesions: a randomized trial. Chest. 2009;136:229–36.
12. Cho JH, Kim J, Kim K, et al. A comparative analysis of video-assisted mediastinoscopy and conventional mediastinoscopy. Ann Thorac Surg. 2011;92:1007–11.
13. Zakkar M, Tan C, Hunt I. Is video mediastinoscopy a safer and

more effective procedure than conventional mediastinoscopy? Interact Cardiovasc Thorac Surg. 2012;14:81–4.
14. Detterbeck F, Puchalski J, Rubinowitz A, et al. Classification of the thoroughness of mediastinal staging of lung cancer. Chest. 2010;137:436–42.
15. Ernst A, Gangadharan SP. A good case for a declining role for mediastinoscopy just got better. Am J Respir Crit Care Med. 2008;177:471–2.
16. Detterbeck FC, Jantz MA, Wallace M, et al. Invasive mediastinal staging of lung cancer: ACCP evidencebased clinical practice guidelines (2nd edition). Chest. 2007;132:202S–20.
17. Little AG, Rusch VW, Bonner JA, et al. Patterns of surgical care of lung cancer patients. Ann Thorac Surg. 2005;80:2051–6. discussion 2056.
18. Deneffe G, Lacquet LM, Gyselen A. Cervical mediastinoscopy and anterior mediastinotomy in patients with lung cancer and radiologically normal mediastinum. Eur J Respir Dis. 1983;64:613–9.
19. Hammoud ZT, Anderson RC, Meyers BF, et al. The current role of mediastinoscopy in the evaluation of thoracic disease. J Thorac Cardiovasc Surg. 1999;118:894–9.
20. De Leyn P, Schoonooghe P, Deneffe G, et al. Surgery for non-small cell lung cancer with unsuspected metastasis to ipsilateral mediastinal or subcarinal nodes (N2 disease). Eur J Cardiothorac Surg. 1996;10:649–54. discussion 654–645.
21. Page A, Nakhle G, Mercier C, et al. Surgical treatment of bronchogenic carcinoma: the importance of staging in evaluating late survival. Can J Surg. 1987;30:96–9.
22. Dillemans B, Deneffe G, Verschakelen J, et al. Value of computed tomography and mediastinoscopy in preoperative evaluation of mediastinal nodes in non-small cell lung cancer. A study of 569 patients. Eur J Cardiothorac Surg. 1994;8:37–42.
23. Leschber G, Sperling D, Klemm W, et al. Does video-mediastinoscopy improve the results of conventional mediastinoscopy? Eur J Cardiothorac Surg. 2008;33:289–93.
24. Schieppati E. Mediastinal puncture thru the tracheal carina. Rev Asoc Med Argent. 1949;63:497–9.
25. Schieppati E. Mediastinal lymph node puncture through the tracheal carina. Surg Gynecol Obstet. 1958;107:243–6.
26. Wang KP, Brower R, Haponik EF, et al. Flexible transbronchial needle aspiration for staging of bronchogenic carcinoma. Chest. 1983;84:571–6.
27. Holty JE, Kuschner WG, Gould MK. Accuracy of transbronchial needle aspiration for mediastinal staging of non-small cell lung cancer: a meta-analysis. Thorax. 2005;60:949–55.
28. Diacon AH, Schuurmans MM, Theron J, et al. Transbronchial needle aspirates: how many passes per target site? Eur Respir J. 2007;29:112–6.
29. Chin Jr R, McCain TW, Lucia MA, et al. Transbronchial needle aspiration in diagnosing and staging lung cancer: how many aspirates are needed? Am J Respir Crit Care Med. 2002;166:377–81.
30. Rusch VW, Asamura H, Watanabe H, et al. The IASLC lung cancer staging project: a proposal for a new international lymph node map in the forthcoming seventh edition of the TNM classification for lung cancer. J Thorac Oncol. 2009;4:568–77.
31. Nakajima T, Anayama T, Shingyoji M, et al. Vascular image patterns of lymph nodes for the prediction of metastatic disease during EBUS-TBNA for mediastinal staging of lung cancer. J Thorac Oncol. 2012;7:1009–14.
32. Nakajima T, Yasufuku K. How I do it–optimal methodology for multidirectional analysis of endobronchial ultrasound-guided transbronchial needle aspiration samples. J Thorac Oncol. 2011;6:203–6.
33. Trisolini R, Cancellieri A, Tinelli C, et al. Rapid onsite evaluation of transbronchial aspirates in the diagnosis of hilar and mediastinal adenopathy: a randomized trial. Chest. 2011;139:395–401.
34. Diette GB, White Jr P, Terry P, et al. Utility of on-site cytopathology assessment for bronchoscopic evaluation of lung masses and adenopathy. Chest. 2000;117:1186–90.
35. Baram D, Garcia RB, Richman PS. Impact of rapid on-site cytologic evaluation during transbronchial needle aspiration. Chest. 2005;128:869–75.
36. Diacon AH, Schuurmans MM, Theron J, et al. Utility of rapid on-site evaluation of transbronchial needle aspirates. Respiration. 2005;72:182–8.
37. Memoli JS, El-Bayoumi E, Pastis NJ, et al. Using endobronchial ultrasound features to predict lymph node metastasis in patients with lung cancer. Chest. 2011;140:1550–6.
38. Lee HS, Lee GK, Kim MS, et al. Real-time endobronchial ultrasound-guided transbronchial needle aspiration in mediastinal staging of non-small cell lung cancer: how many aspirations per target lymph node station? Chest. 2008;134:368–74.
39. Ost DE, Ernst A, Lei X, et al. Diagnostic yield of endobronchial ultrasound-guided transbronchial needle aspiration: results of the AQuIRE Bronchoscopy Registry. Chest. 2011;140:1557–66.
40. Sarkiss M. Anesthesia for bronchoscopy and interventional pulmonology: from moderate sedation to jet ventilation. Curr Opin Pulm Med. 2011;17:274–8.
41. Sarkiss M, Kennedy M, Riedel B, et al. Anesthesia technique for endobronchial ultrasound-guided fine needle aspiration of mediastinal lymph node. J Cardiothorac Vasc Anesth. 2007;21:892–6.
42. Avidan MS, Zhang L, Burnside BA, et al. Anesthesia awareness and the bispectral index. N Engl J Med. 2008;358:1097–108.
43. Stolz D, Chhajed PN, Leuppi JD, et al. Cough suppression during flexible bronchoscopy using combined sedation with midazolam and hydrocodone: a randomised, double blind, placebo controlled trial. Thorax. 2004;59:773–6.
44. Milman N, Laub M, Munch EP, et al. Serum concentrations of lignocaine and its metabolite monoethylglycinexylidide during fibre-optic bronchoscopy in local anaesthesia. Respir Med. 1998;92:40–3.
45. Wahidi MM, Jain P, Jantz M, et al. American College of Chest Physicians consensus statement on the use of topical anesthesia, analgesia, and sedation during flexible bronchoscopy in adult patients. Chest. 2011;140:1342–50.
46. Herth F, Becker HD, Ernst A. Conventional vs endobronchial ultrasound-guided transbronchial needle aspiration: a randomized trial. Chest. 2004;125:322–5.
47. Gu P, Zhao YZ, Jiang LY, et al. Endobronchial ultrasound-guided transbronchial needle aspiration for staging of lung cancer: a systematic review and meta-analysis. Eur J Cancer. 2009;45:1389–96.
48. Huang CT, Chen CY, Ho CC, et al. A rare constellation of empyema, lung abscess, and mediastinal abscess as a complication of endobronchial ultrasound-guided transbronchial needle aspiration. Eur J Cardiothorac Surg. 2011;40:264–5.
49. Moffatt-Bruce SD, Ross Jr P. Mediastinal abscess after endobronchial ultrasound with transbronchial needle aspiration: a case report. J Cardiothorac Surg. 2010;5:33.
50. Steinfort DP, Johnson DF, Irving LB. Incidence of bacteraemia following endobronchial ultrasoundguided transbronchial needle aspiration. Eur Respir J. 2010;36:28–32.
51. Khoo KL, Ho KY. Endoscopic mediastinal staging of lung cancer. Respir Med. 2011;105:515–8.
52. De Leyn P, Lardinois D, Van Schil PE, et al. ESTS guidelines for preoperative lymph node staging for non-small cell lung cancer. Eur J Cardiothorac Surg. 2007;32:1–8.

53. Staples CA, Muller NL, Miller RR, et al. Mediastinal nodes in bronchogenic carcinoma: comparison between CT and mediastinoscopy. Radiology. 1988;167:367–72.
54. Silvestri GA, Gould MK, Margolis ML, et al. Noninvasive staging of non-small cell lung cancer: ACCP evidenced-based clinical practice guidelines (2nd edition). Chest. 2007;132:178S–201.
55. Dales RE, Stark RM, Raman S. Computed tomography to stage lung cancer. Approaching a controversy using meta-analysis. Am Rev Respir Dis. 1990;141:1096–101.
56. Herth FJ, Eberhardt R, Krasnik M, et al. Endobronchial ultrasound-guided transbronchial needle aspiration of lymph nodes in the radiologically and positron emission tomography-normal mediastinum in patients with lung cancer. Chest. 2008;133:887–91.
57. Yasufuku K, Pierre A, Darling G, et al. A prospective controlled trial of endobronchial ultrasound-guided transbronchial needle aspiration compared with mediastinoscopy for mediastinal lymph node staging of lung cancer. J Thorac Cardiovasc Surg. 2011;142:1393–400. e1391.
58. Fujiwara T, Yasufuku K, Nakajima T, et al. The utility of sonographic features during endobronchial ultrasound-guided transbronchial needle aspiration for lymph node staging in patients with lung cancer:a standard endobronchial ultrasound image classification system. Chest. 2010;138:641–7.
59. Satterwhite LG, Berkowitz DM, Parks CS, et al. Central intranodal vessels to predict cytology during endobronchial ultrasound transbronchial needle aspiration. J Bronchol Intervent Pulmonol. 2011;18:322–8.
60. Nakajima T, Shingyouji M, Nishimura H, et al. New endobronchial ultrasound imaging for differentiating metastatic site within a mediastinal lymph node. J Thorac Oncol. 2009;4:1289–90.
61. Sawhney MS, Debold SM, Kratzke RA, et al. Central intranodal blood vessel: a new EUS sign described in mediastinal lymph nodes. Gastrointest Endosc. 2007;65:602–8.
62. Currie GP, Kennedy AM, Denison AR. Tools used in the diagnosis and staging of lung cancer: what's old and what's new? QJM. 2009;102:443–8.
63. Rintoul RC, Tournoy KG, El Daly H, et al. EBUS-TBNA for the clarification of PET positive intrathoracic lymph nodes-an international multi-centre experience. J Thorac Oncol. 2009;4:44–8.
64. Hwangbo B, Kim SK, Lee HS, et al. Application of endobronchial ultrasound-guided transbronchial needle aspiration following integrated PET/CT in mediastinal staging of potentially operable nonsmall cell lung cancer. Chest. 2009;135:1280–7.
65. Bauwens O, Dusart M, Pierard P, et al. Endobronchial ultrasound and value of PET for prediction of pathological results of mediastinal hot spots in lung cancer patients. Lung Cancer. 2008;61:356–61.
66. Yasufuku K, Nakajima T, Motoori K, et al. Comparison of endobronchial ultrasound, positron emission tomography, and CT for lymph node staging of lung cancer. Chest. 2006;130:710–8.
67. Wallace MB, Pascual JM, Raimondo M, et al. Minimally invasive endoscopic staging of suspected lung cancer. JAMA. 2008;299:540–6.
68. Szlubowski A, Zielinski M, Soja J, et al. A combined approach of endobronchial and endoscopic ultrasound-guided needle aspiration in the radiologically normal mediastinum in non-small-cell lung cancer staging–a prospective trial. Eur J Cardiothorac Surg. 2010;37:1175–9.
69. Gasparini S, Zuccatosta L, De Nictolis M. Transbronchial needle aspiration of mediastinal lesions. Monaldi Arch Chest Dis. 2000;55:29–32.
70. Shrager JB. Mediastinoscopy: still the gold standard. Ann Thorac Surg. 2010;89:S2084–9.
71. Hwangbo B, Lee GK, Lee HS, et al. Transbronchial and transesophageal fine-needle aspiration using an ultrasound bronchoscope in mediastinal staging of potentially operable lung cancer. Chest. 2010;138:795–802.
72. Szlubowski A, Kuzdzal J, Kolodziej M, et al. Endobronchial ultrasound-guided needle aspiration in the non-small cell lung cancer staging. Eur J Cardiothorac Surg. 2009;35:332–5. discussion 335–336.
73. Andrade RS, Groth SS, Rueth NM, et al. Evaluation of mediastinal lymph nodes with endobronchial ultrasound: the thoracic surgeon's perspective. J Thorac Cardiovasc Surg. 2010;139:578–82. discussion 582–573.
74. Defranchi SA, Edell ES, Daniels CE, et al. Mediastinoscopy in patients with lung cancer and negative endobronchial ultrasound guided needle aspiration. Ann Thorac Surg. 2010;90:1753–7.
75. Ernst A, Anantham D, Eberhardt R, et al. Diagnosis of mediastinal adenopathy-real-time endobronchial ultrasound guided needle aspiration versus mediastinoscopy. J Thorac Oncol. 2008;3:577–82.
76. Annema JT, van Meerbeeck JP, Rintoul RC, et al. Mediastinoscopy vs endosonography for mediastinal nodal staging of lung cancer: a randomized trial. JAMA. 2010;304:2245–52.
77. Lee BE, Kletsman E, Rutledge JR, et al. Utility of endobronchial ultrasound-guided mediastinal lymph node biopsy in patients with non-small cell lung cancer. J Thorac Cardiovasc Surg. 2012;143:585–90.
78. Campo E, Swerdlow SH, Harris NL, et al. The 2008 WHO classification of lymphoid neoplasms and beyond: evolving concepts and practical applications. Blood. 2011;117(19):5019–32.
79. Young NA. Grading follicular lymphoma on fineneedle aspiration specimens–a practical approach. Cancer. 2006;108:1–9.
80. Young NA, Al-Saleem T. Diagnosis of lymphoma by fine-needle aspiration cytology using the revised European-American classification of lymphoid neoplasms. Cancer. 1999;87:325–45.
81. Caraway NP. Strategies to diagnose lymphoproliferative disorders by fine-needle aspiration by using ancillary studies. Cancer. 2005;105:432–42.
82. Steinfort DP, Conron M, Tsui A, et al. Endobronchial ultrasound-guided transbronchial needle aspiration for the evaluation of suspected lymphoma. J Thorac Oncol. 2010;5:804–9.
83. Marshall CB, Jacob B, Patel S, et al. The utility of endobronchial ultrasound-guided transbronchial needle aspiration biopsy in the diagnosis of mediastinal lymphoproliferative disorders. Cancer Cytopathol. 2011;119:118–26.
84. Kennedy MP, Jimenez CA, Bruzzi JF, et al. Endobronchial ultrasound-guided transbronchial needle aspiration in the diagnosis of lymphoma. Thorax. 2008;63:360–5.
85. Farmer PL, Bailey DJ, Burns BF, et al. The reliability of lymphoma diagnosis in small tissue samples is heavily influenced by lymphoma subtype. Am J Clin Pathol. 2007;128: 474–80.
86. de Tute RM. Flow cytometry and its use in the diagnosis and management of mature lymphoid malignancies. Histopathology. 2011;58:90–105.
87. Fromm JR, Thomas A, Wood BL. Flow cytometry can diagnose classical Hodgkin lymphoma in lymph nodes with high sensitivity and specificity. Am J Clin Pathol. 2009;131:322–32.
88. Nagai S, Izumi T. Bronchoalveolar lavage. Still useful in diagnosing sarcoidosis? Clin Chest Med. 1997;18:787–97.
89. Gilman MJ, Wang KP. Transbronchial lung biopsy in sarcoidosis. An approach to determine the optimal number of biopsies. Am Rev Respir Dis. 1980;122:721–4.

90. Koonitz CH, Joyner LR, Nelson RA. Transbronchial lung biopsy via the fiberoptic bronchoscope in sarcoidosis. Ann Intern Med. 1976;85:64–6.
91. Oki M, Saka H, Kitagawa C, et al. Real-time endobronchial ultrasound-guided transbronchial needle aspiration is useful for diagnosing sarcoidosis. Respirology. 2007;12:863–8.
92. Agarwal R, Srinivasan A, Aggarwal AN, et al. Efficacy and safety of convex probe EBUS-TBNA in sarcoidosis: a systematic review and meta-analysis. Respir Med. 2012;106:883–92.
93. Tremblay A, Stather DR, Maceachern P, et al. A randomized controlled trial of standard vs endobronchial ultrasonography-guided transbronchial needle aspiration in patients with suspected sarcoidosis. Chest. 2009;136:340–6.
94. Nakajima T, Yasufuku K, Kurosu K, et al. The role of EBUS-TBNA for the diagnosis of sarcoidosis–comparisons with other bronchoscopic diagnostic modalities. Respir Med. 2009;103:1796–800.
95. Lin SM, Chung FT, Huang CD, et al. Diagnostic value of endobronchial ultrasonography for pulmonary tuberculosis. J Thorac Cardiovasc Surg. 2009;138:179–84.
96. Lin SM, Ni YL, Kuo CH, et al. Endobronchial ultrasound increases the diagnostic yields of polymerase chain reaction and smear for pulmonary tuberculosis. J Thorac Cardiovasc Surg. 2010;139:1554–60.
97. Navani N, Molyneaux PL, Breen RA, et al. Utility of endobronchial ultrasound-guided transbronchial needle aspiration in patients with tuberculous intrathoracic lymphadenopathy: a multicentre study. Thorax. 2011;66: 889–93.
98. Yasufuku K, Nakajima T, Fujiwara T, et al. Utility of endobronchial ultrasound-guided transbronchial needle aspiration in the diagnosis of mediastinal masses of unknown etiology. Ann Thorac Surg. 2011;91:831–6.
99. Galluccio G, Lucantoni G. Mediastinal bronchogenic cyst's recurrence treated with EBUS-FNA with a long-term follow-up. Eur J Cardiothorac Surg. 2006;29:627–9. discussion 629.
100. Anantham D, Phua GC, Low SY, et al. Role of endobronchial ultrasound in the diagnosis of bronchogenic cysts. Diagn Ther Endosc. 2011;2011:468237.
101. Hergott CA, MacEachern P, Stather DR, Tremblay A. Repair cost for endobronchial ultrasound bronchoscopes. J Bronchol Intervent Pulmonol. 2010;17:223–7.

第 6 章
电磁导航支气管镜

Thomas R. Gildea and Joseph Cicenia

本章提要 电磁导航支气管镜（ENB）自 2004 年开始应用以来，一直不断发展。这个类似于全球定位系统的技术基本包括磁场发生器、与计算机相连接的传感器以及用于三维立体图像成形的计算机断层扫描仪。该技术的一项重大突破是通过标准非引导气管镜使肺外周小结节清晰成像，其价值已被证实。大量国际临床实践阐述了 ENB 融入特定操作流程的方法，并提出了关于 X 线透视、外周超声、活检技术、麻醉技术等辅助技术的应用价值等重要问题。本章对 ENB 及其进展、包括该技术的各方面流程进行相关文献回顾，同时也将归纳文献介绍的及我们经验总结的适合 ENB 检查的理想患者。

关键词 孤立性肺结节，电磁导航支气管镜，气管镜。

引 言

得益于 CT 在很大程度上的广泛使用，偶然发现的孤立性肺结节（SPNs）其发生率逐年升高，CT 在 SPNs 的检查敏感度上比传统的普通胸片更高[1]。自全国肺癌筛查试验（NLST）后 SPNs 的检出率明显增加[2]。多数 SPNs 是良性的，即使在高危患者中也只有 1% 的患者为恶性[2]。因此，减少侵入性而增加精准度的检测方法对于诊断相关的发病率将产生深远的影响。大体上，确定 SPNs 可分成三步策略：①间隔相应时间连续成像检测结节的变化（定期观察）。②创伤性较小的诊断流程（气管镜和经皮细针穿刺活检）。③手术切除。SPNs 潜在恶性的可预测性将增加患者对于疾病的承受能力，这可能会影响已遵循的上述策略[3]。

计算机断层扫描引导下细针抽吸术（CT-FNA）是一种比较常用的获取组织技术，它对恶性肿瘤的敏感度接近 90%[4,5]。然而该技术的并发症如气胸的发生率可高达 30%，其中有 6% 的患者需要放置胸管[5]。气胸的危险因素包括高龄、存在 COPD 或肺气肿、结节与胸膜邻近[6]。在手术切除的 SPNs 中，20% 的患者为良性[6]。高比例的前置胸廓切开术提示会增加患者不必要的发病率和死亡率。

长期以来，常规气管镜对于诊断的价值一直不尽如人意。因为受多种因素的共同影响，其恶性敏感度为 14%~63%[7,8]。这些因素包括结节大小、活检方法、活检组织数量及空气支气管征迹象[9]。

由于辅助性超声探头的使用[10,11]，常规气管镜活检阳性率增加到 70% 左右[12]。但此技术的普及应用高度依赖于操作者的技术和对该技术的熟练程度。此外，活检阳性率随结节大小的减小而显著降低[11]。探针衔接呼吸道入口的能力与结节大小相关。此外，若不借助可操控的导管，仅仅超声引导很难到达小结节区域。

2004 年美国食品及药物管理局 510 K 批准

电磁导航支气管镜（ENB）在美国使用。此项技术的基本原理是通过 CT 扫描重建三维立体图，然后用低能量电磁场下的传感器提供定位信息。导管引导能力和计算机反馈位置的功能与全球定位系统（GPS）技术相似。定位导管从扩展工作通道（EWC）中退出，EWC 留在病灶位置，形成通道，用于治疗装置的进入，直达目标。这在过去一段时间里，已有多项研究，同时大量软件和硬件已经更新。在不同的临床背景下使用不同活检技术、麻醉技术、辅助成像技术不同阈值误差的研究已进行过。尽管有差异，但活检阳性率均在 70% 左右。本章旨在阐述 ENB 的基础知识及我们克利夫兰诊所最新使用的 ENB 技术方法。

系统组件

大型系统由软件和硬件组件组成，组装成类似 iLogic 的系统。该系统包括规划站和程序站。规划站由笔记本电脑组成。笔记本电脑用于编入和消除程序端口需要执行的计划功能。计算机数据以 DICOM 文件的形式储存，可以通过 CD-ROM 下载到笔记本电脑，也可以通过以太网（或者类似的）连接直接下载到电脑中。程序站由中央处理单元（CPU）、电视屏幕、位置放大器、定位板、定位导航和患者传感器组成。程序用的软件由规划部分和程序上的导航部分组成。软件的规划部分位于笔记本电脑的 CPU。CPU 程序端口包括规划和导航软件构件，此外还包括位置放大器，在流程、加工及传递导航数据至 CPU 期间用以联系外部设备。定位板产生如同"感应容积"一样的低频电磁场，在患者胸部区域形成一个磁场（图 6.1）。产生感应容积的定位板大小在 x 轴和 y 轴上接近 40 cm×40 cm，在 z 轴上 20 cm，同时 z 轴高于定位板 5 cm。患者的胸腔必须匹配这个体积，重度肥胖患者在程序启动后可能会出现一些问题。连接在患者身上的传感器三联体用来评估患者的移动，并纠正程序过程中出现的

错误。一般情况下置于由靠近胸骨切迹和双侧沿低肋区组成的三角区域内。定位导航仪（LG）是一种微型传感器，可传递位置信息到 CPU。定位数据包括由 x 轴、y 轴、z 轴组成的空间坐标，辅助探头翻转、前进和偏移。数据以每秒 166 次的频率输送到 CPU。在导航期间，LG 放入一种称之为扩展工作通道（EWC）的管道内（图 6.2A）；EWC 可手动操作。EWC 有 2 次迭代：经典的 EWC 采用手动操控 8 个方向（通过 LG 装置代码接收），同时远端导管的弯度可有 45°、90° 和 180°（图 6.2B）。设计同血管相似的导管远端能更加方便手动调节。假如病变不与气道直接相连，导管远端的弯度同样可用于定向活检。

CT 扫描格式

所有的 ENB 都是从 CT 扫描形成最基本的图像开始的。它需要一些特殊配置用于转换。起初 CT 以每 1.5 秒扫描 3 mm 的层面以呈现最佳的虚拟气道。然而 CT 更换到最新型号后，更多时候选择高分辨率的 CT 扫描。扫描间隔和层面的厚度有 25%~50% 的重叠，而软组织内部最

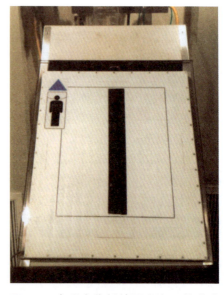

图 6.1　电磁定位板放置在桌面的头端

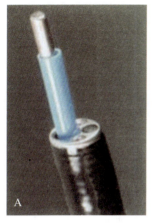
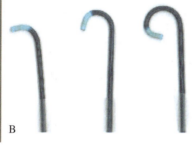

图6.2　A.扩展工作通道（EWC）（蓝色）通过定位导航仪（LG）。气管镜尖端进入已选择的支气管后，EWC和LG均能通过导航找到病变部位；B.导管远端可呈45°、90°和180°弯曲

好减少CT伪影。我们已经注意到一些因剂量减小而导致小气道无法显示的问题，但对最初计划实施和靶目标探测已经足够了。理想的CT采集和图像重建说明书因制造商不同而变化。这些说明书已经由SuperDimension公司确定，并且可以从该公司获取。

程序策划

基于本章节的初衷，我们将介绍当前应用最普遍的策划软件装置，该装置估计有近90%的市场占有率。在过去，策划过程中需要手工标记已经选择好的定位点，而现在标记可以由软件重复自动完成。现在推荐使用自动标记，但需要做好手动标记的准备以防出现自动化应用标记不成功的情况。下面我们会讨论这两种定位技术，不过在编写时我们是从目前应用最普遍的软件装置上展开讨论的。程序策划一般都在独立的装有策划软件的笔记本电脑上开始。策划过程在患者CT数据通过CD-ROM或直接从图像存档和通信系统（PACS）途径从DICOM文件上传到笔记本电脑后就开始启动。如果CT扫描能用合适的格式配置妥当，每个图像系列以及对应的参数将在输入界面出现。符合理想的推荐参数的图像能被软件识别；接收到的不符合理想参数的图像系列也会被罗列出来，不过开始时会有1个警告消息称这些图像可能导致次优的肺部重建。操作者可选择相应的图像系列以进行下一步操作。图像加工过程中，软件会建立一个虚拟的三维气管支气管树让操作者认证。理想气管支气管树应该包含至少四级支气管。一旦三维支气管树确认，屏幕上会显示三个位面的CT多平面重建（水平面、冠状面和矢状面），第四块平板的虚拟气道重建通过标准工具栏联合软件和CT数据完成（图6.3）。

一般情况下，我们下一步需要标记定位点以防操作过程中需要手动标记。标识点在虚拟气管镜上完成，这样在气管镜操作过程中很容易辨别。通常这些点包括右侧隆突、上叶、中叶和下叶；隆突基部将左肺上叶和下叶分隔开来；左肺下叶亚段分叉点。这些标识点应该在空间上分开，并且延伸到肺下叶。定位点选择、标记好后，靶目标也同时予以识别、标记并确认大小。一旦识别出目标区域，软件将生成一条抵达病变部位最近的中央气道通路（图6.4）。从病变部位退出气道的途径在屏幕上会以灰点的形式呈现。在此阶段我们会检查通路，一旦确认，则保存。以下原因可能导致通路无法确认：软件可能无法确定气道末端到病变的路径；某种情况下通向病变部位可能有更近的或者不同的气道路径。如果更近的或者不同的气道路径被识别，我们可以手动添置该气道的中间点，有时被称之为"面包屑"，并通过点击灰点确认

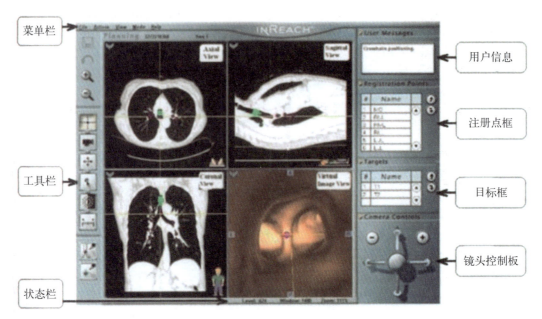

图 6.3 计算机界面显示了胸部 CT 的冠状位、轴状位和矢状位界面以及虚拟气管镜图像

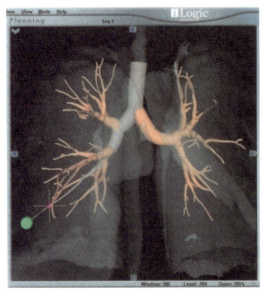

图 6.4 到病变部位的气道路径（绿点代表病变）

生双侧气胸的潜在风险。一旦策划完成，数据将第一时间保存在笔记本电脑上，然后导出到闪存盘中用于下一步程序。

同样，纵隔组织活检也是有可能的。在这个工作流程中直面我们想要活检的纵隔淋巴结放置虚拟摄像头很重要。在选择好靶目标后，靶心大小是很重要的，我们可以通过滑杠使气道透明以获得最佳图像。在程序过程中，图像在导航界面可引导细针活检。

程序定位

一旦规划完成、数据保存好后，就可以开始下一步程序了。患者躺在装有定位板的程序桌或者担架床上后就启动程序。患者躺好使其与定位板平行，其胸廓能容纳感应容积。在我们的研究机构里，事先调整平板与担架床相连的位置，担架床也同样标记好让合适的患者躺下，这样可以将程序进行期间患者重新调整位置的概率减小到最低。一旦患者躺好，确保放置在患者身上的传感器处于感应容积区域内，起到在程序进行过程中检测和纠正患者移

新的退出点。一旦退出点确认，这条通路会变为紫色，之后我们用虚拟气管镜的"飞行模式"检查该通路。此时，其他的靶目标也会选择相似的方式确认。尽管临床上可以选择多个靶点，但我们不会同时选择对侧肺靶点，因为存在发

动的作用。一般情况下这些传感器放在胸骨头端、双侧腋中线。因为程序开始后，所有连向 CPU 的程序必须第一时刻通过软件核查；一旦这一步完成，操作者可以随着程序定位往前操作。

自动化定位

一旦标记元件启动，定位导航可以通过气管镜工作通道观察到它的尖端在视野末端。气管镜在气管中段开始往前进；当气管镜穿过气管时，定位导航放置在每一叶段支气管（为了保证精确，在每个叶段支气管中气管镜应等距推进）。在这个过程中，当 LG 穿过中央气道时要做数百个位点的探测使之与三维虚拟气管支气管树容积匹配。一旦软件有足够的数据以创建一个精准的标记点，那虚拟气管镜成像（其仪表上会列出一条绿色的边框）即可在屏幕上显现。此时，视野应回撤并放在隆突上，虚拟气管镜图像应当手工转动屏幕以对应实时气管镜成像方向。一旦这一步完成，操作者在屏幕上手动按下"标记完成"键，与此同时导航程序开始。

手工标记

某些情况下无法完成自动化标记，或者涉及标记过程中准确性不足的问题，假如出现上述情况，可以采用手工标记。此过程与原先需要软件装置定位的过程相似。此技术中，LG 放在预先设定好的标记点上并在策划过程期间保存（见前述）。每一个在感应容积的坐标点都与 CT 容积内预设点相关。这个过程至少包括 5 个标记点，其中 1 个在隆突上，2 个在每个叶段支气管下端。起到的效果应该是一个能够延伸至隆突外的三角区。由于这不是一个动态过程，这种定位法则可能会引起 CT 变量中的平均基准目标配准误差（AFTRE）的体表误差，当软件定位完成时就会报告。如果 AFTRE 评分是可接受的（<5 mm），那操作者接受定位并继续下一阶段的导航程序。如果 AFTRE 评分不可接受，那需要重新开始手工定位。

AFTRE 是所有变量总数的平均值，是指与那些在真实患者身上操作时相比，在虚拟患者身上每个标记点的观测距离和预期距离。最终结果精确到毫米，因为真实患者和虚拟患者身上探针尖端所在位置呈现的球体并不确定。球外有潜在的两种误差。平移误差可能是定位点在系统同一方向移动引起的误差，且其矫正可能是一个线性调节问题。同样也有可能是旋转误差，这可能是非对称误差：之前一边，之后另一边。这种情况下有放大效应，同时在远离纵隔和中央气道时其误差会增加。最后一种误差源于难以解释的肺部复杂运动。尽管之前有跟踪转至检测胸廓运动，但仍难以解释横膈膜偏移。这有个特别的问题就是肺功能正常的人在 CT 下呼吸时，功能残气量（FRC）在横膈膜向上移动时存在约 5 cm 的变化，同时肺横膈膜病变时，横膈向前或向后移动的情况也是如此。当平移错误在定位结束时检查以确保探针位置在虚拟和实际的气管内成像无差别时，调整并识别错误相对简单。Makris 及其团队指出 CT 体表误差 <4 mm 时与高诊断阳性率相关[13]。

标记过程中的区别

与手工标记相比，iLogic® 引入自动化标记过程具有多个优势。自动化标记过程依赖于良好的虚拟气管镜成像能力及气道内测量的平衡。与手工标记不同，自动化标记不需要手工手动策划及提前获取气管支气管树的解剖标记。自动化标记是用 LG 穿过中央气道时被动进行数百位点的探测并分别定位，使之与虚拟三维气管支气管树匹配取代了个别点单独标记。无自动化定位的实际测量误差的报告，但根据制造商的说明，误差在 3~4 mm，否则它无法标记，以确保此程序只有在准确定位后才能够启动。

麻醉技术

已公布的 ENB 麻醉数据并不统一。欧洲早期的临床试验操作一般是在硬质气管镜下全麻处理[14,15]。美国的第一例临床试验和我们研究的医疗中心的所有流程均在患者清醒状态下使用吗啡、咪达唑仑和利多卡因镇静、麻醉[16]。其他研究中心已经尝试其他技术，如一氧化氮[17]。尽管没有进行对比研究，与常规麻醉相比，两者的潜在获益和风险或并发症无明显差异。理论上无创正压通气下行气管镜活检时有潜在增加气胸的风险；相反的，如果仅仅是温和的镇静，那在气管镜活检过程中患者可能发生咳嗽。另外，镇静状态下的肺与预想的可能有严重出入。因为在步骤计划时获得的 CT 图像，一般在扫描时患者为深吸气状态，而镇静状态下患者呼吸容量接近功能残气量的小潮气量。肺功能正常的患者在胸廓容积和横膈膜移动上有显著差异，特别是病变在下叶的移动幅度大于病变在上叶的。重度阻塞性病变和肺水肿的患者横膈膜移动幅度比较小。全麻期间可以加大通气量以模拟 CT 扫描。在温和镇静下，患者是很难达到这种效果的。总体来说，麻醉方式仍取决于研究中心的选择，这里并没有列举在不同麻醉技术下，相关的预后和并发症。

X 线透视检查和非 X 线透视检查

在使用者手册中，ENB 操作过程中多推荐使用双向透视。我们研究中心发现单向透视比较实用。在大多数欧洲研究中心公布的资料中并没有使用透视，而且显示其效益和并发症相近。我们的经验是假如仪器穿过工作通道会有僵硬性和追踪能力的变化，这可能会增加活检后难以诊断的可能性，因而用透视来代替 EWC 在活检中是有作用的。如果应用透视，需要注意的一点是，透视在定位和导航期间，C 臂机可能会以铁磁性的形式干扰定位板。只有在导航完成后再使用透视应用工作通道和探针定位病变。

辅助成像

使用径向探头支气管内超声（R-EBUS）作为实时成像技术来精准导航很热门。R-EBUS 比透视更有优势，在于其不需要依靠平面成像，并能检测到透视所不能看到的微小病灶。在前瞻性随机试验中，R-EBUS 和透视联合应用其诊断率达 88%[18]，但后续试验显示同组联合后诊断率只有 75%[19]。此外，在美国拥有 R-EBUS 的医学中心不足 5%。尽管如此，我们机构常规使用 R-EBUS 来评价导航成功与否。另外，随着弯曲导管的应用，R-EBUS 能协助合适的导管定向活检（通过旋转导管直到图像显示病灶最大化），尤其是那些难以直接清晰显示的气道病灶等（这些病灶没有支气管空气征）。

导航并获取组织

气管镜嵌入亚段支气管直达靶病灶。EWC 和 LG 同时缓慢向病灶推进。目标在导航期间控制并引导 LG 沿虚拟气管镜成像生成的通道往前推进直至靶目标（图 6.5 紫线显示）。在旧系统中，用仪器直接调控也能使 LG 通过旋转弯曲导管沿通路往前推进。病灶在所有系统观察窗口均呈现为绿色球体（图 6.5）。当 LG 远端靠近病灶时，绿点相对应地持续增大。一旦 LG 接近距离病灶理想的位置时，EWC 或弯曲导管通过气管镜活检通路的末端由闭锁结构切入，同时 LG 后撤。透视可用来协助 LG 在其移动时观测最佳位置。气管镜配件如活检钳、经气管镜抽吸针和气管镜毛刷可通过 EWC 进入以获取组织标本。气管内超声探头可进入辅助确认位置。EWC 可容纳所有标准气管镜活检工具。如果需要在 EWC 弯曲时，或需要成角度进入上叶或者下叶亚段的话，标准式细针将比较困难。多个研究中心已经报道基于单独 TBBx 而其他应用多种工具如细胞刷、细胞细针、经气管镜活检钳、细针毛刷和细胞抽出物的诊断率比较。没有明显的最佳设备，它们的作用是互补的，而且在不同的情况下需要联合应用不同的设备。该方法已经使我们获取很多类型的样本。有一份关于导管抽吸与经气管镜活检的效益比较。导管抽吸有明显的获益，即使在缺乏明确 EBUS 成像的情况下，其效益可达 50%[19]。

诊断阳性率。有大量的变量可能会影响诊断的阳性率，并且多个研究中心之间有极大的相似之处。最近的一项荟萃分析显示，在 2010 年前合并阳性率是 70%[12]。最近的文献显示阳性率增高的趋势，这可能与多种技术的更新、活检工具的改变及选择支气管征阳性的患者相关[9]。表 6.1 总结了相关研究结果，明确了 ENB 在孤立性肺结节的诊断地位。

ENB 在介入治疗中的应用

ENB 在气管镜检查中越来越有取代原先基准标记的趋势，特别是对立体定向放射手术治疗或射波刀治疗。这种治疗通常为那些有局限性肺癌但不适合外科手术切除的患者准备[28]。

使用这种技术，可以将肿瘤周边组织结构留空，而将肿瘤暴露在相当集中的射线剂量下，减少辐射导致的损害风险。对于精准肿瘤消融，射波刀需要肿瘤的基准位置。传统标记的方法是通过 CT 引导下经胸廓路径进行，但这也与气胸的高风险相关。例如，有研究显示 47% 的患者在经胸廓基准标记后进展为气胸，并需要行胸导管引流[29]。当基准点采用气管镜路径标记时气胸发生率显著降低。然而，气管镜标记基准点需要导航工具对外周肿瘤进行精确定位[30]。多个研究已经证实使用 ENB 更能准确标记基准点。一项研究中，9 例患者有 8 例应用 ENB 引导下标记，共 39 个基准点而未出现任何明显的并发症[31,32]。另一项研究中，15 例患者采用经胸廓路径标记基准点，8 例患者在 ENB 引导下经支气管镜路径标记。结果经胸骨路径标记基准点的 15 例患者中有 8 例发展为气胸，其中 6 例需要胸管引流。而经 ENB 引导的气管镜标记的患者均无气胸发生[33]。

经气管镜放置的基准点有可能会从初始位

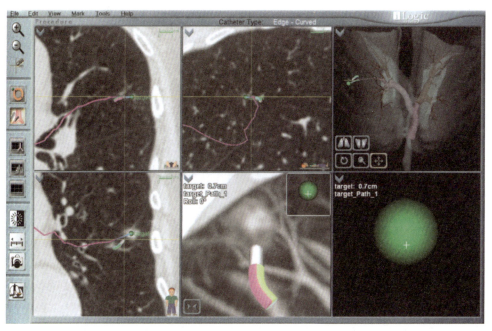

图 6.5 这 6 块导航界面显示应用弯曲导管可有多维 CT 图像，同时加强投影 MIP（底部中心）最大化的选择。右上角动态气管图像、标准目标窗口标记形象地描述了病灶中心距离探针尖端的距离

表 6.1 电磁导航支气管镜的诊断率

文献	技术	N	病灶大小 (mm) 范围或均值	诊断率	RE/NE	气管镜操作时间（分钟）	麻醉方式	气胸发生率 (%)
Becker (2005)[15]	ENB + fluoro	29	12~106	69%	RE: 6.1 ± 1.7	N/A	GA	3.3
Hautmann (2005)[20]	ENB + fluoro	16	22 ± 6	未获得	4.2	N/A	CS	0
Schwarz (2006)[21]	ENB + fluoro	13	15~50	69%	NE: 5.7	46分钟	CS	0
Gildea (2006)[16]	ENB + fluoro	58	PPL: 22.8 LN: 28.1	PPL: 74 % LN: 100 %	RE: 6.6 ± 2.1 NE: 9 ± 5	(51 ± 6) 分钟	CS	3.4
Wilson (2007)[22]	ENB + fluoro + ROSE	248	PPL: 2.1 LN: 1.8	70%~86 %	RE: 0.5 ± 0.02	N/A	CS	1.2
Makris (2007)[13]	ENB	40	23.5	62.5 %	RE: 4 ± 0.15 NE: 8.7 ± 0.8	N/A	GA	7.5
Eberhardt (2007)[14]	ENB	89	24	67%	RE: 4.6 ± 1.8 NE: 9 ± 6	(29.9 ± 6.5) 分钟	GA 或 CS	2.2
Eberhardt (2007)[18]	ENB	39	26	88%	N/A	N/A	GA 或 CS	6
Lamprecht (2009)[23]	ENB + PET-CT + ROSE	13	30	76.9%	N/A	60分钟	—	0
McLemore (2007)[24]	ENB + EBUS	48	23 (6~60)	90%	N/A	N/A	—	2.1
Bertoletti (2009)[17]	ENB	53	31.2	77.3%	RE: 4.7 ± 1.3 NE: 10 ± 5.9	29.5 分钟	Nitrous oxide	4
Seijo (2010)[9]	ENB + ROSE	51	25 (15~35)	67%	RE: 4	N/A	—	0
Eberhardt (2010)[19]	ENB + EBUS	53	23.3 (11~29)	75.5%	RE: 3.6 (1.8~5.7)	25.7分钟 (16~45)	—	1.9
Mahajan (2011)[25]	ENB + fluoro	48	20 ± 13	77%	N/A	N/A	CS	10
Lamprecht (2012)[26]	ENB + PET-CT + ROSE	112	27.1 ± 1.3	83.9%	N/A	45 分钟	GA	1.8
Pearlstein (2012)[27]	ENB + ROSE	104	28	85%	RE: 4.0 (2.4~7)	70分钟 (25~157)	GA	5.8

注：CS. 镇静麻醉；ENB. 电磁导航支气管镜；EBUS. 超声支气管镜；GA. 全身麻醉；LN. 淋巴结；PPL. 肺外周病灶；ROSE. 床旁快速检测；RE. 注册误差；NE. 导航误差；N/A. 空缺

置移出。线性黄金基准标记表面平滑，有报道称，经 ENB 引导放置的基准点有 10%~30% 移出[32,34]。有报道称，使用线圈基准标记的难以手术的肺癌患者接受射频刀治疗也有较好的结果[35]。在一项研究中，共 52 例患者连续接受 ENB 引导下的基准标记放置。其中 4 例患者接受 17 例线性基准标记，49 例患者共 56 个肿瘤接受 217 个线圈基准标记。射频刀计划中，217 个线圈基准标记有 215 个（99%）仍在原位，而 17 个线性基准标记中有 8 个（47%）还在原位置（P=0.000 1）。4 例患者中有 2 例最初接受线性基准标记后需要进行额外的基准标记，而接受线圈基准标记的患者没有 1 例需要额外操作程序。有 3 例（5.8%）患者发展为气胸。上述结果提示 ENB 引导下经气管镜放置线圈标记比线性黄金基准标记更加合适。

ENB 也曾用于胸膜附近小的肺结节术前放置定位标记，这对于那些在电视胸腔镜外科治疗中不易发现的、不显眼的病灶的定位也很有帮助[36]。

近年来，同位素间质内放射治疗已作为对于局部难以手术切除肺癌的一种治疗选择。有研究显示，ENB 已用于辅助近距放疗治疗那些临床上难以手术切除治疗的孤立性非小细胞肺癌患者[37]。研究者第一次在 ENB 引导下定位右肺上叶肿瘤。成功定位病灶后，EBUS 辅助并将近距放疗导管直接放在肿瘤内。对大剂量近距放疗显示部分消除而组织学显示肿瘤完全消除时再用 EBUS 和 CT 复查。类似的，在 ENB 和 EBUS 引导下，Becker 及其团队应用同位素间质内放疗治疗了 18 例难以手术的孤立性肺癌患者。18 例中有 9 例（50%）完全缓解，剩下大部分患者部分缓解[38]。

并发症

不同研究显示气胸是 ENB 最常见的并发症，其发生率在 0~10% 不等（表 6.1）。没有研究证实 ENB 是患者气胸风险增加的相关因素。

理论上，气胸发生可能受 AFTRE 影响，因为几毫米的误差可能是至关重要的，特别是小的孤立性或胸膜下病灶。尤其是在操作中没有透视引导的情况下，误差无疑是可能的。

自限性出血在一些病例中发生[15,22]。也许，EWC 的应用对控制出血很有帮助，这有助于在操作过程中使亚段支气管视野保持清晰[16,18]。在 1 例病例中，通过 EWC 活检钳可重复进入和移出[14]。

局限性

尽管有高端导航软件和定位引导系统的辅助，该技术仍只有 70% 左右的诊断阳性率。不能获得较高的阳性率的原因可能有以下几点。第一，基于 CT 虚拟构建的结构和真实患者解剖结构仍有差异。第二，该技术下的活检未能实时动态引导。尤其是透视未能应用。第三，呼吸运动可能阻碍活检，特别是病灶在肺叶较低处时。第四，肺有些区域可弯曲气管镜和导航导管难以到达。第五，有一种可能是组织取样时，EWC 已从原位移出。气管镜操作者必须考虑到这种可能性，如果有怀疑，则导航过程重复进行。

另外，很重要的一点涉及该技术的学习曲线。这项技术的应用需要一个包括气管镜操作者及其助手的训练有素的团队。操作程序相当复杂，并需要一份谨慎的预程序计划。然而，部分研究已经报道了该技术十分陡峭的学习曲线[13]。气管镜操作者精通此技术前需要多长的学习过程仍不清楚。令人鼓舞的是，此技术已成功地在社区医院应用[22,27]。明显地，在 ENB 应用于气管镜操作前训练并掌握基本的气管镜技能是很重要的。众所周知，当气管镜操作者能够更熟练地应用此技术后，其诊断阳性率也有可能提高。

另外一个热点是关于 ENB 用于获取孤立性肺结节组织标本时所需要的总操作时间。正如表 6.1 所示，平均气管镜操作时间为 25~70 分钟。

多数研究没有明确报道在策划阶段额外需要的时间，但根据经验，这至少可以减少10分钟。

患者装有起搏器和自动植入心脏除颤器（AICD）被认为是ENB使用的相对禁忌证，因为在操作过程中的磁场下，可能会有使装置失灵的潜在风险。在最近的一项研究中，ENB用于装有起搏器或者AICD的24例患者，在操作期间有电生理学家参与[38]。操作期间没有一例患者出现心律失常或者起搏器功能失常。由此作者认为ENB应用于装有起搏器或者AICD的患者是安全的。尽管在这些病例中需要高度警惕，我们仍相信需要进一步的研究来证实此结论。

最后，最重要的是ENB是一项费用较高的技术。初始设备就需要大量的装置。定位板和EWC都是一次性用品，而且每一个流程都需要很高的花费。就此而言，该流程不足以由第三方支付者完全偿还。如果在全麻下操作或为了使诊断阳性率最高，将径向探头EBUS与ENB联合应用，费用可能会进一步增加。常规加入ROSE也会增加费用。显然，在资源不足的区域该技术是没有条件使用的。

总　结

ENB是用来提高孤立性肺结节诊断率的一种最新的气管镜诊断技术。这被认为是标准而又安全的流程，特别是对于我们研究所中那些有CT-FNA高危风险的患者，或者是那些无法手术但是需要活检的患者。现在不断有关于对高度选择性患者（比如有支气管征）行ENB检查的文章发表，有新型软件的开发使用和更好的定位设计。让人兴奋的是，最新研究表明对于那些患局限性肺癌不能接受手术切除治疗的患者，使用ENB可辅助最新内科治疗。我们相信这一领域在应用ENB诊断、治疗上能不断创新。

参考文献

1. Henschke CI, McCauley DI, Yankelevitz DF, Naidich DP, McGuinness G, Miettinen OS, et al. Early lung cancer action project: overall design and findings from baseline screening. Lancet. 1999;354:99–105.
2. Aberle DR, Adams AM, Berg CD, Black WC, Clapp JD, Fagerstrom RM, et al. Reduced lung-cancer mortality with low-dose computed tomographic screening. N Engl J Med. 2011;365:395–409.
3. Ost D, Fein AM, Feinsilver SH. Clinical practice. The solitary pulmonary nodule. N Engl J Med. 2003;348:2535–42.
4. Gould MK, Ananth L, Barnett PG. A clinical model to estimate the pretest probability of lung cancer in patients with solitary pulmonary nodules. Chest. 2007;131:383–8.
5. Wiener RS, Schwartz LM, Woloshin S, Welch HG. Population-based risk for complications after transthoracic needle lung biopsy of a pulmonary nodule: an analysis of discharge records. Ann Intern Med. 2011;155:137–44.
6. Davies B, Ghosh S, Hopkinson D, Vaughan R, Rocco G. Solitary pulmonary nodules: pathological outcome of 150 consecutively resected lesions. Interact Cardiovasc Thorac Surg. 2005;4:18–20.
7. Popovich Jr J, Kvale PA, Eichenhorn MS, Radke JR, Ohorodnik JM, Fine G. Diagnostic accuracy of multiple biopsies from flexible fiberoptic bronchoscopy. A comparison of central versus peripheral carcinoma. Am Rev Respir Dis. 1982;125:521–3.
8. Rivera MP, Mehta AC. Initial diagnosis of lung cancer: Accp evidence-based clinical practice guidelines (2nd edition). Chest. 2007;132:131S–48.
9. Seijo LM, de Torres JP, Lozano MD, Bastarrika G, Alcaide AB, Lacunza MM, et al. Diagnostic yield of electromagnetic navigation bronchoscopy is highly dependent on the presence of a bronchus sign on CT imaging: results from a prospective study. Chest. 2010;138:1316–21.
10. Kikuchi E, Yamazaki K, Sukoh N, Kikuchi J, Asahina H, Imura M, et al. Endobronchial ultrasonography with guide-sheath for peripheral pulmonary lesions. Eur Respir J. 2004;24:533–7.
11. Paone G, Nicastri E, Lucantoni G, Dello Iacono R, Battistoni P, D'Angeli AL, et al. Endobronchial ultrasound-driven biopsy in the diagnosis of peripheral lung lesions. Chest. 2005;128:3551–7.
12. Memoli JS, El-Bayoumi E, Pastis NJ, Tanner NT, Gomez M, Huggins JT, et al. Using endobronchial ultrasound features to predict lymph node metastasis in patients with lung cancer. Chest. 2011;140:1550–6.
13. Makris D, Scherpereel A, Leroy S, Bouchindhomme B, Faivre JB, Remy J, et al. Electromagnetic navigation diagnostic bronchoscopy for small peripheral lung lesions. Eur Respir J. 2007;29:1187–92.
14. Eberhardt R, Anantham D, Herth F, Feller-Kopman D, Ernst A. Electromagnetic navigation diagnostic bronchoscopy in peripheral lung lesions. Chest. 2007;131:1800–5.
15. Becker HD, Herth F, Ernst A, Schwarz Y. Bronchoscopic biopsy of peripheral lung lesions under electromagnetic guidance: a pilot study. J Bronchol Intervent Pulmonol. 2005;12:9–13.
16. Gildea TR, Mazzone PJ, Karnak D, Meziane M, Mehta AC. Electromagnetic navigation diagnostic bronchoscopy: a prospective study. Am J Respir Crit Care Med. 2006;174:982–9.
17. Bertoletti L, Robert A, Cottier M, Chambonniere ML, Vergnon

JM. Accuracy and feasibility of electromagnetic navigated bronchoscopy under nitrous oxide sedation for pulmonary peripheral opacities: an outpatient study. Respiration. 2009;78:293–300.
18. Eberhardt R, Anantham D, Ernst A, Feller-Kopman D, Herth F. Multimodality bronchoscopic diagnosis of peripheral lung lesions: a randomized controlled trial. Am J Respir Crit Care Med. 2007;176:36–41.
19. Eberhardt R, Morgan RK, Ernst A, Beyer T, Herth FJ. Comparison of suction catheter versus forceps biopsy for sampling of solitary pulmonary nodules guided by electromagnetic navigational bronchoscopy. Respiration. 2010;79:54–60.
20. Hautmann H, Schneider A, Pinkau T, et al. Electromagnetic catheter navigation during bronchoscopy: validation of a novel method by conventional fluoroscopy. Chest. 2005;128:382–7.
21. Schwarz Y, Greif J, Becker HD, et al. Real-time electromagnetic navigation bronchoscopy to peripheral lung lesions using overlaid CT images: the first human study. Chest. 2006;129:988–94.
22. Wilson DS, Barlett RJ. Improved diagnostic yield of bronchoscopy in a community practice: a combination of electromagnetic navigation system and rapid on-site evaluation. J Bronchol. 2007;14:227–32.
23. Lamprecht B, Porsch P, Pirich C, Studnicka M. Electromagnetic navigation bronchoscopy in combination with PET-CT and rapid on-site cytopathologic examination for diagnosis of peripheral lung lesions. Lung. 2009;187:55–9.
24. McLemore TL, Bedekar AR. Accurate diagnosis of peripheral lung lesions in a private community hospital employing electromagnetic guidance bronchoscopy (EMB) coupled with radial endobronchial ultrasound (REBUS). Chest. 2007;132:452S.
25. Mahajan AK, Patel S, Hogarth DK, Wightman R. Electromagnetic navigational bronchoscopy. An effective and safe approach to diagnose peripheral lung lesions unreachable by conventional bronchoscopy in high-risk patients. J Bronchol Intervent Pulmonol. 2011;18:133–7.
26. Lamprecht B, Porsch P, Wegleitner B, Strasser G, Kaiser B, Studnicka M. Electromagnetic navigation bronchoscopy (ENB): increasing diagnostic yield. Respir Med. 2012;106:710–5.
27. Pearlstein D, Quinn CC, Burtis CC, Ahn KW, Katch AJ. Electromagnetic navigation bronchoscopy performed by thoracic surgeons: one center's early success. Ann Thorac Surg. 2012;93:944–50.
28. Sherwood JT, Brock MV. Lung cancer: new surgical approaches. Respirology. 2007;12:326–32.
29. Pennathur A, Luketich JD, Heron DE, et al. Stereotactic radiosurgery for the treatment of stage I non-small cell lung cancer in high-risk patients. J Thorac Cardiovasc Surg. 2009;137:597–604.
30. Linden PA. Use of navigation bronchoscopy for biopsy and endobronchial fiducial placement. Innovations (Phila). 2011;6:271–5.
31. Anantham D, Feller-Kopman D, Shanmugam LN, et al. Electromagnetic navigation bronchoscopyguided fiducial placement for robotic stereotactic radiosurgery of lung tumors: a feasibility study. Chest. 2007;132:930–5.
32. Kupelian PA, Forbes A, Willoughby TR, et al. Implantation and stability of metallic fiducials within pulmonary lesions. Int J Radiat Oncol Biol Phys. 2007;69:777–85.
33. Harley DP, Krimsky WS, Sarkar S, et al. Fiducial marker placement using endobronchial ultrasound and navigational bronchoscopy for stereotactic radiosurgery: an alternative strategy. Ann Thorac Surg. 2010;89:368–74.
34. Schroeder C, Hejal R, Linden PA. Coil spring fiducial markers placed safely using navigation bronchoscopy in inoperable patients allows accurate delivery of cyberknife stereotactic radiosurgery. J Thorac Cardiovasc Surg. 2010;140:1137–42.
35. Andrade RS. Electromagnetic navigation bronchoscopy-guided thoracoscopic wedge resection of small pulmonary nodules. Semin Thorac Cardiovasc Surg. 2010;22:262–5.
36. Harms W, Krempien R, Grehn C, et al. Electromagnetically navigated brachytherapy as a new treatment option for peripheral pulmonary tumors. Strahlenther Onkol. 2006;182(2):108–11.
37. Becker HD, McLemore T, Harms W. Electromagnetic navigation and endobronchial ultrasound for brachytherapy of inoperable peripheral lung cancer. Chest. 2008;134:S396.
38. Khan AY, Berkowitz D, Krimsky WS, et al. Safety of pacemakers and defibrillators in electromagnetic navigation bronchoscopy. Chest 2013;143:75–81.

第 7 章
虚拟支气管镜临床应用

Fumihiro Asano

本章提要　对于肺周围型病灶（PPLs），经支气管肺活检（TBBx）的并发症要少于经皮穿刺活检。但是使用 TBBx 的诊断率并不高，这与操作者的技术有关。虚拟支气管镜导航（VBN）是一种利用虚拟支气管镜（VB）沿支气管走形观察外周病变的方法。这个系统可以对目标自动搜索路径，产生 VB 图像，与真实图像相匹配的显示图像已经被开发出来。该系统可用于诊断外周病变、标记手术或放疗部位、教学和培训。VBN 可与 CT 引导下超细支气管镜、含引导套管的超声支气管镜（EBUS-GS）、包括或不包括 X 线荧光透视的支气管镜相结合。一项前瞻性研究显示，VBN 对所有 PPLs 的诊断率为 74%，对 ≤ 2 cm 病灶的诊断率为 68%。最近的一项随机对照研究表明，VBN 联合 EBUS-GS 将 ≤ 3 cm 病变的诊断率从 67% 提高至 80%，并且缩短了检查时间。一项 meta 分析则显示了 VBN 的有效性。VBN 有许多优势，即使是初学者也可以很容易地使用这项技术检测周围病灶，并能得到较高的检测率。为了提高 VBN 的诊断率，明确病变与外周支气管的关系，选择合适的内镜技术与 VBN 结合十分重要。CT 需要在适当的时候使用。VBN 是支持支气管镜检查的有效方法。我们对它的广泛应用和进一步发展翘首以待。

关键词　CT 引导超细支气管镜，超声支气管镜，导航系统，肺外周病变经支气管肺活检，超细支气管镜，虚拟支气管镜，虚拟支气管镜导航。

肺周围型病灶（PPLs）可在胸部 CT 中经常被发现。由于胸部 CT 在临床实践中的广泛应用，胸部 CT 常可偶然发现较小的 PPLs[1]。全国肺癌筛查试验（NLST）显示，许多医师期望在临床实践中使用 CT 进行肺癌筛查[2]。CT 上发现的大部分肺部结节为微小病灶。在这些小结节中发现早期肺癌仍具有挑战性，这是个艰巨的任务。病理信息对诊断肺癌是必要的。肺结节标本获取方法包括手术活检，经皮穿刺活检和支气管镜活检（TBBx）[3]。手术活检虽然最准确，但创伤最大。由于大部分偶然发现或者筛查出的 PPLs 为良性，并不需要切除，对于这些患者，胸外科手术伴随的费用和并发症是难以接受的。美国胸科医师学会（ACCP）指南推荐经皮穿刺活检为小病变的首选诊断方法，其敏感性为 90%，特异性为 97%[4]。然而，经皮穿刺活检的敏感性会受到是否有 CT 定位、病灶大小及性质的影响[4]。且经皮穿刺活检的并发症发生率较高，21% 发生气胸，5% 发生咯血[5]。Tomiyama 等人研究了日本 124 个机构 9 783 例 CT 引导下的穿刺活检，死亡率为 0.07%，严重并发症（张力性气胸、血气胸、空气栓塞、病灶播散）率 0.75%，气胸发生率 35%[6]。相比之下 TBBx 更为安全。根据日本呼吸内镜协会对 37 485 例病例的调查，TBBx 死亡率为 0.003%，并发症发生率 1.79%（出血 0.73%，气胸 0.63%）[7]。尽管这些研究没有直接的可比性，但它们是在相似的条件及相似的患者群体中进行的，结果暗示 TBBx 比 CT 引导下经皮穿刺活检更安全。然而，使用标准支气管镜下的方法诊断周围型病灶是不充分的。根据 ACCP 的循证医学证据，TBBx 对所有病变的诊断率为 78%，对 ≤ 2 cm 病变的诊断率为 34%[4]，故 ACCP 不推荐使用支气管镜检查这些病灶。影响气管镜对周围型孤立性病变诊断率的疾病相关因素包括：病变大小[8,9]、位置[8]、是否累及支气管[10]，病变性质[9] 等。术者相关因素主要则是操作者的技能和经验[11]。目前，外径 5~6 mm 的气管镜在 X 线荧光透视的引导下可至 PPLs。限制 TBBx 应用的主要因素是引导气管镜和活检器械至病变部位的难度。为了到达周围型病灶，对气管镜和活检器械正确的引导是必需的，因为这些装置必须经过很多支气管分支。因此，气管镜操作者在检查过程中通常根据操作前获得的经二维轴层 CT 数据重建的三维支气管图来选择通往病灶的支气管路径。但这种方法并不准确[12]，太靠近外周的病灶无法用 CT 观察到，只能通过细支气管镜或者超细支气管镜观察。为此，我们需要更准确的导航方法直通外周病变。

虚拟支气管镜（VB）可以根据三维（3D）螺旋 CT 产生的图像来模拟真实气管镜图像[13]。VB 为无创检查，已用于评估和治疗中央气道狭窄[14,15]，但尚未用于 PPLs。虚拟支气管镜导航（VBN）是根据支气管树 VB 图像引导操作者通往外周病变的技术[16]。直接观察呈现在 VB 图像的支气管路径，这种方法可以使气管镜在较短时间内被引导至病灶，而不受操作者技术的影响。此外，目标设置后系统会自动搜索通向目标的支气管路径，产生路径的 VB 图像，并呈现与真实图像相匹配的 VB 图像，产生相应的 VB 图像。此系统已投入临床[17,18]。VBN 可与 CT 引导的超细支气管镜和 EBUS-GS 结合使用，反应良好[17-22]。一项随机试验显示，VBN 结合 EBUS-GS 使用可提高诊断率，减少引导时间及操作时间[23]。同样，先前的一项 meta 分析也表明了 VBN 的有效性[24]。本章节将从科学基础、临床应用、临床结果、操作步骤、提高诊断率的方法、应用限制等方面介绍 VBN。

科学基础

虚拟支气管镜

螺旋 CT 提供连续的三维立体数据，这些数据有多种显示方式。VB 是一种对支气管和管腔图像三维显示并模拟真实气管镜检查的方法[13]。

VB 图像可以反映真实的解剖结果，并为引导支气管镜提供通过观察支气管腔得到的支气管模型等重要信息。这些信息还包括支气管口形状、分叉处支气管大小、分叉角度和分叉后的走形等。

VB 有以下优点：①无创。②可从任意角度或方向观察。能够发现普通气管镜无法观察到的细支气管和远端支气管狭窄。③支气管壁半透明化可显示管壁外的结构。④能精确测量支气管长度、面积、体积。VB 的缺点如下：①图像分辨率取决于 CT 图像。②无法检测黏膜褶皱里的细小改变。③无法获取用于确诊的组织标本。

VB 已用于气道狭窄的评估[14,15]、支架置入等介入治疗[26]、气道异物检测[27] 和气管镜训练[28,29]。然而，VB 因为外周支气管显像困难，之前并未用于 PLLs 诊断。除了 CT 性能的限制，VB 也无法利用可到达外周区域的细支气管镜及超细支气管镜。目前，多排螺旋 CT 已能够在胸部单一呼吸相进行高速详细的扫描，同时能消除呼吸和心脏收缩的影响，提高时间和空间分辨率。在大多数情况下，利用多排螺旋 CT 的数据可建立通向周围病变的气道路径。

超细支气管镜

近年来，气管镜已经变得越来越细。尤其

是超细支气管镜，可以进入更远端的支气管直接观察[30]。2.8 mm 外径、1.2 mm 允许活检的工作通道的超细支气管镜已投入商业应用[31]。超细支气管镜用于诊断 PPLs 时，因为它们可更加接近病灶，因而能更加精确地指导活检[32]。传统支气管镜难以到达的部位，例如肺尖纵隔侧病灶，可用超细支气管镜检查[33]。2010 年的一项研究称，44% 的日本呼吸内镜协会会员机构使用了超细支气管镜。

虚拟支气管镜导航

虚拟支气管镜导航对外周型病灶而言是比 VB 更先进的临床技术。这项技术产生通往病灶路径的 VB 图像，并与相应支气管图像同时显示，帮助操作者控制支气管镜到达选择的靶点。我们在 2002 年报道了我们最初的经验[16]。在这项报告中，VB 可产生 10 级支气管图像并描绘出通往靶点的支气管路径。VB 图像与真实图像同时显示，超细支气管镜可根据提示路径接近病变部位[16]。日本及我们的研究都使用了日本术语命名的支气管分叉。这一系统中，所有的肺亚段支气管被称为第 3 级支气管，随后的分支级数相应加 1[34]。因此，与西方国家相比，研究日本的文献更需要谨慎。

VB 可在每个机构 CT 系统提供的软件中运行，但是临床应用 VBN 时需注意一些问题。VB 分为表面绘制和体积绘制。VB 图像产生时设定的阈值很重要。选择阈值可以决定空气与支气管壁间的界限。阈值改变，VB 图像也随之变化。因此有时操作者会因一些分支的缺失而得到错误的信息，有时并非真实存在的类似于分支开口的孔洞会在 VB 图像中呈现出来，这在外周气道尤为常见[15,35]。每当 VB 图像和真实图像气道路径中分支数量存在差异时，支气管镜都有可能进入错误的位置。当使用实时浏览模式显示虚拟支气管镜通往病灶时，产生正确反映支气管分支的 VB 图像至关重要。分支是否存在需要通过轴向、矢状面或冠状面图像确认。其他需要注意的是气管镜旋转时图像的变化。不同于 VB 能够多种方式操作，气管镜只能上下移动，因此前进时适当的旋转是必要的。当气管镜旋转，真实的图像会根据之前产生的 VB 图像转变。由于外周区域经常能观察到通往两个细支气管的分叉，所以旋转 ≥ 90° 后很难确定通向目标的支气管镜应该进入哪根支气管。这种分叉在路径中可被反复观察到。因此，为了避免进入错误的支气管路径，常需要在分支处调整 VB 图像以实现 VB 图像与实际图像间的协调。

VBN 系统

VBN 使用的传统 VB 软件存在两个严重问题。首先，虚拟支气管镜朝着目标前进时采用实时浏览模式产生 VB 图片是耗时的，而且需要技巧选择阈值。其次，如上讨论引进误差的旋转并不推荐。为了克服这些问题，我们开发了一个允许支气管路径中自动产生 VB 图像的导航系统（称为 VB 图像自动生成功能）[18]，并显示与真实图像对比的 VB 图像[17]。该系统于 2008 年在日本发售（BF Navi®），2010 年日本 12% 的认证机构使用该系统。2009 年，美国 Lungpoint® 系统发售，随后便成为医保覆盖的导航气管镜检查[36]。

该导航系统有两大重要功能。一是 VB 图像产生和信息准备，即编辑或规划功能。BF Navi® 和 Lungpoint® 都能自动选择路径生成 VB 图像，但后者只在设置目标后搜索路径，因此更容易操作。三个不同位面（轴向，矢状面，冠状面）CT 和支气管树综合显示也是可行的[37]。使用 BF Navi® 需设置终点而非靶点。设置终点后，管腔自动生成，并在三个位面 CT 中显示为蓝色，同时可确认支气管的获取。因为尚未获取的支气管及其分支在 VB 图像上无法显示，故无法精确定位。因此确认已获取的支气管是提高定位精度的重要前提。此外，当支气管未能自动获取时（如邻近病变或狭窄的周围支气管），利用 BF Navi® 可以手动获取支气管。以这种方式，终止点可确定为病变附近已获取支气管的准确位点。设置这样的终止点看似复杂，但能使病灶周围的路径更加精确地显示。如果终止点确定的范围包括目标，但是半径比目标大，BF Navi®（Lungpoint）®会自动获取终点范围内的支气管。这样做是为了增加到病变的距离，并显示多条路径。尽管 VB 图片在气管镜前生成，图像生成速度取决于 CT 质量和运行计算机的规格。

VBN 系统的另一个重要功能是导航功能，也称作浏览或操作功能。导航功能可为手动或自动。手动导航系统在每一分叉处都显示 VB 图像，根据参考的图片为气管镜显示通向病变的合适支气管。气管镜操作者可手动匹配 VB 图像和真实图像。当两者图像匹配显示后，气管镜尖端会显示在支气管树和对应 CT 图像中。BF Navi® 是具有代表性的人工导航系统。自动导航系统自动获取支气管镜位置信息，并在 CT 图像上实时显示气管镜位置。为了自动追踪支气管镜，需要根据可靠方法对气管镜尖端准确定位。目前，有两种位置追踪方法：图像登记[38-41]和磁性位置传感器[42]。图像登记能基于真实和虚拟图像的相似性预测气管镜的移动。最接近真实图像的 VB 图像能根据样式识别自动选择。根据 VB 图像视点和视线方向的信息可以预测和追踪气管镜的移动。Lungpoint® 具备这个功能。VB 图像上到病变的路线和距离、支气管名称、支气管旁主要的血管能叠加在系统获取的气管镜视野里。这种方法较磁性传感器法更直观，更精确。然而，与真实图像匹配时，由于电脑的处理需要时间，气管镜操作相对缓慢。此外，当支气管管腔视野因咳嗽无法观察时，追踪将被打断，其中仍有许多问题需要改进。此系统也可使用手动导航。安装在支气管镜尖端或专门设计的磁性传感器配件能够提供位置信息。具体而言，VB 图像通过真实气管镜的磁性传感器获取坐标信息，磁感受器位置和 CT 数据相整合，使支气管镜尖端实时显示在 CT 图像上。这种方法称为电磁导航（EMN），在 2004 年获得 FDA 批准[44]。EMN 不同于 VBN。在 EMN 的图像中，中央支气管只用于校准而非导航，并通过磁性位置传感器进行引导。主要问题是误差校准和呼吸运动的影响。近年来 EMN 已经使用 CT 图像而非 VB 图像的支气管中线进行校准。假设气管镜沿着支气管中线前进时，磁性传感器获取的位置信息会和 CT 图像具体匹配。目前 EMN 系统的商用品牌有 iLogic™ 和 Spin Drive™。

临床应用

VBN 的临床应用包括周围型病变的诊断，手术和放疗位置的标记和培训。

外周病变的诊断

因为 VBN 无法确认活检器械是否到达病变部位，故通常结合 CT、X 线透视或支气管内超声（EBUS）。以往用 VBN 诊断 PPLs 的研究总结在表 7.1 中，并附上简要的讨论。

CT 引导的超细支气管镜

即使 X 线透视无法观察，气管镜检查时的实时 CT 成像能确认活检器械是否到达病变部位。一些研究证实此方法有助于诊断 PPLs[45,46]。自从 VBN 和 CT 同时运行后，CT 检查的同时也能确定 VBN 的准确性。VBN 结合 CT 引导的超细支气管镜对所有病变和直径≤2 cm 病变的诊断率分别是 65%~86% 和 65%~81%[17,19,20,22]。回顾性研究显示，VBN 系统能缩短检查时间[22]。磨玻璃影（GGO）靠透视或 EBUS-GS 难以发现。相比之下，CT 则容易识别。因此，VBN 结合 CT 引导的超细支气管镜对于从 CT 上主要表现为磨玻璃样改变的病变中获取活检标本，可能是最适合的技术。然而，由于辐射暴露和 CT 相关的额外费用，这类确诊方法仅限于少数选择性的病例。有报道认为：支气管征是否可见和超细支气管镜的推进范围是影响诊断的因素[47]。此外，超细支气管镜收集的样本量有限，可能

表 7.1　VBN 的相关研究结果

研究者	VBN 系统	活检前确认方法	检验病变数目	诊断率(%)	<2 cm 病变数目	<2 cm 病变诊断率(%)	检测时间（分钟）
Asano 等[19]	无	CT 和 X 线	36	86.1	26	80.8	无
Shinagawa 等[20]	无	CT	26	65.4	26	65.4	29.3
Asahina 等[21]	无	EBUS	30	63.3	18	44.4	25.7
Asano 等[17]	Bf-NAVI	CT 和 X 线	38	81.6	26	80.8	24.9
Shinagawa 等[22]	Bf-NAVI	CT	71	70.4	71	70.4	24.5
Tachihara 等[52]	Bf-NAVI	X 线	96	62.5	77	54.5	24.1
Asano 等[18]	Bf-NAVI	EBUS	32	84.4	15	73.3	22.3
Eberhardt 等[37]	LungPoint	无透视	25	80.0	无	无	15
Ishida 等[23]	Bf-NAVI	EBUS	99	80.8	58	75.9	24
总结			453	74.0	317	67.5	

只会满足细胞学诊断[48]。

EBUS-GS

近年来，有研究表明径向 EBUS 在气管镜检查中明确外周病变的有效性[49]。EBUS-GS 确定到达病变，并通过病灶处引导套管活检[50]。VBN 联合 EBUS-GS 对所有病变和直径 ≤ 2 cm 病变的诊断率分别是 63%~84% 和 44%~73%[18,21,23]。为客观确认 VBN 联合 EBUS-GS 的有效性，我们进行了一项多中心随机对照研究[23]。200 例直径 ≤ 3 cm 的 PPLs 患者进行 EBUS-GS 活检，随机分为 2 组：联合 VBN（VBNA）和非联合 VBN（NVBNA）。VBNA 组：超细支气管镜在 VBN 系统引导下活检，作为对照，NVBNA 组则在轴位 CT 图像引导下活检。VBNA 组，VB 图像获取了第 4~12 级（平均第 6 级）支气管，和真实图像的匹配度达 98%。VBNA 组诊断率（80%）明显高于 NVBNA 组（67%）。此外，活检前所耗时间和气管镜总时间，VBNA 组（8.1 分钟；24 分钟）少于 NVBNA 组（9.8 分钟；26.2 分钟）。

在这种方法中 EBUS 是需要的，价格易接受，操作也不复杂。而且，透视观察不到的病变标本可以通过引导管准确、重复获取。上述随机对照研究的高诊断率提示，VBN 联合超细支气管镜和 EBUS-GS 可能成为检查 PPLs 的常规方法。最近还有不用 X 线透视的 EBUS-GS 的相关报道[51]。由于使用 VBN 系统替代 X 线透视可准确引导气管镜，即使不使用 X 线透视也可获得较高诊断率。

X 线透视

Tachihara 等[52] 对 96 例直径 ≤ 3 cm 的 PPLs 应用导航系统，所有病变和直径 ≤ 2 cm 病变的诊断率分别是 63% 和 55%，检查时间为 24.1 分钟。他们只研究透视下的 VBN。然而，由于透视引导的气管镜检查 TBBx 简单易行，气管镜联合 VBN 的效果需要进一步研究。

无透视辅助

Eberhardt 等[37] 利用 VBN 引导超细支气管镜（无 X 线透视辅助）获取 25 例 PPLs 活检标本，平均直径 28 mm，诊断率达 80%。

VBN 对外周病变的诊断率

VBN 的前瞻性研究显示，对所有病变和直径≤2 cm 病变的诊断率分别为 74% 和 68%[53]。由于诊断率受病变部位大小、疾病进展、病变位置、是否累及支气管等因素影响，故很难与传统方法比较。不过较 ACCP 指南中 34% 的诊断率还是高出不少[4]。Memoli 等对单用气管镜或联合电磁导航气管镜（ENB）、VB、径向支气管内超声、超细支气管镜和引导套管对肺结节的总体诊断率进行了 meta 分析。分析包含了 39 项研究，共 3 004 例患者，3 052 个病变。VB 的诊断率为 72%（95% 可信区间为 66%~79%），包含一项对纵隔及肺门病变研究（非外周病变）和一项回顾性研究。

外周病变标记位置

VBN 不仅用于诊断，也用于治疗[54]。在胸腔镜手术时，我们对 31 例 X 线无法透视 GGO 表现的病变（≤1 cm）进行 CT 引导的经支气管标记显示病变位置和切除范围[55]。VBN 引导的超细支气管镜可平均至第 6 级支气管，再在 CT 引导下在病变附近通过特制导管放置钡标记。病变部位和标记的平均距离为 4 mm，其中 27 个病变部位与标记的距离 < 1 mm。31 例患者均无明显并发症。胸腔镜下所有病变均可沿着标记被切除。本方法不引起气胸或出血，可用于多发性病变；由于方法简单易行，可对单个病变放置多个标记以 3D 显示切除范围。VBN 也可定位基准标记，用于定向放疗。

教学和培训

显示支气管树和命名有益于教学。VBN 也可用于患者教育，帮助他们了解气管镜的概要。对操作者而言，VBN 模拟了气管镜，提高了对病变和气道联系的理解。

与其他方法的比较

如上所述，EMN 是另一种导航方法[43,44,56]（见第 6 章）。在 EMN 系统中，确认病变部位的活检装置包含在活检装置而非气管镜中。然而，EMN 传感器的位置信息和 CT 图像上存在的误差，可根据检查前的 CT 图像确认是否到达活检位置。因此，EMN 联合实时检测病变部位的方法，如 EBU，据报道可增加诊断敏感性[57]。一项 meta 分析显示，EMN 的诊断率为 67%（46%~88%），与 VBN 相似[24]。因为 EMN 需要一次性电磁传感器，故成本较高。此外，不像传统的气管镜，使用电磁传感器需要一定的培训。相比而言，VBN 只需承担相应系统的费用，且更容易掌握。即使是初学者也能容易地应用气管镜检查周围病变，并有较高的诊断率。

步　骤

患者选择：需要 TBBx 的外周病变患者建议使用 VBN。大部分合适的病灶是那些能够在 CT 图像上清楚显示受累支气管的。外周病变需要胸腔镜手术或化疗前标记位置的也适用 VBN。

设备

VBN 引导的气管镜需要螺旋 CT 的 DICOM 数据、VBN 系统（LungPoint 或 Bf-NAVI）、气管镜（最好是超细支气管镜）和一套标准的气管镜配件。必要时，VBN 也可联合径向 EBUS 探头和系统，对 PPLs 进行活检。

步骤

1. CT DICOM 数据准备。CT 在推荐的 VBN 系统条件下工作并重建图像。图像推荐厚度（以及重建间隔）≤1 mm。通常，图像越薄，越可以产生更靠近外周的 VB 图像。呼吸运动可致 VB 图像精确度下降。

2. 病变路径 VB 图像的产生

LungPoint

（1）输入 CT 扫描：薄层 CT 的 DICOM 数据输入支气管自动提取的系统。

（2）定义目标：定义病变部位为目标时，可半自动跟踪（图 7.1）。

（3）回顾交互式 VB 动态图像和通向病变

的气道路径：最大化显示通向病变的 3 条路径。路径上的每一条分支都会自动记录。3D CT 断层图像（轴向，矢状面和冠状面）、三维支气管树和虚拟气管镜位置对应的 VB 图像同时显示，屏幕可以切换（图 7.2）。通过观察这些图像，确定最接近病变的路径。尽量避免明显弯曲的路径，因为气管镜和活检设备难以操作。当病变远离路径终点，导航系统无法在此区域操作，会导致诊断率下降（图 7.3）。第 3 代 LungPoint 适用于基准位置的立体定向放疗。目标及路径可显示在透视图像中（虚拟透视图像）（图 7.4）。

Bf-NAVI

（1）CT 的 DICOM 数据导入系统。

（2）目标设定：设定目标以使它能在每个层面环绕病灶。当设定目标后，自动获取的支气管显示为蓝色。

（3）终点设定：终点一般设定在离病变最近的支气管内。当通向病变的支气管显示但未自动获取时，有必要手动获取。屏幕滚动显示，从终点追踪选取的支气管以确认选定支气管的分支是否都被获取。如果未被获取，它们的分支就无法在 VB 图像上识别，因此，下面描述

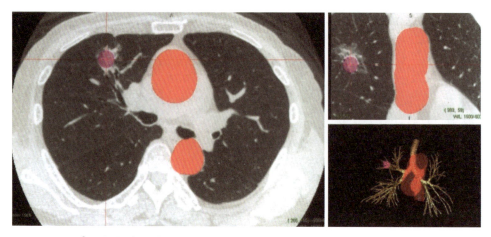

图 7.1　LungPoint® 目标设定。右侧 S3 段 2.5 cm 大小的病变设为目标，用紫色表示。右下图为提取的支气管树。主动脉显示为红色

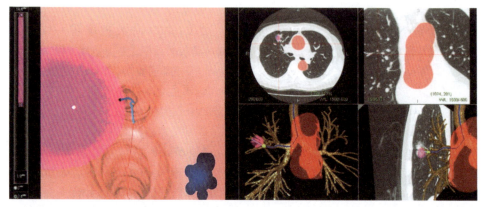

图 7.2　路径显示。左图为 VB 图像。至病变的支气管中线显示为淡蓝色，病变目标为粉色。右下图为病变区域的矢状位 CT、支气管树、虚拟气管镜位置的复合图像，有助于理解病变与支气管树的关系

的提取方法是必要的。

(4) 路径确认（图 7.6）：设置终点后，通向终点的路径立即显示在每个轴面上。这条路径也会在支气管树上得到确认。

(5) 标注缩略图（图 7.7）：当起点至终点的路径被移除，每个分支点会以缩略图标注显示。在进行 VB 导航时，VB 图向前推进，在每个缩略图的地方暂停。根据操作者的偏好，每个分支点都会被标注。当观察到多分支时，标记最里面的分支继续前进。

(6) 支气管的额外提取（图 7.8 和 7.9）：当提取支气管的末端离病变距离较长时，这段距离的 VB 图像信息是缺失的，导致诊断率下降。Bf-NAVI 系统可通过额外提取获取靠近病变的 VB 图像。自动提取从选取的支气管末端开始。手动强制提取用于狭窄或弯曲的区域。例如，当路径中 1 条支气管的分支到达病变部位时，关于这条分支的信息是不可或缺的。如果这个信息不存在，VB 图像不显示此分支，会导致 VB 图像和真实支气管分支的不一致。然而，支气管分支周围的信息可有可无。因此，支气管分支后应立即手动强行提取。手动提取增加

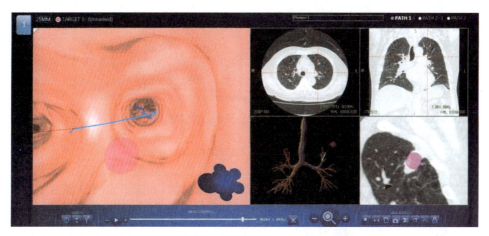

图 7.3　病变与路径终点的间隔。当病变远离路径终点（中间下图所示）时，此段区域将无法导航，诊断率因此下降

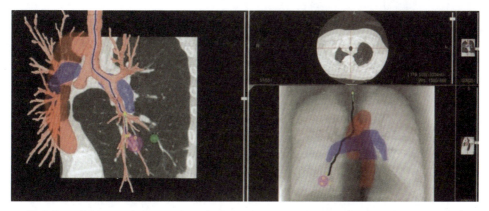

图 7.4　基准位置的标记。紫色圆圈表示病变，周围的 4 个黄色小圆圈提示基准标记的放置位置。虚拟的透视图显示在右侧

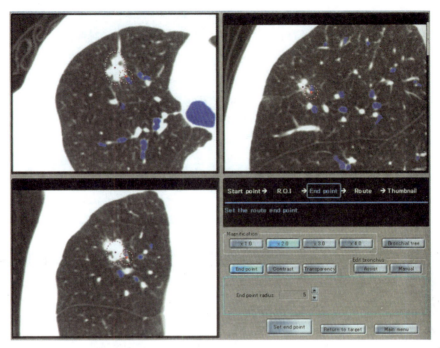

图 7.5　Bf-NAVI 的终点设置。较大的红色虚线表示目标。较小的红色虚线代表终点。提取的支气管显示为蓝色

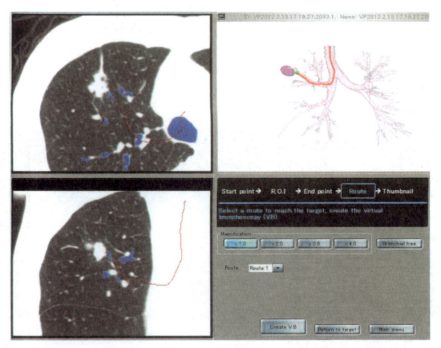

图 7.6　路径确认。红线为指向终点的路径。绿点是虚拟气管镜的位置,一同显示的还有相应的轴面

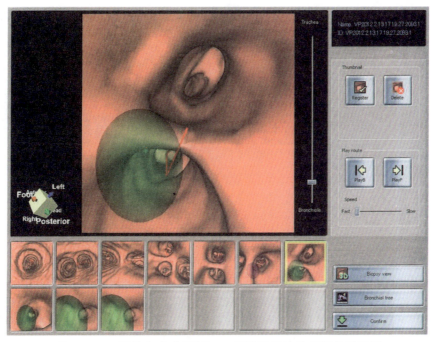

图 7.7　VB 图像和缩略图标记。下栏显示的为标记的缩略图

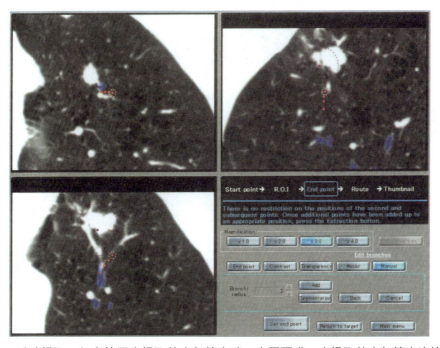

图 7.8　手动提取。红点放置在提取的支气管末端，在需要进一步提取的支气管中连续显示

介入支气管镜临床指南

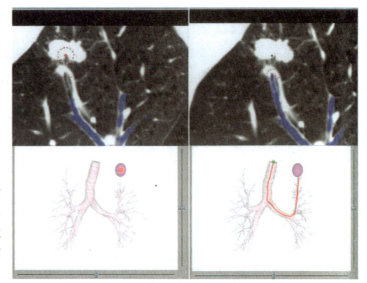

图 7.9　附加提取。左图为附加提取之前，右图是提取之后。附加提取可以在到达病变部位（支气管树终点与病变接触）前立即提取

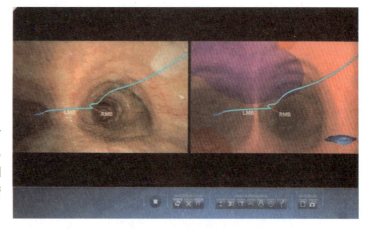

图 7.10　导航。左图和右图分别显示 VB 图像和真实图像。两者同步显示，前者与后者相匹配。在真实图像上，支气管中心线和路径是叠加的

的图像显示为黄色。

3. 气管镜引导（导航）

LungPoint

应用 VBN 时，气管镜根据叠加在虚拟或真实图像上的路径信息前进。关于手动导航，可参照 Bf-NAVI 的操作步骤。

Bf-NAVI

在检查室，Bf-NAVI 显示器尽量靠近气管镜显示屏。VB 数据编辑后导入显示器，助手（导航操作者）使用前进、后退或旋转按钮可调整 VB 图像。在每个分支点，前进和旋转 VB 图像以匹配真实图像对提高图像质量至关重要。熟悉操作步骤后，操作者应帮助助理了解旋转方向和气管镜的位置，以助于和真实图像匹配。操作者和助理配合默契后，VB 和真实图像能够同步显示。

4. TBBx。在目标区域活检（如钳活检、针吸活检、刷检、灌洗细胞学）。详见第 4 章节 EBUS-GS 步骤。

提高诊断率的技巧

VBN 对显示为 I 型或 II 型肿瘤-支气管关系的病变有较高的诊断率[58,59]。评估病变和选定支气管在 CT 上的关系，并确认病变附近区域 VB 图像的正确产生很重要。尤其应该从每一轴

面图像中确认路径中提取的支气管分支。若使用 Bf-NAVI，当提取不恰当时，必须额外提取，而且终点应该尽可能离病灶近些。VB 图像生成时，需要选择联合使用的方法，难度取决于涉及支气管的有无、靠近目标的支气管分支数和弯曲程度。对于 VBN，气管镜越细越好，但获取的标本量也随着活检钳通道变细而减少。在我们医院，用于 EBUS 的外径为 4 mm，工作通道为 2 mm，并可容纳外径 2 mm 引导套管的超细支气管镜（P260，Olympus）已作为常规检查。当气管镜下只见少数分支时，支气管弯曲程度较轻，病变在仅插入 EBUS 探头后就可以观察到，进而活检。随机研究中提到[23]，VBNA 组用 EBUS 能看见 92% 的病变。某些病例，根据 VBN 选择了正确的支气管路径、使用了超细支气管镜进入病变后，EBUS 探头引导可能就没有必要了。然而，第 6 级及更细的支气管，和明显弯曲的支气管（如 B6），应在 X 线透视下使用超细支气管镜。

并发症

既往的 453 病例有 2 例发生气胸。发生率和传统的 TBBx 相近。VBN 本身无明显并发症。

限 制

CT 条件：VB 图像显示的解剖细节取决于胸部 CT 数据。因此，需要适时采用个体化 VBN 系统进行 CT 扫描。不同的扫描仪获取的 CT 参数数据量不同，但是极小化的校准和至少 50% 的重叠图像适合使用 VBN 系统。

价格：CT 是唯一需要重复的检查。由于患者暴露于射线，CT 检查越少越好。

检查时间：有 VBN 引导，气管镜的检查时间明显缩短[23]。然而，VB 图像需要在气管镜检查前 10~15 分钟生成。

学习曲线：由于 VB 成像只需要一个气管镜引导，故无须专门的培训。但在某些情况下熟悉 VB 图像的生成和程序还是有必要的。

禁忌证：对于气管镜和 TBBx 适应的患者，VBN 没有禁忌证。

适应证：即使没有在 CT 上选定支气管，气管镜仍可借助 VBN 引导至最接近病灶的支气管。但有些患者，随后的活检钳引导较为困难，而且诊断率低。这些患者，经支气管针吸活检可能有用，但没有数据支持。此外，对于已证实支气管及肺动脉未受病灶累及的患者，CT 引导的经皮穿刺活检或手术活检都可考虑。

展 望

随机对照研究和 meta 分析表明，VBN 提高了诊断率，缩短了检查时间。由于 VBN 成本低，未来可能得到广泛应用。支气管镜检查比经皮穿刺活检并发症少。然而，需要研究进一步确定 VBN 和经皮穿刺活检诊断率的高低，及确定哪些病变采用 VBN 最合适。还需要更多的工作来提高 VBN 系统的自动追踪和图像标注功能。

结论和总结

使用 TBBx 处理 PPLs 较经皮穿刺活检的并发症少。然而，TBBx 的诊断率是不充分的，并且依赖于操作者的技术水平。VBN 是一种利用支气管路径到外周病灶的图像进行气管镜引导的方法，系统能自动搜索通向目标的路径，生成 VB 图像，并匹配真实图像。该系统用于诊断外周病变，标记手术或放疗位置，教学和培训。VBN 可与 CT 引导的超细支气管镜、EBUS-GS、有或者无 X 线透视的气管镜相结合。前瞻性研究指出，VBN 对所有病变和直径 ≤ 2 cm 病变的诊断率分别是 74% 和 68%。最近的一项随机对照研究指出，VBN 联合 EBUS-GS 将 ≤ 3 cm 病变的诊断率从 67% 提高至 80%，并缩短了检查时间。一项 meta 分析也证实了 VBN 的有效性。VBN 有诸多优点。即使是初学者也可以容易地应用，并能得到较高的诊断率。为了增加 VBN 的诊断率，明确病变和提取支气管的关系，并联合合适的气管镜技术是很重要的。适当条件下需要使用 CT。VBN 是一种支持气管镜检查的有效方法；期待 VBN 的进一步发展和广泛应用。

参考文献

1. Kaneko M, Eguchi K, Ohmatsu H, Kakinuma R, Naruke T, Suemasu K, et al. Peripheral lung cancer: screening and detection with low-dose spiral CT versus radiography. Radiology. 1996;201:798–802.
2. Aberle DR, Adams AM, Berg CD, Black WC, Clapp JD, Fagerstrom RM, et al. Reduced lung-cancer mortality with low-dose computed tomographic screening. N Engl J Med. 2011; 365:395–409.
3. Yung RC. Tissue diagnosis of suspected lung cancer: selecting between bronchoscopy, transthoracic needle aspiration, and resectional biopsy. Respir Care Clin N Am. 2003;9:51–76.
4. Rivera MP, Mehta AC. Initial diagnosis of lung cancer: ACCP evidence-based clinical practice guidelines (2nd edition). Chest. 2007;132:131S–48S.
5. Manhire A, Charig M, Clelland C, Gleeson F, Miller R, Moss H, et al. Guidelines for radiologically guided lung biopsy. Thorax. 2003;58:920–36.
6. Tomiyama N, Yasuhara Y, Nakajima Y, Adachi S, Arai Y, Kusumoto M, et al. CT-guided needle biopsy of lung lesions: a survey of severe complication based on 9783 biopsies in Japan. Eur J Radiol. 2006;59:60–4.
7. Asano F, Aoe M, Ohsaki Y, Okada Y, Sasada S, Sato S, et al. Deaths and complications associated with respiratory endoscopy: a survey by the Japan society for respiratory endoscopy in 2010. Respirology. 2012;17:478–85.
8. Chechani V. Bronchoscopic diagnosis of solitary pulmonary nodules and lung masses in the absence of endobronchial abnormality. Chest. 1996;109:620–5.
9. Baaklini WA, Reinoso MA, Gorin AB, Sharafkaneh A, Manian P. Diagnostic yield of fiberoptic bronchoscopy in evaluating solitary pulmonary nodules. Chest. 2000;117:1049–54.
10. Naidich DP, Sussman R, Kutcher WL, Aranda CP, Garay SM, Ettenger NA. Solitary pulmonary nodules. CT-bronchoscopic correlation. Chest. 1988;93:595–8.
11. Minami H, Ando Y, Nomura F, Sakai S, Shimokata K. Interbronchoscopist variability in the diagnosis of lung cancer by flexible bronchoscopy. Chest. 1994;105:1658–62.
12. Dolina MY, Cornish DC, Merritt SA, Rai L, Mahraj R, Higgins WE, et al. Interbronchoscopist variability in endobronchial path selection: a simulation study. Chest. 2008;133:897–905.
13. Vining DJ, Liu K, Choplin RH, Haponik EF. Virtual bronchoscopy. Relationships of virtual reality endobronchial simulations to actual bronchoscopic findings. Chest. 1996;109:549–53.
14. Hoppe H, Dinkel HP, Walder B, von Allmen G, Gugger M, Vock P. Grading airway stenosis down to the segmental level using virtual bronchoscopy. Chest. 2004;125:704–11.
15. De Wever W, Vandecaveye V, Lanciotti S, Verschakelen JA. Multidetector CT-generated virtual bronchoscopy: an illustrated review of the potential clinical indications. Eur Respir J. 2004;23:776–82.
16. Asano F, Matsuno Y, Matsushita T, Seko A. Transbronchial diagnosis of a pulmonary peripheral small lesion using an ultrathin bronchoscope with virtual bronchoscopic navigation. J Bronchol. 2002;9:108–11.
17. Asano F, Matsuno Y, Shinagawa N, Yamazaki K, Suzuki T, Ishida T, et al. A virtual bronchoscopic navigation system for pulmonary peripheral lesions. Chest. 2006;130:559–66.
18. Asano F, Matsuno Y, Tsuzuku A, Anzai M, Shinagawa N, Yamazaki K, et al. Diagnosis of peripheral pulmonary lesions using a bronchoscope insertion guidance system combined with endobronchial ultrasonography with a guide sheath. Lung Cancer. 2008;60:366–73.
19. Asano F, Matsuno Y, Takeichi N, Matsusita T, Ohoya H. Virtual bronchoscopy in navigation of an ultrathin bronchoscope. J Jpn Soc Bronchol. 2002; 24:433–8.
20. Shinagawa N, Yamazaki K, Onodera Y, Miyasaka K, Kikuchi E, Dosaka-Akita H, et al. CT-guided transbronchial biopsy using an ultrathin bronchoscope with virtual bronchoscopic navigation. Chest. 2004;125:1138–43.
21. Asahina H, Yamazaki K, Onodera Y, Kikuchi E, Shinagawa N, Asano F, et al. Transbronchial biopsy using endobronchial ultrasonography with a guide sheath and virtual bronchoscopic navigation. Chest. 2005;128:1761–5.
22. Shinagawa N, Yamazaki K, Onodera Y, Asano F, Ishida T, Moriya H, et al. Virtual bronchoscopic navigation system shortens the examination time—feasibility study of virtual bronchoscopic navigation system. Lung Cancer. 2007;56:201–6.
23. Ishida T, Asano F, Yamazaki K, Shinagawa N, Oizumi S, Moriya H, et al. Virtual bronchoscopic navigation combined with endobronchial ultrasound to diagnose small peripheral pulmonary lesions: a randomised trial. Thorax. 2011;66:1072–7.
24. Wang Memoli JS, Nietert PJ, Silvestri GA. Metaanalysis of guided bronchoscopy for the evaluation of the pulmonary nodule. Chest. 2012;142(2):385–93.
25. Rodenwaldt J, Kopka L, Roedel R, Margas A, Grabbe E. 3D virtual endoscopy of the upper airway: optimization of the scan parameters in a cadaver phantom and clinical assessment. J Comput Assist Tomogr. 1997;21:405–11.
26. Ferretti GR, Thony F, Bosson JL, Pison C, Arbib F, Coulomb M. Benign abnormalities and carcinoid tumors of the central airways: diagnostic impact of CT bronchography. AJR Am J Roentgenol. 2000;174:1307–13.
27. Adaletli I, Kurugoglu S, Ulus S, Ozer H, Elicevik M, Kantarci F, et al. Utilization of low-dose multidetector CT and virtual bronchoscopy in children with suspected foreign body aspiration. Pediatr Radiol. 2007;37:33–40.
28. Colt HG, Crawford SW, Galbraith 3rd O. Virtual reality bronchoscopy simulation: a revolution in procedural training. Chest. 2001;120:1333–9.
29. Ost D, DeRosiers A, Britt EJ, Fein AM, Lesser ML, Mehta AC. Assessment of a bronchoscopy simulator. Am J Respir Crit Care Med. 2001;164:2248–55.
30. Tanaka H, Takizawa H, Satoh M, Okada Y, Yamasawa F, Umeda A. Assessment of an ultrathin bronchoscope that allows cytodiagnosis of small airways. Chest. 1994;106:1443–7.
31. Saka H. Ultra- fine bronchoscopy: biopsy for peripheral lesions.

Nippon Rinsho. 2002;60 Suppl 5:188–90.
32. Asano F, Matsuno Y, Komaki C, Kato T, Ito M, Kimura T, et al. CT-guided transbronchial diagnosis using ultrathin bronchoscope for small peripheral pulmonary lesions. Nihon Kokyuki Gakkai Zasshi. 2002;40:11–6.
33. Asano F, Kimura T, Shindou J, Matsuno Y, Mizutani H, Horiba M. Usefulness of CT-guided ultrathin bronchoscopy in the diagnosis of peripheral pulmonary lesions that could not be diagnosed by standard transbronchial biopsy. J Jpn Soc Bronchol. 2002;24:80–5.
34. Fujisawa T, Tanaka M, Saka H. Report by the Bronchus Nomenclature Working Group. J Jpn Soc Bronchol. 2000;22:330–1.
35. Seemann MD, Seemann O, Luboldt W, et al. Hybrid rendering of the chest and virtual bronchoscopy [corrected]. Eur J Med Res. 2000;5:431–7.
36. Edell E, Krier-Morrow D. Navigational bronchoscopy: overview of technology and practical considerations—new current procedural terminology codes effective 2010. Chest. 2010;137:450–4.
37. Eberhardt R, Kahn N, Gompelmann D, Schumann M, Heussel CP, Herth FJ. LungPoint—a new approach to peripheral lesions. J Thorac Oncol. 2010;5:1559–63.
38. Mori K, Deguchi D, Sugiyama J, Suenaga Y, Toriwaki J, Maurer CR, Jr., et al. Tracking of a bronchoscope using epipolar geometry analysis and intensity-based image registration of real and virtual endoscopic images. Med Image Anal. 2002;6:321–36.
39. Higgins WE, Helferty JP, Lu K, Merritt SA, Rai L, Yu KC. 3D CT-video fusion for image-guided bronchoscopy. Comput Med Imaging Graph. 2008;32:159–73.
40. McLennan G, Ferguson JS, Thomas K, Delsing AS, Cook-Granroth J, Hoffman EA. The use of MDCTbased computer-aided pathway finding for mediastinal and perihilar lymph node biopsy: a randomized controlled prospective trial. Respiration. 2007;74:423–31.
41. Merritt SA, Gibbs JD, Yu KC, Patel V, Rai L, Cornish DC et al. Image-guided bronchoscopy for peripheral lung lesions: a phantom study. Chest. 2008;134:1017–26.
42. Mori K, Deguchi D, Kitasaka T, Suenaga Y, Hasegawa Y, Imaizumi K, et al. Improvement of accuracy of marker-free bronchoscope tracking using electromagnetic tracker based on bronchial branch information. Med Image Comput Comput Assist Interv. 2008;11:535–42.
43. Schwarz Y, Mehta AC, Ernst A, Herth F, Engel A, Besser D, et al. Electromagnetic navigation during flexible bronchoscopy. Respiration. 2003;70:516–22.
44. Schwarz Y, Greif J, Becker HD, Ernst A, Mehta A. Real-time electromagnetic navigation bronchoscopy to peripheral lung lesions using overlaid CT images: the first human study. Chest. 2006;129:988–94.
45. Wagner U, Walthers EM, Gelmetti W, Klose KJ, von Wichert P. Computer-tomographically guided fiberbronchoscopic transbronchial biopsy of small pulmonary lesions: a feasibility study. Respiration. 1996;63:181–6.
46. Kobayashi T, Shimamura K, Hanai K. Computed tomography-guided bronchoscopy with an ultrathin fiberscope. Diagn Ther Endosc. 1996;2:229–32.
47. Shinagawa N, Yamazaki K, Onodera Y, Asahina H, Kikuchi E, Asano F, et al. Factors related to diagnostic sensitivity using an ultrathin bronchoscope under CT guidance. Chest. 2007;131:549–53.
48. Matsuno Y, Asano F, Shindoh J, Abe T, Shiraki A, Ando M, et al. CT-guided ultrathin bronchoscopy: bioptic approach and factors in predicting diagnosis. Intern Med. 2011;50:2143–8.
49. Herth FJ, Ernst A, Becker HD. Endobronchial ultrasound-guided transbronchial lung biopsy in solitary pulmonary nodules and peripheral lesions. Eur Respir J. 2002;20:972–4.
50. Kurimoto N, Miyazawa T, Okimasa S, Maeda A, Oiwa H, Miyazu Y, et al. Endobronchial ultrasonography using a guide sheath increases the ability to diagnose peripheral pulmonary lesions endoscopically. Chest. 2004;126:959–65.
51. Yoshikawa M, Sukoh N, Yamazaki K, Kanazawa K, Fukumoto S, Harada M, et al. Diagnostic value of endobronchial ultrasonography with a guide sheath for peripheral pulmonary lesions without X-ray fluoroscopy. Chest. 2007;131:1788–93.
52. Tachihara M, Ishida T, Kanazawa K, Sugawara A, Watanabe K, Uekita K, et al. A virtual bronchoscopic navigation system under X-ray fluoroscopy for transbronchial diagnosis of small peripheral pulmonary lesions. Lung Cancer. 2007;57:322–7.
53. Asano F. Virtual bronchoscopic navigation. Clin Chest Med. 2010;31:75–85.
54. Asano F, Matsuno Y, Ibuka T, Takeichi N, Oya H. A barium marking method using an ultrathin bronchoscope with virtual bronchoscopic navigation. Respirology. 2004;9:409–13.
55. Asano F, Shindoh J, Shigemitsu K, Miya K, Abe T, Horiba M, et al. Ultrathin bronchoscopic barium marking with virtual bronchoscopic navigation for fluoroscopy-assisted thoracoscopic surgery. Chest. 2004;126:1687–93.
56. Gildea TR, Mazzone PJ, Karnak D, Meziane M, Mehta AC. Electromagnetic navigation diagnostic bronchoscopy: a prospective study. Am J Respir Crit Care Med. 2006;174:982–9.
57. Eberhardt R, Anantham D, Ernst A, Feller-Kopman D, Herth F. Multimodality bronchoscopic diagnosis of peripheral lung lesions: a randomized controlled trial. Am J Respir Crit Care Med. 2007;176:36–41.
58. Tsuboi E, Ikeda S, Tajima M, Shimosato Y, Ishikawa S. Transbronchial biopsy smear for diagnosis of peripheral pulmonary carcinomas. Cancer. 1967;20:687–98.
59. Gaeta M, Pandolfo I, Volta S, Russi EG, Bartiromo G, Girone G, et al. Bronchus sign on CT in peripheral carcinoma of the lung: value in predicting results of transbronchial biopsy. AJR Am J Roentgenol. 1991;157:1181–5.

第 3 篇

治疗性介入支气管镜

Therapeutic Interventional Bronchoscopy

第 8 章
中央气道阻塞的气管镜治疗

Sarah Hadique, Prasoon Jain, and Atul C. Mehta

> 有两种理念，科学和观念，前者带来知识，后者则是无知。
>
> 希波克拉底

本章提要 中央气道阻塞（CAO）是中央气道内恶性和良性变化结果导致的。进展期肺癌是最常见的病因。临床表现一般由缓慢进展的咳嗽和呼吸困难到急剧变化的呼吸窘迫和窒息不等。对此，介入呼吸病学医师、放射科医师、麻醉师及胸外科医师之间的亲密协作是解决这一类难关的最佳途径。治疗的近期目标是保证气道安全和恢复气管腔的通畅，有多种气管镜介入治疗技术通过可弯曲或硬质气管镜来实现这一目标。相关介入技术的选择依赖于疾病的基本病因、阻塞类型、中央气道阻塞的严重程度及仪器和专业知识的运用。可以通过机械清创、激光切除、电凝止血、氩离子凝固术、冷冻切除和球囊扩张（球囊支气管成形术）等来即刻解除症状。近距放疗、光动力治疗和冷冻治疗均会使疗效延迟，因此对需要即刻解除症状来说并不适合。气管支架对于外压性气道压迫患者来说是很有帮助的。上述规范治疗通常能成功地快速解除气道症状并为后续进一步治疗如外照射、化疗及手术做铺垫。

关键词 中央气道阻塞，气管镜介入治疗，气管狭窄，肺癌，硬质气管镜。

引 言

中央气道是指气管、主支气管和肺支气管。中央气道阻塞是中央气道内恶性或良性疾病变化的结果（表 8.1）。阻塞病变可分为腔内型、外压型或混合型（图 8.1）[1]。原发性肺癌是中央气道阻塞最常见的病因。肺癌发生率的增加意味着介入肺科医师在未来可能会面对越来越多的中央气道阻塞患者。中央气道阻塞会引起一系列症状，包括呼吸困难、咳嗽、咯血、哮喘、肺不张、阻塞性肺炎。患者呼吸困难是由于气流受限和呼吸做功增加。这些患者当中，在严重呼吸窘迫或即将窒息时呼吸困难非常严重。在其他如哮喘和慢性阻塞性肺病（COPD）患者中临床表现多缓慢进展。由此，内科医师通常不能在中央气道阻塞的早期予以识别并正确诊断。

中央气道阻塞

对 CAO 的管理揭示了问题的独特性并需要多学科综合治疗[2-4]。拥有一个专门的气道团队对快速评估和治疗这一类患者非常有效，但这样的团队只在完备的医疗中心才有[5]。中央气道阻塞的解除应该快速并保证气道安全[6]。一旦气道安全，则应用介入治疗恢复气道腔的

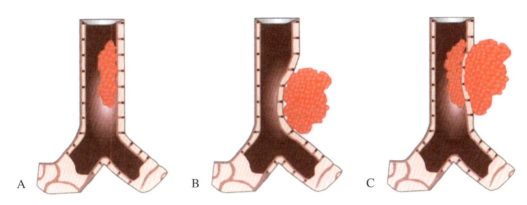

图 8.1 中央气道阻塞类型。A. 腔内型；B. 外压型；C. 腔内外压混合型

通畅。

相关介入治疗的技术多种多样，包括机械切除、球囊支气管成形术、冷冻治疗、激光切除、电烙术、氩离子凝固术、近距放疗、光动力治疗和支架置入术[7-9]。介入治疗的选择取决于病变类型和部位及相关流程的紧迫性。此外，患者临床稳定性、疾病可能的诊断、总预后及生活质量也将影响介入治疗的选择。目前仍缺乏这一领域的大量随机对照研究来指导治疗。治疗的选择也取决于训练有素的人员和仪器设备，个人喜好及机构的操作流程。很多时候通过优化组合以达到最佳结果。

这一章我们回顾恶性疾病引起次级中央气道阻塞的诊断和治疗方法。通过探讨病因、临床评估、影像学和治疗方式选择使介入肺脏科医师更好地治疗恶性疾病引起的中央气道阻塞。同样我们也高度关注这一领域当前的发展趋势和最新的进展。

中央气道阻塞的病因

恶性气道阻塞多见于原发气道肿瘤、气道毗邻恶性肿瘤侵犯或者气管转移（表 8.1）。

肺癌是导致恶性中央气道阻塞最主要的原因。据估计，近 20%~30% 的肺癌患者有中央气道阻塞，同时高达 40% 患者的死因与进展性局部或毗邻疾病相关[10]。其他常见病因包括食管癌、甲状腺癌和原发性恶性纵隔肿瘤。很多气道区域的恶性肿瘤不仅可以包绕并压迫气管引起外压性气道改变，而且侵犯气管全层引起腔内气道改变。更多时候，中央气道阻塞是腔内、腔外压力共同导致的结果[2]。

气管内转移在乳腺癌、结肠癌、黑色素瘤和肾细胞癌患者中最容易观察到[11]。尸检研究发现，2% 的胸外恶性肿瘤患者仅仅气管内转移而无肺实质转移[12]；与此相反，约 18%~42% 的肺转移患者有气管内病变[13,14]。由此，当患者出现咳嗽、呼吸困难、咯血或肺不张时，临床医师必须想到运用气管镜检查以明确诊断。

卡波西肉瘤（KS）是人类免疫缺陷病毒（HIV）感染后最常见的恶性并发症。20% HIV 感染的皮肤卡波西肉瘤可能与肺相关[15]。大多数情况下，KS 累及气道并出现中央气道阻塞的症状[16]。通过气管镜可以观察到，气管黏膜上可有多个圆形樱桃红或紫癜样凸起损伤，有时可引起全肺叶或部分气管腔内阻塞[17]。

原发气道肿瘤比较少见，也给诊断和治疗带来困难。美国每年估计有 600~700 例[2]。近 1/3 的气管、隆突原发肿瘤是鳞状细胞癌和腺样囊性癌。得克萨斯州马里兰安德森癌症中心 60 岁的气管肿瘤患者中，74 例诊断为原发性气

表 8.1　中央气道阻塞（CAO）的良恶性病因

恶　性	良　性	
原发性肺肿瘤	获得性	先天性
原发气道肿瘤	气管插管后	气管软化
鳞癌	气管切开术后	支气管软化
腺样囊性癌	热或化学呼吸道烧伤	血管骑跨
黏液表皮样癌	异物	膜状蹼
类癌	外科吻合术后	多发性软骨炎
转移性肿瘤	放疗后纤维化	
甲状腺源性	**系统性疾病**	
结肠源性	结核病	
乳腺源性	结节病	
肾源性	淀粉样病变	
黑色素瘤	纵隔纤维化	
卡波西肉瘤	韦格纳肉芽肿病	
气管邻近肿瘤	人乳头瘤状病毒所致的乳头瘤病	
食管癌	**其他**	
喉癌	黏液栓	
纵隔肿瘤	血凝块	
淋巴瘤	血管瘤	
	会厌炎	
	甲状腺肿	
	特发性疾病	

管肿瘤。其中 34 例（45.9%）是鳞状细胞癌，19 例（25.7%）是腺样囊性癌，另外还有 21 例（28.4%）是其他组织类型[18]。鳞状细胞气管肿瘤通常发生在 60~70 岁患者中，多见于男性吸烟患者；相反，腺样囊性癌见于较年轻患者，与吸烟无关，而且男女比例相近[19]。

类癌是隆突下肿瘤最常见的类型[20]。很多气管内类癌患者多表现为咳嗽、咯血、单侧肺哮鸣音，并不伴有类癌综合征。

气管肿瘤生长缓慢，临床表现和发作隐匿，在确诊前患者通常易被误诊为成人哮喘发作数月[21]。当对呼吸困难和气喘通过常规哮喘治疗后无效果时，临床医师必须敏锐地想到气管肿瘤引起的可能性。

中央气道阻塞也可以由很多非恶性疾病引起（表 8.1）。成人中最常见的非恶性疾病是肉芽组织形成和长时间气管插管后或气管切开术后引起的纤维性狭窄，其他常见原因包括异物和气管支气管软化症。与恶性中央气道阻塞相比，当病变引起不利和危及生命的体征和症状时，用"非恶性疾病"一词形容要比"良性疾病"更为恰当。关于非恶性中央气道阻塞细节的讨论会在其他章节中谈到，在此不做赘述[22-25]。

临床评价

气道阻塞的临床表现取决于其严重程度及阻塞部位。此外，某种程度上患者潜在的健康状态和气流受限的代偿能力也将影响症状的出现。临床表现可从无症状的影像学异常到危及生命的气道阻塞。

呼吸困难是最常见的症状。早期症状不易被重视，因为大多数患者在日常活动受限中慢慢适应劳力性呼吸困难或咳嗽。典型的劳力性呼吸困难不会发生，直到气管狭窄到约 8 mm 或气管直径的 50%。休息时出现呼吸困难通常气管狭窄到约 5 mm 或气管直径的 25%[26,27]。因此多数患者出现中央气道阻塞症状时，气道疾病已加重。当面临黏液栓、血块或气道炎症时，气道狭窄更容易向完全性气道阻塞转变。由此可见大部分中央气道阻塞的患者表现为急性呼吸窘迫并不奇怪[25]。

咯血是第二大常见症状，约在 50% 的中央气道阻塞患者中可出现[28]。中央气道阻塞的临床表现还包括咳嗽、气喘、喘息、反复发作的气道感染和肺不张。近 1/3 的患者在早期可发现阻塞性肺炎。当出现声音嘶哑或吞咽咳嗽时，多提示声带麻痹、喉功能障碍或食管癌。

多数患者被诊断为哮喘或慢性阻塞性肺病急性加重。事实上，一些患者经长期频繁使用类固醇类药物而表现出库欣综合征特征。当出现包括不典型或临床上的难治性成人型哮喘和慢性阻塞性肺病急性加重在内的上述任何一种症状时，需要高度怀疑中央气道改变，并做进一步影像学和气管镜检查。

患者详尽的个人史和家族史通常能提供疾病的关键因素及其早期临床表现形式。这类信息对评估患者预后很有帮助。尽管在一些患者中急性气道阻塞是其最先的恶性表现，大部分恶性中央气道阻塞患者多已告知有胸腔肿瘤。因此，新发及陈旧性恶性肿瘤的患病史，以及接受化疗或放疗的治疗史都必须收集。由于很多中央气道阻塞的患者因心肺储备受限而病情很重，严谨的手术风险评估对每位患者来说都很重要。在规范的诊疗计划中，合并症评估包括心脏病（可能影响麻醉管理）、凝血障碍、肾功能衰竭、阻塞性睡眠呼吸暂停综合征和颈椎炎（可能行硬质气管镜操作比较困难）。在气管插管或气管检查中，寻找以往可能的任何疾病很重要，因为这有助于治疗团队在介入操作过程中提高警惕。

体格检查在早期可能并不受重视。胸部检查可能会找到气管偏移、喘鸣、局限性或弥漫性哮鸣音、声音嘶哑、呼吸音减弱或分泌物残留、阻塞性肺炎的体征。此外，少数患者可表现为皮下气肿或面部、上肢浮肿和胸壁静脉曲张等上腔静脉综合征。急性呼吸窘迫的患者可以看到用肋间肌辅助呼吸，并有心动过速、呼吸急促、出汗、坐立不安的体征表现。心动过速、发绀和意识不清等先兆，一般提示气管腔严重受累。为避免窒息和死亡，这类患者需要立即行介入治疗。

肺功能检查

很多患者身体太虚弱，不能在紧急情况下完成肺功能检测。用力呼气试验可能使气流阻塞加重，当重要的大气道狭窄时不应该尝试此操作。对这类患者而言，详细的病史、体格检查联合胸部影像学和气管镜检查有利于诊断和指导治疗。

对病情稳定的患者而言，肺功能检查能提供有用的信息。肺量测定法在中央气道阻塞早期的敏感性较低。相反，呼吸流速可以帮助识别气道阻塞部位，并能提供可贵的临床资料[29]。吸气末呼吸流速高提示可变性胸外气道阻塞，一般由声带麻痹、胸外甲状腺肿或喉癌引起（图 8.2A）。呼吸循环中呼气末曲线扁平提示可变性胸内气道阻塞（图 8.2B）。混合性大气道阻塞见于气管狭窄、较大肿瘤压迫气管，多表现为吸气和呼气流速曲线中段扁平（图 8.2C）[30]。

胸部影像学

影像学检查在诊疗准备和气管镜规划中起着重要的作用。放射学领域的技术进步，特别是计算机断层扫描（CT）成像为中央气道无创成像带来革新。尽量获取 CT 影像资料，但对急性病情较重的患者，呼吸困难或难以平卧的患者而言，该操作就难以进行[31]。

胸片虽然敏感性低，但在某些情况下仍能提示中央气道或支气管阻塞。气管狭窄或柱状气管，气管变形或重度偏移均高度提示中央气道阻塞（图 8.3）。另外胸片可提示大的融合或纵隔淋巴结肿大。影像学上远端气管阻塞可提示肺不张、实变、渗出和膈肌抬高。在完成介入操作前，也必须通过胸片评估结果，以排除操作相关的不良事件如气胸或肺不张。术后胸片对日后对比也很有用。

1991 年首先出现螺旋 CT，而最近的多层螺旋 CT（MDCT）扫描仪可以显著提高轴成像的图片质量，并且二维或三维重建成像能显著减少运动伪影。最新的 CT 扫描仪能在极短时间内获得中央气道的薄层图像。它的主要特点是能显示气管镜无法探测到的气管远端狭窄。静脉注射造影剂不是必需的，但其能很好地区别气管旁肿大淋巴结与甲状腺占位。

横断面 CT 中央气管及相关胸腔内结构成像在早期评价和治疗中至关重要（图 8.4）。然而需注意其诸多不足。第一，横轴位成像不能很好地显示真正颅底范围内的疾病。第二，发现早期气管狭窄仍有局限性。第三，横轴位成像不能展示阻塞部位和复杂气道的三维联系。上述提及的诸多横轴位成像的局限性均可通过 CT 多层三维重建成像来克服[32]。中央气道横轴位成像和重设多维成像可提供补充信息[33]。CT 三维重建检测能为气管支架长度和大小的选择提供有用信息[34]。多项研究已经证实 MDCT 在评价支架相关并发症上的价值[35,36]。在一项研究中，MDCT 发现了 29/30（97%）支架相关并发症，最后通过气管镜检查明确诊断[36]。多层螺旋 CT 三维重建对提前评估早期中央气道阻塞患者进行的其他介入治疗或手术治疗也很有帮助[37]。

三维重建有两种基本方式：外渲染和内渲染。三维外渲染可显示气管外表及其与相邻结构的关系（图 8.5）。诸多研究已证实了三维外渲染对中央气道阻塞患者进行介入治疗操作前的应用价值。研究显示横轴位成像联合三维外渲染成像能为 1/3 非恶性气管支气管狭窄患者在形状、长度和气管狭窄程度等方面提供详细信息，并纠正了 10% 患者的横轴位成像结果[38]。

如传统气管镜检查术中所见一样，用于螺旋 CT 成像后的内渲染成像可显示气管腔内结

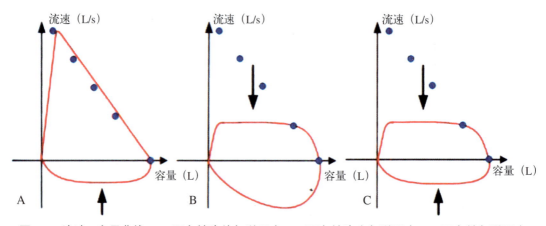

图 8.2　流速 - 容量曲线。A. 可变性胸外气道阻塞；B. 可变性胸内气道阻塞；C. 固定性气道阻塞

第 3 篇　治疗性介入支气管镜

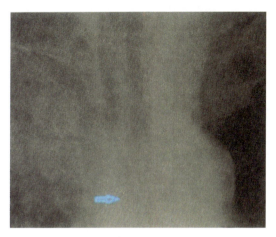

图 8.3　胸部 X 线片提示二级气管狭窄系被右上叶肺癌压迫所致

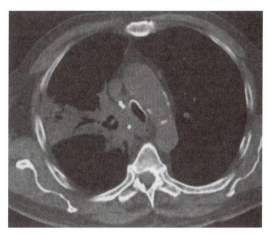

图 8.4　胸部 CT 提示外压引起气管狭窄、变形

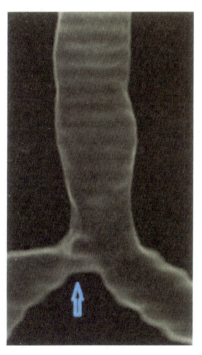

图 8.5　外部三维渲染成像提示气管远端及右主支气管狭窄

构。仿真气管镜检查可探测到标准气管镜检查不到的较深部位病灶[39]。有研究显示仿真气管镜检查在 19/20 例气管高度狭窄的患者中可做出明确诊断，而在轻微外压的 25% 的患者中仍不能明确诊断[40]。另一则报道显示，仿真气管镜对腔内或阻塞性病变有 90%~100% 的敏感性，而对黏膜病变的敏感性只有 16%[41]。最近有一项研究对比了 50 例气管支气管病变患者进行的仿真气管镜检查和可弯曲气管镜检查的结果：仿真气管镜检查在显示气管远端阻塞病变上比可弯曲气管镜更有优势，而可弯曲气管镜在检测早期肿瘤浸润和轻微黏膜改变上比仿真气管镜有优势[42]。仿真气管镜因假阳性而使实用性受限，特别是当气管内分泌物稠厚或者是血凝块时，易被误认为气管内肿瘤[43]。然而仿真气管镜在肺段支气管的假阳性率要比中央气道的更高，而前者是介入治疗的主要部位[44]。

光学相干断层成像术（OCT）是一种与超声成像相似，但采用红外线代替声波获取图像的影像学技术。初步经验显示与超声相比，OCT 有更高的空间分辨率，因此能提供更多的细节，比如肿瘤侵犯气道的深度[45]。解剖光学相干断层成像术（aOCT）是 OCT 的一个分支，用来精确地实时测量中央气道的大小和直径。aOCT 从气管镜的工作管道进入，探测到气管镜所不能到达的阻塞病变部位，从而评估狭窄程度。aOCT 导管通过气管镜缓慢伸缩而获得图像。该技术已经通过测量气管模型、猪离体气管及正常人气管直径而被证实可行[46]。就 CAO 的临床经验而言，仅存在一项通过 aOCT 获取

115

到 3 例患者有用信息的单独报道[47]。第一例患者应用 aOCT 指导支架选择，第二例患者应用 aOCT 评价左主支气管肿瘤阻塞程度，第三例患者的 aOCT 则是被用于在重度气管支气管软化下评估呼吸道的动态属性。aOCT 还有个潜在功能，即用于协同 CT 影像评估患者能否采用气管镜治疗，但这一领域仍需进一步的研究。最重要的问题在于解决联合 aOCT 获得的额外视角能否转化为患者的切身利益。

气管镜检查术

气管镜检查为中央气道阻塞患者介入操作前的评估提供了基本信息。直视观察不仅可以识别病灶、部位及气管累及范围，而且突显病变血管的分布及脆性（图 8.6）。此外，还能提供组织病理诊断，让术者能够评价黏膜浸润程度和肿瘤引起的任何气管外源性压迫。同样，气管镜检查可被用来判断狭窄气管的直径，从而选择合适的支架[48]。然而气管镜检查并非毫无风险。仍有部分严重中央气道狭窄的患者接受气管镜检查后可能发展为完全性气道阻塞。

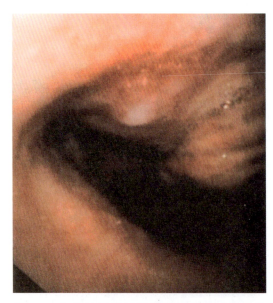

图 8.6 气管镜图像显示外源性压迫引起气管明显缩小、变形及右侧部位肿瘤浸润

气管镜检查引起的气管腔内局部渗血和黏膜损伤可能会进一步增加突发性通气障碍和窒息的风险。因此，整个过程尽可能由最有经验的、具备及时进行心肺复苏能力的人员来操作是至关重要的。

某些情况下，常规气管镜不能通过严重狭窄的气管。这类患者可采用超细支气管镜，它可到达直径约 2.8~3.5 mm 的气管远端部位。常规气管镜无法通过阻塞病变以下气管，而采用超细支气管镜后近 80% 的患者成功探测到气管远端部位[49,50]。

可弯曲气管镜或硬质气管镜的选择对介入治疗很重要。该领域的众多资深医师更倾向于使用硬质气管镜来介入治疗多数 CAO 患者。但很遗憾，只有部分三级医疗中心才能使用硬质气管镜，而且只有部分肺脏学专家接受过训练，或者说有硬质气管镜的操作经验。然而，这种现象在慢慢改变。实际上，硬质气管镜在 CAO 中的应用受到越来越大的重视，以致那些不为人知的功能得以重现[51]。

气管镜介入治疗中，与可弯曲气管镜相比，硬质气管镜有诸多优点（表 8.2）[52]。它可以较好地保护气管并同时通气。它有一个更宽的工作管道，不会使气道闭塞，使吸痰和器械操作更加有效。因上述工作管道可用于扩张狭窄的气道，对于一些患者，可通过硬质气管镜使气道立即再通，并找到病变。当操作过程中伴发大出血而使情况变得复杂时，硬质气管镜相对于可弯曲气管镜来说更有用。最后，一些介入治疗（如硅胶支架置入和微吸切器减瘤等）只有硬质气管镜才能完成。

硬质气管镜在介入治疗中的实用性在一篇对 32 例需要介入治疗 ICU 患者的回顾性文献中已经证实。紧急介入治疗如气管扩张、激光切除或硅胶支架置入，可在手术室全麻下操作。10/19（52.6%）的机械通气患者可以在介入治疗前紧急拔管，20/32（62.5%）的患者可在介入治疗后立即改变为更低级别的护理[53]。

不像硬质气管镜，可弯曲气管镜可在清醒

表 8.2　气管镜介入治疗中硬质气管镜和可弯曲气管镜的比较

	硬质气管镜	可弯曲气管镜
实用性	有限制	无限制
气道保护	++	无
工作管道	宽	窄
抽吸能力	强	弱
止血	更有效	欠佳
麻醉	全麻	清醒镇静
范围	仅适用于气管和主支气管	还包括叶、段支气管
机械减瘤	迅速	欠佳且耗时
独特性	硅胶支架置入和微吸切器	超细支气管镜和超声支气管镜
LPR 时出现火花的风险	低	高

镇静下操作，开展也更广泛。很多介入治疗如激光切除、电凝止血、氩离子凝固术、冷冻治疗、光动力治疗和金属支架置入都能通过可弯曲气管镜操作。然而，在重度 CAO 下操作也会带来严重风险。正如上述讨论的，气管镜检查同样可能使不完全中央气道阻塞转变为完全气道阻塞。此外，在可弯曲气管镜检查中，因应用镇静药物导致呼吸肌松弛和中枢神经系统抑制，从而使呼吸道变得不稳固。所以有必要进一步加强呼吸道管理，包括硬质气管镜在这些患者中应用的准备工作。如果没有这类设备可利用，需慎重考虑在最初复苏后将患者转移到有专业气道团队的专门机构。

在对 CAO 患者的管理中气管镜超声检查（EBUS）作为气管镜检查的重要组成部分正快速发展。EBUS 可以较好地评估黏膜下和气管周围肿瘤，而在气管镜检查中是很难评估其真实范围的。EBUS 可以很好地估算气管内肿瘤患者气管支气管壁的侵犯深度。有研究显示，23/24（95.8%）的这类患者 EBUS 结果已经证实与外科手术标本接近。也有研究表明 EBUS 结果可能不一样，比如曾将淋巴细胞的软骨环浸润误解为肿瘤浸润[54]。在另一个研究中，EBUS 在选择合适的早期中央型肺癌候选人时很有帮助，这类患者可进行光动力根除治疗[55]。基于 EBUS 可探测到肿瘤在软骨外播散的证据，研究者选择对 9 例患者做替代治疗，后者最初是 PDT 合适的候选者。采用 EBUS 评估肿瘤侵犯深度的精确度，在 9 份外科手术标本中有 6 份相同。同样 EBUS 在气管支架置入前也很有帮助。Miyazawa 等通过流速 - 容量曲线、可弯曲气管镜、EBUS、CT 和超细支气管镜分别检测咽喉部位支架置入患者的功能预后[56]。咽喉部是气流受限最厉害、通常也是呼吸道最容易狭窄的区域。在此研究中，所有手术不能切除合并气管外压的肺癌患者需用球囊扩张，再用硬质气管镜支架置入。这些介入治疗都能快速改善受试者的呼吸困难和流速 - 容量曲线。气管广泛狭窄的患者则有部分缓解，同时反复评估显示最初咽喉部支架位点已经下移。EBUS 在咽喉处新的位置显示有软骨破坏。额外支架在这些区域的置入可以改善呼吸困难、流速 - 容量曲线和肺功能。研究表明 EBUS 在 CAO 患者气管支架置入后具有改善气管功能的潜在作用。

EBUS 也同样对正在接受气管镜治疗的进展期 CAO 患者有帮助。Herth 和他的团队在 3

年时间里用 EBUS 检查了 2 446 例气管镜治疗中的 1 174 例[57]。EBUS 与机械肿瘤清创术、气道支架置入、激光切除、氩离子凝固术、近距放疗、异物移除和内镜脓肿引流联用。在 EBUS 引导下改变治疗方法的总共占 43%。最常见的治疗变化在于气管支架尺寸的调整和当发现很靠近大血管时操作中止。一些病例的 EBUS 结果提示需要外科介入治疗而不是选择内镜治疗。在操作过程中，运用 EBUS 后没有患者出现严重出血或者瘘管。

麻醉和通气

合适的麻醉是气管镜介入治疗的重要组成部分。深入探讨这个话题超出本章范围，对于一些细节，读者可以阅读相关文献[58,59]。多数因中央气道狭窄需要紧急介入治疗的患者都有麻醉相关并发症的高危风险，多数合并严重呼吸窘迫、低氧血症、肺相关败血症和上腔静脉阻塞。按美国麻醉医师协会的身体状况分级，多数患者处于Ⅳ级或Ⅴ级高危（表 8.3）。对于经验丰富的麻醉师而言，进行呼吸道管理很有效，它对调节氧合、通气、循环也很有帮助，同时也强烈推荐给气管镜介入治疗的这类患者。

表 8.3 美国麻醉医师协会（ASA）身体状况分级

ASA 分级	描述
Ⅰ级	患者正常，无系统性疾病
Ⅱ级	患者有轻微系统性疾病
Ⅲ级	患者有严重系统性疾病以致活动受限，但未丧失工作能力
Ⅳ级	患者因系统性疾病失去工作能力，以致经常面临生命安全的威胁
Ⅴ级	濒危患者活不过 24 小时或者失去手术机会
E	需要紧急手术，数字前标注"E"

在计划介入治疗前，必须开始实行积极的支持治疗。很多患者经氧气湿化和吸入支气管扩张剂处理后症状缓解。尽管类固醇治疗应用很普遍，但在这类患者中并没有应用价值。已经有过报道称有症状的严重 CAO 患者吸入 70% 氦气和 30% 氧气（氦氧混合剂）可得到暂时性的缓解[60]。

病情不严重的患者在清醒镇静下可通过可弯曲气管镜进行多种介入治疗，如冷冻疗法、电凝止血、APC 和气管支架置入。某些情况下，深度镇静或全麻是为了使患者舒适和更好地控制咳嗽。全麻在某些可弯曲气管镜的介入治疗中也同样需要，比如激光切除时全麻是为了使患者在相当长的时间内保持静止。对这类患者可用 8 号或大的气管内导管或者喉罩建立呼吸道。硬质气管镜检查通常在全麻状态下施行。硬质气管镜对麻醉师在复杂、较长时间的气管镜介入治疗中保持通气而言，是最可靠的气道。

气管插管既可用于清醒状态下的浅表麻醉，也可用于吸入或静脉给药联用（或不联用）非去极化骨骼肌松弛药的麻醉。用各种各样的方法研究关于呼吸道管理失控，关于这方面已经有过报道。由专门培训过的操作者在紧急情况下需要气管插管时马上进行硬质气管镜操作以保障气道安全是很有必要的[61]。

一些麻醉师更喜欢用静脉麻醉，因为作用快速、对呼吸道刺激少且温和[62]。其他麻醉师可能喜欢用吸入性药物如氟烷[63]或七氟烷来诱导患者[64]。很多吸入性药物有支气管扩张的效果，能帮助合并气道高反应疾病的患者。

麻醉维持既可以通过药物吸入也可以由静脉内给药完成。介入治疗中最近流行的是采用静脉全麻（TIVA）[65]。在吸气引流、支气管扩张及支架置入期间采用持续静脉给药以维持麻醉是可行的，而在上述操作中吸入给药肯定会中断麻醉[66]。丙泊酚在静脉麻醉中最受欢迎，因为它起效时间短（30 秒）且在输液 2 小时后用 15 分钟即可快速恢复。芬太尼也因它 60 秒后就快速发挥效应，同时持续时间短（3~10 分钟）而应用得较多。尽可能避免使用长效阿片类药物，以防止术后患者呼吸抑制。

高度中央气道狭窄的患者很难维持通气。可弯曲气管镜通过气管内导管（ETT）接合器的侧孔时运用正压通气可以解决这一难题。气管镜穿过自封闭的接合器以尽量减少潮气量损失。因为气管镜的存在会增加气流阻力，气管镜介入治疗时会选择最小的 8 号和更大的 ETT。

硬质气管镜有侧壁接合器，能注入麻醉药，并在气管镜介入治疗时辅助通气。气管镜近端由一个目镜封堵，能协助控制通气，但当目镜移除时漏气难以避免，因此在操作过程中术者会有一定吸入麻醉药的风险。

高频喷射通气（HFJV）在硬质气管镜检查过程中不间断地通气。2 mm 大小的导管能提供安全水平的氧合作用。HFJV 导管常放在患者气管阻塞狭窄处的远端[67]。在 HFJV 期间有可能出现肺动态过度膨胀，因为气流阻力在呼气时比吸气时增加更多。然而，在硬质气管镜操作过程中 HFJV 的气道压力（Paw）通常不会超出安全界限，同时在肺正常的人群中也不大可能引起严重肺膨胀或气压伤[68]。

麻醉师和气管镜操作者必须随时准备处理介入过程中发生的并发症，比如大出血、气压伤或者气管穿孔。尽管很少需要紧急开胸术，但胸外科医师需在一旁严阵以待[69]。术后应立即予以仔细监护，因为中央气道阻塞可能因黏液栓塞、水肿、吸气、血块、脱落的组织或支架移位而出现再次发生的危险。

气道内火花在激光切除、电凝止血和氩离子凝固术中需要重点关注。潜在因素包括易燃麻醉药的使用、操作过程中存在高 FiO_2 和气管内有如 ETT 之类的易燃材料。将 FiO_2 降低到 0.4 及以下，以及在上述操作期间中止喷射通气数秒，可以减少气管内着火的风险[70,71]。

中央气道阻塞的管理

所有中央气道阻塞患者都应归为高危患者。最新数据表明这类患者气管镜介入治疗后并发症发生率有 19.8%，30 天内死亡率有 7.8%，反映疾病的严重程度和糟糕的身体状况[72]。拥有有经验的、专业的气道治疗团队很重要，这对处理此类有难度的患者来说并没有夸大。

从一开始，每一个患者的治疗目标都必须因人而异。气管镜治疗的基本原则是缓解症状。毫无疑问，成功的介入治疗在于快速解除症状和提高生活质量。比如，在一项前瞻性研究中，85% 的受试者呼吸困难有改善，65% 的因恶性肿瘤引起中央气道阻塞进展患者在接受气管镜治疗后生活质量改善[73]。相似的结果在另一个研究中也有报道，进展期恶性肿瘤引起中央气道阻塞的患者在接受气管镜介入治疗 30 天后，6 分钟步行增加了 99.7 m，FEV1 增加了 448 ml，FVC 增加了 416 ml[74]。更重要的是，多数患者在治疗后呼吸困难可改善。中央气道肿瘤的患者在接受介入治疗后咯血得到暂时控制的达到 94%[75]。

另外，关于气管镜介入治疗能否提高恶性中央气道阻塞患者的总生存期仍有争议。这问题引发了很多讨论，但因缺乏前瞻性随机研究仍然悬而未决。在这类患者中开展前瞻性、双盲、随机试验既不可行也违背伦理。由于缺乏前瞻性随机试验提供的高质量证据，本文中大多数信息都是通过病例分析、回顾性研究和病史对照的数据推断获得[75,76]。尽管如此，我们讨论介入治疗时，生存期是一个不恰当的研究终点，因为最初的研究设计是为了解除窒息、呼吸窘迫那些不愉快和很痛苦的症状。此外，期望通过局部解除阻塞进而提高总生存期是不切实际的，因为多数恶性中央气道阻塞的患者不仅有已经进展、难以手术切除的恶性肿瘤，而且有严重的并发症，比如 COPD 急性加重和冠心病。

尽管如此，令人鼓舞的是大多数最初为进展期的中央气道阻塞患者在接受气管镜治疗改善症状和卡氏评分后仍有能力接受额外的抗肿瘤治疗[77]。介入治疗后控制肺脓毒症对提高患者承受化疗的能力很有帮助。有研究显示在非小细胞肺癌患者化疗前接受气管镜介入治疗中央气道阻塞和进展期肺癌接受化疗但最初无中央气道阻塞依据的患者之间,生存率无明显差异[78]。有报道指出早期、快速使用内镜介入治疗缓解症状、随后化疗可以使一些患者能接受手术治疗以达到治疗目的[79,80]。经严格筛选的患者在接受手术治疗后获得较长的生存期已成为可能。例如,诱导化疗后手术治疗的3年存活率为52%,而在另一个研究中仅接受姑息治疗的中位生存期为12.1个月[80]。

简易治疗法则在图8.7中已有总结。明显地,烧蚀技术归类到即刻起效和延迟起效的方法中。机械减瘤、激光切除(LPR)、电凝止血和氩离子凝固术(APC)有即刻起效的作用[81],而冷冻治疗、近距放疗和光动力治疗(PDT)一般是延迟起效[81],多适用于不需紧急缓解的症状。气管支架主要用于外源性气道压迫,可以快速撑开并增加气管内径。球囊扩张在支架置入前的气道准备,金属支架置入后的撑开,放置近距放疗导管(使其不被高度狭窄处阻碍)等方面也特别有效。多数情况下,多种介入治疗联合应用是最理想的方式。在下一部分,我们将简单讨论科学原则,临床应用,并发症和

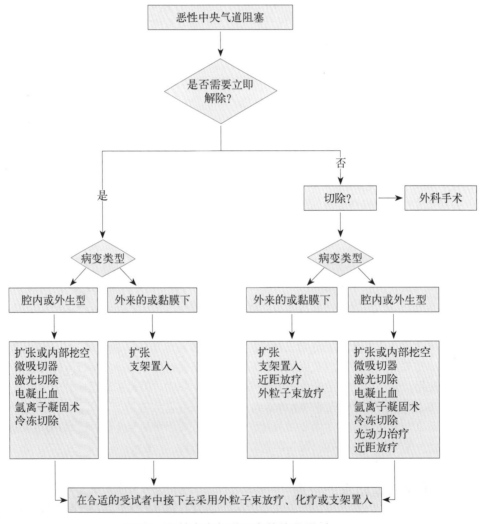

图8.7 恶性中央气道阻塞的处理原则

多种介入治疗恶性中央气道阻塞患者的局限性。

机械减瘤

机械减瘤术即通过硬质气管镜使中央气道迅速再通，是一种很有效的方法。在这项技术中，硬质气管镜末端的斜坡当作一个凿子用来削去大部分阻塞的气管内肿瘤。这个过程也被称为"挖空"。这项技术最适用于气管及主支气管内源性肿瘤引起的重要气道狭窄的患者。硬质气管镜是进行这项操作的理想选择，因为它能控制气道，有更好的吸引能力，能使大号钳子通过，可用来抓取肿瘤碎片，与可弯曲气管镜相比能更加有效地控制出血。

多数患者在操作时因为重要气道狭窄而产生急性呼吸窘迫。气道管理团队必须在场，在尝试诱导麻醉下准备进行硬质气管镜操作使气道通畅。在很多情况下没有时间进行影像学检查。诚然，在操作前观察病灶、评估病变并且检查远端气管非常重要。同时，让积累的分泌物和血块尽可能多地从气道内清除以增加能见度。可弯曲气管镜利用硬质镜头管道操作可达到上述目的。在尝试挖空病灶前决定气道轴线是必要的。肿瘤中机械挖空可通过气管镜尖端切除肿瘤基部、剥除病变完成。为了减少打穿气管和邻近血管的风险，在操作过程中操作者必须让硬质气管镜与气管纵轴平行。肿瘤碎片可通过抓钳、吸引清除，某些情况下可用冷冻治疗探针协助。可弯曲气管镜可用于清除阻塞气管近端病变的肿瘤碎片。出血一般很少发生，且可通过冰冻生理盐水灌洗、局部注射肾上腺素或硬质气管镜直接定向压迫止血。如果应用上述方法后仍有渗血，可用氩离子凝固术。球囊压迫可用于气管远端出血。在某些情况下，可应用热能阻断肿瘤血流供应以减少肿瘤挖空操作中出血的风险。

多数患者在这一操作后能快速解除症状。比如在一项研究中，内窥镜检查出现后能显著改善症状，51/56 的患者在接受治疗后其主观症状和影像学结果均有获益[63]。在这项研究中肿瘤减瘤后接受外科介入治疗的有 16 例（29%），其他干预治疗如外粒子束放疗或化疗的有 34 例（62%）。

采用硬质气管镜减瘤最大的优势在于它费用低、起效快。一个成功的操作为可控的后续干预和日后提供安全的操作环境做铺垫。该操作最显著的局限性在于是否拥有受过硬质气管镜培训的操作者。机械减瘤曾被描述为用一个旋转的气道微吸切器，指一个有旋转叶片和抽吸能力的电动设备。它既可以和硬质气管镜联用，又可以同支撑喉镜合用。最初的经验是令人鼓舞的，但被广泛使用仍需要更多的研究[83,84]。

球囊支气管成形术

球囊扩张是一个很简单的技术，即用一个加压球囊快速解除中央气道阻塞引起的症状。在恶性气管支气管狭窄中，球囊扩张常常在支架置入前用于扩张由外源性压迫引起的气管狭窄患者的气管[85]。也用于扩开先前放置的气管支架，也可用于打开折叠的 Dumon 支架[86]。球囊扩张也被用于帮助近距放疗导管更好地通过阻塞的部位。球囊扩张在对不同良性原因如肺移植后吻合口狭窄、气管插管后狭窄和肺结核等引起的气管狭窄继而引起的气道狭窄的处理中有明确的地位[87-89]。

过去，球囊扩张通常在硬质气管镜或透视下由导丝引导完成[85]。然而，多个研究已经证实非危重患者在镇静清醒状态下运用可弯曲气管镜的可行性和安全性[88,90]。这里，泄气的球囊通过工作管道越过阻塞部位放置，在直视下注压使之膨胀。膨胀球囊直径的波动在 4~20 mm，球囊长度在 4~8 cm。在很多情况下，操作者不得不用多个球囊增加其内径以获得理想的结果。

多数患者在气管球囊扩张后症状可获得快速缓解[87,90]。很多情况下，阻塞性肺炎和肺不张会得到解决。在一组病例中,气管扩张操作1个月后FEV1平均提高10%[91]。有效的气管扩张有助于气管支架的放置,也可以帮助其他治疗方式有效地运用,如近距放疗。球囊扩张对那些不适合手术或先前手术尝试失败的良性气管狭窄患者也很有用。这项操作费用低,技术也容易学习。不幸的是,尽管最初效果很好,但获益不持久,多数患者需要进一步的气管扩张或者额外的操作来缓解症状,如放置支架[87,88,91]。一般说来,这个操作安全,不会出现重大并发症,但少数情况下会发生出血、气管穿孔或纵隔气肿。在一项研究中,60例患者发生浅表黏膜撕裂,球囊扩张后124例患者中有4例出现深部黏膜撕裂[92]。所有的黏膜撕裂痊愈而未出现严重的临床后果。很多专家认为连续球囊扩张损伤要比硬质气管镜下机械扩张损伤小。

电烙术

电烙术因其可以快速缓解恶性中央气道阻塞患者的症状正成为介入治疗比较普遍的选择,因为它有能力通过快速消融肿瘤恢复正常气道腔。电烙术通过热能加热组织来获得想要的结果,如低温下凝固性坏死或高温下组织汽化。通过硬质或可弯曲气管镜,用各种各样的探头使电能传递到气管腔内组织。由于电压不同,电流可通过探头向靶组织传递。电流在经过高电阻抗的组织时产生热能。组织中的生物学效应依赖于热能产生的多少,反过来也取决于电流类型,接触面积,电量,接触持续时间及组织特性。在电凝模式中,当组织体温接近70℃时,低电压、低电量和高强度电流都会引起凝固性坏死。相反,切割模式涉及高电压、低电流的应用,使组织温度接近200℃,这会引起汽化或炭化。很多时候,凝固和切割模式的混合应用会取得理想的结果。一个有效的电烙术可以发现黏膜表面的改变和凝固性坏死的范围。血管丰富的病灶由于"散热"效果好需

要更高的参数。分泌物或任何形式的体液覆盖的病灶也需要更高的热能,因为这样可以减少电流阻力。

这项技术需要高频发电机、绝缘支气管镜和传递电流到组织的一系列配件。接地极板贴近治疗部位以使电路完整。放置地极板远离治疗部位需要更高的参数使电路循环,并需要金属绝缘。

电烙术附属配件包括息肉摘除术套圈,凝固探针,切割器和热活检钳。配件选择依赖于内镜下肿瘤的外表。套扎最常用于带蒂病变。用套圈环绕在病灶上并慢慢收紧,当电烙术开始启动时能切除、凝固病灶基部。组织可被电流离断而不是通过机械套扎用力摘除。凝固探针用于处理无柄或平整的病灶。切割器用于放射状切削在气管或主支气管上的网状狭窄。机械减瘤可能需要电凝、切除、汽化来实现气道的快速再通。组织碎片可以通过活检钳、吸引器或冰冻探头移除。为尽可能地保持手术视野清晰,需要频繁清除出血、炭化组织和碎片。

多个研究已经明确电烙术在快速解除中央气道阻塞患者症状中的实用性。Sutedja和他的团队运用可弯曲气管镜施行气管镜下电烙术处理镇静清醒状态下的局限性进展期中央型肺癌患者[94]。11例患者气管内径开放超过75%,17例中有8例呼吸困难缓解。Coulter和Mehta用可弯曲气管镜为38例中央气道肿瘤或良性网状病变的患者实施了47次电烙术操作[95]。达到满意效果的有89%,因此避免了激光切除(LPR)的需要。有一点需要注意,濒危患者不在此研究范围内,纳入研究的包括气道阻塞内径<50%的患者,肿瘤最大径<2 cm的患者。然而,研究者发现,对一些严格筛选的患者,电烙术可作为LPR的替代治疗。最近来自杜克大学医学中心的大型回顾性研究解决了良恶性中央气道阻塞患者行电烙术的实用性和安全性问题[96]。在这个研究中,过去5年有94例患者接受了117次电烙术操作,其中的62%用到硬质支气管镜。94%的患者在内镜下病变获得改

善，71% 的患者症状缓解，同时也有相当比例的患者影像学上改善明显。这些结果清晰地显示了电烙术为进展期的中央气道阻塞患者快速解除症状的重要性。有些情况下，电烙术还用于治疗不能手术根治的隐匿性中央气道肿瘤[97]。

在相当比例的严格筛选 CAO 患者中，电烙术治疗效果同 LPR 相似[98]。前者比后者更具优势在于其费用低，而且可在清醒镇静下行可弯曲气管镜操作。事实上，多数时候电烙术已取代 LPR 成为 CAO 患者的一线热疗方式。电烙术操作过程安全，主要并发症很少发生[99]。然而，该技术也存在一些不足。如果没有合适的预防措施，仍有风险，如气管腔内着火。为了降低这一风险，FiO_2 必须在 0.4 及以下，同时确保气道内无易燃物，如气管内插管或硅胶支架。如果需要用高流量氧气维持足够氧合，那么不能使用此项操作。有永久起搏器或除颤器的患者，应避免使用电烙术。电烙术不适用于控制气道出血，同时在严重气道出血时电烙术会失去治疗效果。

氩离子凝固术

氩离子凝固术（APC）是非接触式的电烙治疗，用于治疗中央气道阻塞和明显来源于气管内的咯血[100]。等离子，有时候被认为是物质的第四种状态，是有特殊物理性质的带电粒子的气体。当有一个高频、高压电流传递到钨电极电离，而氩气以 0.3~2 L/min 的频率通过聚四氟乙烯导管时，氩离子可在导管中产生。氩离子自导管尖端产生并由喷射电极电离获取，从而引起最靠近的基底组织凝固性坏死。与标准电烙术相似，地极板放置在靠近治疗位置以中止电流循环。电流通过支气管黏膜使组织发热、脱水、凝固。当组织凝固时电阻抗会增加，以阻止电流流通，因此一般使用 2 秒后组织凝固深度限制在 2 mm 左右。APC 在组织凝固方面的自身局限，限制了它快速解除大气道肿瘤的功效，但也减少了气管支气管壁穿孔的风险。

APC 有一个很重要的优势，它可以通过探针到达气管侧面的病灶，以及不适合 LPR 操作的气道拐弯处和角落的病变。

主要病灶在气管或主支气管的、气管腔远端或肺功能正常的患者最适合行 APC 治疗。APC 通过可弯曲气管镜到达支气管内组织。对于病情不稳定的患者，可以通过硬质气管镜或气管插管导管保护气道，通过人工气道将可弯曲气管镜导入气管支气管树。标准的可弯曲支气管镜技术很适合病情稳定的患者。电流由高频电流发电机产生。可弯曲探针直径在约 1.5~2.3 mm，并通过气管镜的工作管道导入气道。为了防止仪器的热损害，需确保的一点就是等离子熔射启动前探针距离靶病灶 1 cm 以内。初步设定氩气流速在 0.8~1 L/min，电压在 30 W。氩等离子需连发 1~3 秒以获得理想的结果。在支气管肿瘤减瘤术中，APC 术后需要定期用活检钳或冰冻探针清除凝固组织和焦痂。APC 将会重复应用于存活的下属组织，周而复始，直到获得理想的治疗结果。

多个病例已经证实 APC 在气道疾病中的实用性。Reichle 和他的团队对有各种各样适应证的 364 例患者施行了 482 次 APC 治疗[100]。对 186 例中央气道肿瘤患者成功地施行了 APC 治疗。气道重新开放的患者占总人数的 67%。90% 的患者硬质气管镜与 APC 联用。APC 用于治疗支气管源性咯血患者的有 119 例，其中 118 例得到充分止血。在 34 例患者中，研究者成功用 APC 使气管支架再通，支架闭塞多数由于肿瘤或肉芽组织在其内生长。同样地，Morice 和他的团队为 60 例患者因肿瘤引起气道阻塞及控制出血实施了 70 次 APC 治疗[101]。唯独 4 个流程操作在清醒镇静下完成，没有使用气管插管。31 例有咯血的患者气道内出血可以看得很清晰。处理前气道内阻塞有 76%，整个操作结束后残留的阻塞减少到 18%。所有中央气道阻塞的患者接受 APC 治疗后症状均有改善。类似地，APC 治疗良恶性中央气道阻塞的结果也已经有过报道[102-104]。

APC 的主要优点在于费用不高以及能很好地控制腔内病变表面出血。另一个引人注目的特点是通过可弯曲气管镜传递氩等离子体。然而，因可能引起严重气管狭窄，APC 不适合腔内肿瘤减瘤。还有，操作过程中 FiO_2 浓度不能维持在 0.4 以下，否则会有气管腔内着火的风险。此外，最近的一则报道引起广泛关注，即 3 例 APC 治疗 3 年后引起气体栓塞，预计其发生率为 1.5%~2%[105]。操作过程中维持尽可能低的氩气流，可以使气体栓塞的风险最小化。

激光切除

激光切除（LPR）对快速解除中央气道阻塞引起的症状来说是一种高效的技术。尽管因为电烙术和 APC 的实用性使得 LPR 的应用有所下降，但在临床实践中仍留有重要地位。激光通过电磁辐射人工产生，因而在自然界中并不存在。激光在活跃物质的电子向高能级转移时产生。当电子回落到低能级时，能量以光子的形式释放出来并组成激光束。用于产生激光的物体称为媒介。激光的波长取决于使用的媒介。激光不同于普通光线，体现在以下三方面。①白光属于混合光，其波长在 390~800 nm，而激光是单色的，并且所有光波均有相同的波长。②所有激光光波的波峰和波谷都是同相的，这一性质称为相干性。③激光波传播方向相同的窄束散度很小，这一性质称为准直性。基于这些特性，激光携带的能量以窄电子束的形式集中在强电源靶点上。

由于这些特性，激光在医学上有很多用途。激光能量可以切除、凝固或汽化生物组织。在气管镜介入治疗中，多用于中央气道阻塞的治疗。掺钕钇铝石榴石（Nd:YAG）是气管镜检查中最常用来激发产生激光的媒介。Nd:YAG 激光的波长为 1 064 nm，在红外线区域，可以使人失明。因此操作者需要佩戴飞行员红灯，这样才能在应用到气管支气管树时看到激光束。由于 Nd:YAG 激光很少被石英材料吸收，以至可以通过可弯曲气管镜传递到气管支气管树。侵透到 10 mm 后可被 Nd:YAG 吸收，而很难被血红蛋白和含水量多的组织吸收。Nd:YAG 激光在低功率背景下即可凝固组织，在高功率下可汽化组织。用 CO_2 激光可精准切除组织，而 Nd:YAG 激光难以达到。最近，很多气管镜介入治疗师在气管镜检查中开始使用掺钕钇铝钙钛石（Nd:YAP）激光，因为它比 Nd:YAG 激光更便宜、便携，组织凝固性更好。前期研究显示 Nd:YAP 激光在治疗中央气道阻塞上疗效与 Nd:YAG 激光相当。

缓解不能切除的有症状的外生型中央气道肿瘤最常见的治疗方法是 LPR 治疗。气管镜治疗最常见的良性指征是声门下及气管狭窄。LPR 偶尔也用于治疗支气管内肉芽肿、细支气管炎和炎症性息肉。在中央气道肿瘤的姑息治疗中，认识到与 LPR 治疗相关的有利和不利因素很重要（表 8.4）。其中最重要的因素是阻塞的部位和阻塞以下气道的状态。病变位于气管或主支气管比那些位于气道远端的病变更适合 LPR 治疗。肺段和亚段支气管的肿瘤行 LPR 成功率相当低。最适合行 LPR 的是肿瘤 <4 cm 的、气道远端无肿瘤的患者。LPR 对那些肿瘤在气管远端和肺实质广泛浸润的患者没有多大作用。在这种情况下清除邻近气管的肿块对患者来说并没有实际获益。胸部 CT 扫描结果可以为 LPR 的疗效提供相应的信息。胸部 CT 显示的肿瘤直接侵犯或压迫相应的肺动脉是 LPR 的禁忌证，因为重新开放气道会增加无效通气，可能会进一步加重而不是改善呼吸困难或低氧血症。类似地，为了避免产生瘘管，如果 CT 显示食管、气管同时侵犯，那也不能尝试操作 LPR。同样，当纵隔解剖结构严重变形或胸部大血管靠近病灶部位时也应高度警惕。气管外压也是 LPR 的禁忌证。

LPR 既可以通过硬质气管镜操作，也可以采用可弯曲气管镜操作。两种方式的最终结果和并发症发生率相近[106]。因此，选择哪种方式

表 8.4 影响 LPR 预后的相关因素

因 素	有 利	不 利
部位	气管和左右主支气管	叶、段支气管
病变类型	腔内型为主	外压型为主
气管镜下表现	外生型	黏膜下型
病变长度	<4 cm	>4 cm
气管腔内远端	可视、无瘤	不可视、肿瘤广泛浸润
肺不张持续时间	<4~6 周	>4~6 周
纵隔解剖	正常	变形
肺血管供应	完整	被浸润和压迫的肿瘤盗用
血流动力学状态	稳定	不稳定
PS 评分	好	差
心肺储备	足够耐受麻醉	不能耐受麻醉
需氧量	≤ 40%	>40%
凝血功能检查	正常	不正常

主要取决于操作者的个人喜好和熟练程度。因其操作视野固定及方便机械减瘤和抽吸,操作者更青睐硬质气管镜[107]。在操作过程中,采用硬质气管镜能更好地处理气道内出血和并发症。所以,对血管病变严重的,更多时候用到的是硬质气管镜而不是可弯曲气管镜。而在很多医疗中心,多数 LPR 过程由可弯曲气管镜进行,因为它可以通过气管插管导管或喉罩。可弯曲气管镜另一个很重要的优势在于它能处理叶支气管远端的肿瘤,而硬质气管镜很难到达此区域。然而,采用可弯曲气管镜进行 LPR 操作时持续时间相当长,因为用活检钳夹取肿瘤碎片耗时巨大。同样,与硬质技术相比,可弯曲技术引起气管内着火的风险更高,因为气管镜、气管插管导管和激光纤维都是易燃物,而硬质气管镜不是易燃物。

当使用硬质气管镜时,常用低功率设置凝固肿瘤后再用硬质气管镜的斜面进行机械减瘤[108]。清除大部分肿瘤后,激光可进一步汽化残留组织、控制出血。运用可弯曲技术,机械减瘤后运用活检钳和激光凝固同样可以获得类似的结果。为了使气管穿孔风险最小化,激光束必须沿着气管壁而不是直接对准气道[109]。激光尖段必须一直保持离靶病灶 4 mm。烟雾、碎片、出血必须定期清除以尽可能保持视野清晰。吸入氧必须一直限制在 0.4 以下以减少气管内着火风险。对可弯曲气管镜进行 LPR 操作,研究者制定了一般准则,设定了"4 规则"以获取最佳效果及尽量减少操作过程中并发症的出现(表 8.5)。

研究报道 LPR 后有 70%~90% 的患者可改善气管口径和缓解症状[110-114]。操作的成功率依赖于肿瘤在气管支气管树的部位。例如,Cavaliere 和他的团队对肿瘤侵犯气管或主支气管 LPR 操作的成功率超过 90%,而肿瘤累及叶支气管处理后的成功率只有 50%[108]。类似结果 Hermes 和他的团队也有报道:肿瘤侵犯气管的 LPR 成功率有 95%,侵犯主支气管的有 80%,而侵犯叶支气管的只有 68%[115]。成功的 LPR 操作可以明显地改善关键气管狭窄及多数中央气

表 8.5　Nd:YAG 激光联合可弯曲气管镜治疗的 Mehta 4 规则

病变长度	<4 cm
肺不张持续时间	<4 周
初始设定	
功率（无触点）	40 W
脉冲持续时间	40 秒
距离	
气管内导管距离病灶	>4 cm
光纤头距离病灶	4 mm
纤维尖段的远端视野	4 mm
吸入氧浓度	≤0.4
清理的脉冲数目	<40
操作时间	<4 小时
激光总治疗次数	<4
预期寿命	>4 周
激光团队	>4

道阻塞患者引起的窒息症状[116,117]。有报道显示，17 例中有 9 例是因急性呼吸衰竭需要辅助通气且无法手术切除的中央气道肿瘤患者，经成功 LPR 后撤管，这些患者中有很多能够接受进一步的肺癌治疗。成功的 LPR 操作也与控制咯血、改善肺功能、肺通气弥散、肺不张的影像学表现、卡氏 PS 评分和生活质量等方面相关[119-121]。在行 LPR 解除中央气道阻塞症状后，很多患者接受了外科手术治疗和肺癌姑息治疗[122]。LPR 治疗后的生存率仍停留在推测阶段，因其缺乏前瞻性随机研究。然而，一些学者已有报道，通过历史对照研究，成功操作 LPR 的患者有较好的生存期[123]。例如，有报道显示既往无 LPR 治疗的患者生存期不超过 7 个月，而 LPR 术后患者的 7 个月存活率达 60%，1 年存活率接近 28%[123]。也有报道称成功 LPR 治疗的生存期比那些不成功的要长[124]。然而，这可能与高肿瘤负荷的患者在初始 LPR 术后难以获得较好的治疗结果相关。也有研究报道，接受 Nd:YAG 激光治疗患者的生存期显著长于既往仅仅接受外照射的患者[125]。此外，另一项研究报道，患者接受近距放疗联合 Nd:YAG 激光治疗的生存期要比仅仅接受激光切除的好[126]。

14 组病例分析文章显示超过 4.4% 的患者 LPR 术后有并发症[127]。影响并发症发生率和患者预后的关键因素在于对患者的精心照料和由有经验的操作者操作。大组分析数据显示并发症包括大出血（占 1%）、LPR 术后气胸（占 4.4%）[111]。一些数据显示近 1%~2% 的患者出现死亡[112,116]。激光束引起胸部主要血管穿孔导致的大出血是 LPR 术后最严重的并发症[113]。这种情况使所有控制出血的方法失效，在大多数病例中患者都马上死亡。气管内导管燃烧也是一类严重而少见的并发症。预防火灾至关重要[128,129]。FiO_2 维持在 0.4 以下、用单脉冲激光、尽可能地保持视野和激光纤维的清洁、操作过程中避免易燃麻醉药的使用等均能降低气管内着火的风险。硅胶管比标准 PVC 气管内套管更能抵抗火花。尽可能拉大气管内导管与手术范围的距离也可以降低着火风险[128]。气管热灼伤的患者必须密切随访，因为以后可能向肉芽组织增生和气管狭窄发展[128,130]。LPR 的设备很昂贵，难以广泛应用[131]。所有进行 LPR 操作的人员都需要进行激光安全的系统教育和培训。一名专业气道团队队员和一个有经验的麻醉师就可以很好地进行此操作。

冷冻疗法

生物组织暴露在反复冰冻和解冻环境下会引起细胞损伤和死亡。气管镜冷冻治疗采用一氧化氮气体和硬质或软质探针冰冻气管内组织。在 Joule-Thompson 原则指导下冷却相应的区域，即气体膨胀的温度从高压区到低压区逐渐降低。这一技术用于将一氧化氮储存在室温环境下的高压气缸内。探针尖段释放出来的气压快速降低可以使温度快速冷却到 −70℃ 以下，使得探针周围的组织在数秒内快速冷冻。

　　反复冰冻、解冻的细胞损伤机制有多条。细胞内结冰将损害重要的细胞结构如线粒体。细胞外结冰可引起渗透性损伤和细胞脱水，这主要由于穿过细胞膜的离子浓度发生改变。组织反复冰冻、解冻也会延长缺血再灌注损伤，因为在操作6~12小时后会发生血管收缩、血小板聚集和血栓形成。因此进一步推测，通过激活自然杀伤细胞，冷冻疗法可使组织的免疫功能受损。

　　细胞死亡程度依赖于冰冻、解冻的速度。细胞损伤随与操作中心的距离而变化。冷冻治疗后效应的其他重要决定因素是冰冻、解冻次数和冷冻治疗时组织的含水量。由于组织含水量低，纤维组织和软骨自然而然能抵抗冷冻伤害，这也解释了为何冷冻治疗后气管穿孔率低。

　　硬探针和可弯曲冷冻探针都能应用，如何选择全凭个人喜好。两者的重要区别之一在于解冻过程中，硬技术比较灵活而可弯曲技术则相对迟钝。基于此，与硬质设备相比，操作时应用软探针需要花费更多的时间。运用可弯曲技术进行冷冻治疗是在镇静清醒状态下完成的。可弯曲探针可通过工作管道。探针尖段进入浸润的肿瘤或者直接插入外源性病变的大块肿瘤。踩脚踏板开始冷冻，持续20~30秒直到在探针周围能看到一个冰球。当脚离开踏板时组织马上开始解冻。1~3个冷冻、解冻周期最常见，每一个区域持续约60秒。探针大概退出5 mm距离，然后在肿瘤邻近区域进行相同的操作。尽可能地覆盖整个肿瘤。在操作的最后，肿瘤看上去没有变化。传统的冷冻治疗，操作过程中不能移除肿块的任何一部分，操作后马上出血很少见。肿瘤迟发性坏死一般发生在操作后的5~10天。这一阶段需要气管镜活检钳或者气管镜下吸引清理干净。有时，自然而然的咳嗽能清除肿瘤比较大的部分。

　　冷冻治疗适用于破坏外生型肿瘤和黏膜下及浸润生长的肿瘤。目前已报道的治疗有效率在75%~80%[132-134]。大多数患者在呼吸困难、运动量、肺功能和PS评分方面都能获得改善[135-137]。有报道称90%的患者咯血问题得到解决[138]。然而，冷冻治疗起效一般都要延迟数天，因此并不适用于大气道肿块引起的急性和严重中央气道阻塞的减瘤治疗。冷冻治疗适用于处理血管丰富的肿瘤和支气管类癌[139]。冷冻治疗也适用于原位癌和微浸润癌。比如在一个研究中，35例早期肺癌的患者接受了冷冻治疗。1年有效率达91%。治疗后4年内有10例患者（28%）肿瘤复发[140]。冷冻治疗可用于控制支架放置后产生的肉芽肿，也可用于气管异物和阻塞血块的清除。含水量丰富的有机异物最适合用此项技术清除。一项小型临床研究已经显示出不能手术切除的肺癌患者采用冷冻治疗联合外照射治疗的协同疗效[141]。但仍需要其他独立研究证实这些数据。动物实验研究已经证实冷冻治疗联合化疗治疗非小细胞肺癌模型的增敏可能[142,143]。人体实验还有待证实。

　　气管镜下冷冻治疗有个很好的安全记录。并发症如出血、支气管痉挛和心律失常很少发生。若是有的话，气管穿孔的风险是最低的。无气管内导管自燃风险，与此同时不管需不需要高流量给氧治疗均能进行冷冻治疗。初始设备和个人程序都比多数气管镜介入治疗程序便宜。主要缺点在于治疗起效慢，使得想要快速得到疗效的时候并不是很适合选用冷冻治疗。最近，冷冻治疗的分支技术即冷冻切除，在即刻解除中央气道阻塞方面疗效显著。

冷冻切除

　　旧版的可弯曲探针并不用来牵拉大片的肿瘤组织。新版的冷冻探针具有较强的冷冻能力，能稳定地衔接气体管道和探针，这可以扛住50 N的牵拉而不出现组织瓦解。运用这类探针可以使阻塞的气道再通。探针直径约2.3 mm，能用于任一气管镜治疗。操作可在气管插管镇静清醒状态下进行。冷冻探针进入工作管道并导入肿瘤组织中。探针尖段需要冷却5~20秒。

一旦冰球形成，用推进的探针将冷冻的肿瘤连同气管镜一起从周围组织中拔除。可放在水池中将肿瘤从探针尖段移除。这个过程需要重复进行直到大部分肿块都提取出来，同时气道重新恢复开放状态。疗效立竿见影，也不需要在气管镜下清除干净。

Hetzel 及其团队用此项技术对 60 例患者进行冷冻切除[144]。37 例（61%）患者的气道完全再通。另外 13 例（22%）患者部分气道再通。严重气管内出血需要用氩离子凝固术止血的患者有 6 例（10%）。他们已经更新了冷冻切除技术的经验，同时对 225 例患者中的 205 例（91%）成功进行了此项操作[145]。在这个研究中，对肿瘤浸润引起的长亚段气管二级狭窄患者进行此操作是有效的。用冰生理盐水或局部肾上腺素处理的轻微出血患者有 9 例（4%）。中度出血需要球囊压迫或 APC 控制的有 18 例（8%）患者。

冷冻切除有多个优点。操作成本不昂贵，不需要硬质气管镜协助或者全麻，也不需要通过气管镜清理干净，同时即刻见效。操作持续时间比 LPR 需要的时间还要短。然而，安全性需要重点关注。气道出血是主要考虑的问题，操作者需要做好解决出血相关并发症的准备，预计大约 10% 的患者会有这类问题。

光动力疗法

光动力疗法（PDT）是利用光敏感剂暴露在无热效应激光的合适波长中，来破坏中央气道肿瘤的一种疗法。卟吩姆钠是实现这一目的最常用的光致敏剂。静脉给药后，卟吩姆钠会在 72 小时内从主要脏器中排出，但会在支气管肿瘤、肝脏、脾脏及皮肤保留相当长的时间。肿瘤选择性在根本上是基于肿瘤细胞和支气管黏膜之间光致敏剂浓度的差异。卟吩姆钠暴露在波长合适的光线下，即相当于在吸收光谱下时能吸收光线，并在Ⅱ型光氧化作用下诱导快速激活单线态氧。细胞内产生高度激活的活性氧，从而产生毒素直接破坏肿瘤细胞[146]。内皮损伤和局部缺血同样可使肿瘤退化。也有免疫系统及补体诱导途径损伤肿瘤细胞的依据[147]。最终，肿瘤在数日后发生衰退。一般说来，PDT 不适合用于快速解除中央气道阻塞引起的症状。

卟吩姆钠静脉给药剂量是 2 mg/kg。差不多 48 小时后，用可弯曲气管镜进行操作，同时将肿瘤置于光线中以激活光致敏剂。为此，光线在红光区的波长为 630 nm，这能渗透至距肿瘤表面约 5~10 mm 深处[148]。磷酸氧钛钾（KTP）泵送染料激光器最常用作光线来源。作为一种无热效应的激光，可以通过石英纤维输送，也适用于可弯曲气管镜。标准的激光防护措施，比如护目镜是很有必要的，但没有气管内导管燃烧的风险。有两种不同技术可实现照明。圆柱形扩散器能让光线 360° 围绕圆周扩散。石英纤维尖段直接置入肿瘤间质进行照射。相反，显微镜头能向前发射光线，能用于表面处理扁形或体表肿瘤。初始治疗部分推荐 200 J/cm 的光能，相当于 400 mW/cm 扩散 500 秒[149,150]。这一剂量的曝光时间大概 8 分钟一个周期。坏死的肿瘤和碎片会在初始治疗后的 48 小时内积累。有些患者可能会发展为肺不张或阻塞性肺炎或者需要气管镜紧急治疗。初始治疗 48 小时后用气管镜清除坏死的肿瘤组织、黏液和组织碎片。有时，坏死的肿瘤呈一种胶冻状，很难清理干净[151]。对于这一情况，需要用坚固的仪器或冷冻探针清理气道。清除坏死肿瘤和黏液后，需要对气道内残留肿瘤再次评估。如果残留肿瘤找到，需要再次进行光照。这期间不再需要光致敏剂给药，因为肿瘤能保留卟吩姆钠 7 天时间。

PDT 在进展期气道肿瘤的姑息治疗中有重要地位。晚期不能手术切除的和以气管腔内肿瘤为主的患者是 PDT 治疗最合适的受试者。成功的 PDT 疗效为显著解除症状，减少腔内阻塞和改善肺功能。在一组 PDT 用于治疗 100 例难以手术治疗患者的研究中，腔内阻塞从 86% 降到 18%，FVC 和 FEV1 分别增加了 430 ml 和 280 ml[149]。WHO PS 评分 <2 的患者接受 PDT 治疗后其生存期显著长于 WHO PS 评分 >2 的患者。PDT 治疗晚期中央型肺癌的结果也有类似报道[152,153]。PDT 也与其他治疗方式如 LPR[154] 和近距放疗[155]（治疗后有良好临床反应的恶性中央气道阻塞患者）联用。尽管序贯治疗以 4~6 周为一阶段分隔，但仍需进一步研究最有效的顺序及不同气管镜下治疗的最佳间隔时间。很少有点对点的比较研究进行 LPR 治疗结果和 PDT 治疗结果的对比。与 LPR 相比，PDT 临床起效虽然缓慢，但能在较长一段时间内获益[156]。在一个随机研究中，PDT 治疗后的患者有一个相当长的稳定时间直到治疗失败，同时其中位生存期也显著长于 LPR 治疗后的患者[157]。然而，此研究受限于样本量太小和不同肿瘤分期上的随机化，同时 PDT 组中晚期中央型肺癌患者不多。多个研究也已经证明了 PDT 能用于早期中央气道肿瘤不能手术切除的患者[158,159]。实际上，PDT 已被 2003 年的 ACCP 肺癌循证临床实践指南推荐作为治疗此类患者的一线治疗方法[160]。

PDT 治疗后最常见的不良反应是呼吸道症状如咳嗽、咳出坏死的肿瘤组织、呼吸困难和肺不张[161]。有时候有必要施行紧急气管镜检查。已报道 18% 的患者有非致命性的咯血。PDT 最重要的副作用是皮肤光过敏。不过这可以预防，在另一个研究中只有 4% 的患者在接受 PDT 治疗后出现轻微光过敏[149]。

对于中央气道阻塞，PDT 与其他气管镜下治疗相比有多个优势。流程技术简单，且可在镇静清醒状态下行可弯曲气管镜操作。操作过程安全性高。气道穿孔和出血风险低。然而 PDT 的不足之处也很突出。操作流程涉及的设备很昂贵，需要重复清理气管镜。有些患者需要用硬质气管镜做呼吸道灌洗。最重要的是，光过敏严重的在近 6 周内不能参加室外活动，这对一些患者来说是难以接受的。患者必须穿防护服和护目镜 4~6 周以避免直接暴露在阳光下。这对预期寿命有限的患者来说是一个严重弊端。

近距离放射治疗

近距离放射治疗是一种将放射源放在靶目标中或靠近靶目标，从而使肿瘤接受最大剂量而周边正常组织接受较少剂量辐射的技术。对于中央气道肿瘤，通过可弯曲气管镜协助，将放射源直接放在靠近肿瘤的支气管树中。对周边组织的放射剂量通过平方反比定律计算，对此，根据随中心放射源距离的平方成反比，放射剂量逐渐降低。相应地，这种治疗模式，与周边正常组织如肺实质和纵隔相比，肿瘤接受相当高的放射剂量。一般说来，放疗后肿瘤衰退需要 3 周的时间。因此近距离放射治疗不适合快速解除中央气道阻塞的症状。

近距放疗的基本目标是缓解不能接受有效手术中央气道肿瘤患者的症状，如咳嗽、呼吸困难和咯血。近距放疗很适合有黏膜下或支气管周边病变的气管内肿瘤。对那些肿瘤复发并能接受最大次数外照射治疗的患者来说也是个有用的选择。为能接受近距离放疗，气管镜需要通过导管越过阻塞病变区域。气道接近完全狭窄的患者，接受近距放疗前，气道部分再通需要用到其他技术如 LPR、电烙术或球囊扩张。近距离放射治疗适用于前文提及的气管镜下技术无法解决的位于软骨和气管壁外的肿瘤，对支气管内转移的治疗也有效。但并不适合气道明显外压的患者，对于后者气管支架置入是最合理的选择。我们也需高度警惕气管壁和毗邻结构发生瘘管的可能。

肿瘤的放疗剂量依赖于放射源的选择和放射源在肿瘤中或其附近的时间。放疗剂量从距离源轴 10 mm 开始估计。低放射剂量率 (LDR)、中放射剂量率 (IDR)、高放射剂量率 (HDR)，对应距离靶目标 10 mm 的剂量分别是 <2 Gy/Hr, 2~12 Gy/Hr 和 >12 Gy/Hr。多数医学中心采用高放射剂量率近距放疗，其中以铱-191 (Ir-192)

作为放射源。美国近距放射疗法协会推荐当 HDR 近距放疗作为缓解症状的主要治疗手段时，3 周一个阶段每次 7.5 Gy，2 周一个阶段每次 10 Gy 或 4 周一个阶段每次 6 Gy[162]。每个治疗阶段持续 5~30 分钟，这对门诊患者很容易进行操作。

近距放疗需要气管镜检查者和放射肿瘤医师的相互协助。气管镜检查者的工作是筛选合适的患者，放置导管至支气管树以方便放射源传递。放射肿瘤医师主要估算放射剂量，以及估算实际到达肿瘤需要的放射剂量，即放置装有放射源的后装导管靠近肿瘤的区域。近距放疗操作通过鼻下镇静清醒表面麻醉。在气管镜检查过程中，透视引导用于布置皮肤上射线无法穿透的标记物，相当于肿瘤的远端和近端，以帮助放射肿瘤医师描绘放射长度。一个后装导管的外径有 2~3 mm，运用导丝钩放到肿瘤远端，然后气管镜撤出。后装导管在鼻下时是安全的。放射肿瘤医师将模拟放射源放进射线无法穿透标记过的导管，得到正交直线胸片以模仿放射源的路径。一旦最终治疗计划确定，患者转至屏蔽室并将模拟放射源取出。然后放射源导入后装导管并在计算机控制下进入目标位置。放射长度由第一次和最后一次放射源停留的时间确定，以气管镜检查者所做的皮肤标记为指导。在每个肿瘤末端放射距将延长 1 cm。放疗剂量输送完毕后撤去导管，患者在接受短期观察后再出院。HDR 后装技术的使用消除了医务人员暴露在放射源下的风险。

近距放疗显示了对先前没有接受治疗[163-165]和已经接受治疗[166]的中央气道阻塞肺癌患者都有很好的缓解效果。研究显示在改善症状上的效果与气管镜检查相近[164]。据报道，咳嗽改善的有 20%~70%，呼吸困难改善的有 25%~80%，咯血改善的有 70%~90%[167]。正如所预料的那样，气管镜检查能反映近距放疗结果与症状解除相关[168]。有 25% 的患者肺不张已解除[166]。研究报道近距放疗后能改善患者生活质量、肺功能和肺通气—灌注[169,170]。近距放疗后生存获益并没有显示出来。然而，在一项随机研究中，无症状期从单独 LPR 治疗的 2.8 个月增加到 LPR 与 HDR 近距放疗联合治疗的 8.5 个月[171]。如果患者没有接受早期治疗，接受外照射治疗的有效持续时间和生存期要比近距放疗治疗来得好[172]。因此在 EBRT 前，近距放疗并不作为一线治疗。然而近距放疗可以为那些已经接受 EBRT 最大限度治疗的和复发的患者提供治疗。外照射与近距放疗联合治疗已经与仅仅接受外照射治疗不能手术切除的患者进行过比较。有研究报道，主支气管肿瘤阻塞的患者，接受外照射和近距放疗联合治疗的患者中有 57% 的患者肺复张，而仅仅接受外照射治疗的只有 35% 的肺复张[173]。此外，外照射后加用近距放疗对肿瘤局部控制的研究发现正常肺实质暴露在辐射环境下能降至 32%[174]。

早期阶段隐匿的中央气道肿瘤如果无法进行手术，那近距放疗将是一个不错的选择。有报道指出近距放疗后的患者气管内完全起效的有 60%~90%，5 年生存率有 30%~80%[163,175,176]。最近的病例研究显示不符合手术治疗而接受近距放疗的中央型肺癌患者，其中位生存期接近 2 年[177,178]。近距放疗也可以用于治疗肺移植后肉芽组织过度增生[179-182]。

腔内近距放疗有比较多的副反应，其中最需要关注的是咯血和气管瘘管的形成。近距放疗后致命性咯血的发生率为 5%~10%[163,164,178]。近距放疗后存在的恶性肿瘤、直接与近距放疗装置和气管壁接触、邻近区域有主要大血管及联合 LRP 治疗，这些是近距放疗后大咯血的高危因素[183,184]。每次剂量 >10 Gy 也是出血并发症的高危因素[185]。有其他研究提示近距放疗治疗肺上叶肿瘤也是咯血高危因素，这可能是因为过于靠近右肺上叶前段的肺动脉和左肺上叶舌尖段肺动脉[186]。有时候，出血仅仅反映疾病正常发展。近距放疗后有 10% 的患者会发生放射性气管炎和气管狭窄[187]。组织学变化可以是黏膜炎症甚至严重的支气管壁纤维化。放射性气管炎的高危因素有病理为大细胞肺癌、既往行 LPR 治疗、有联合外照射治疗的应用及近距放疗作为治疗[188]。

近距放疗与其他气管镜技术相比有以下优势。对于气管镜检查者而言，是一个简单的操作流程。近距放疗用于在大角度或者支气管亚段的病变部位，而对于 LPR 来说很多时候难以进入。该流程对支气管周围肿瘤也同样有效。主要劣势在于有潜在的严重不良反应及需要昂贵的仪器将放射源送至支气管腔内病变部位。因此，近距放疗的相关设备仅大型三甲医疗中心才有。此外，气管镜检查医师和放射肿瘤医师紧密联系是必要的，但也会引起学科之间的安排冲突。

气管支架

对于气管外源性压迫引起气管狭窄的患者，气管支架在维持气道开放上面占有很重要的地位[189-191]。成功部署气管支架可以快速解除呼吸困难和窒息。很多时候，支架置入可以使呼吸机依赖的患者成功脱机和拔除气管插管[192]。气管腔内肿瘤用其他气管镜介入技术如 LPR 或电烙术处理后，再用支架置入，而支架通常用于外源性气管压迫引起的气管狭窄[193]。对于气管支架的讨论，读者可以阅读第 9 章。

外照射

外照射治疗是晚期、不能手术治疗患者的一种很重要的治疗手段。最近有项研究共 125 例患者，症状缓解的咯血有 68%，咳嗽有 54%，疼痛有 51%，呼吸困难有 38%[194]。然而治疗起效缓慢，放疗后黏膜水肿和炎症可能会使已经有严重中央气道狭窄的患者有潜在进一步恶化的风险。外照射仅仅在气管镜治疗后气管腔重新开放的情况下使用。多个研究已经证实了外照射在腔内肿瘤阻塞引起的肺不张方面的实用性。外照射治疗 21%~74% 的患者有放疗应答和不张的肺再通[195-197]。其中的一项研究中，71% 的患者在接受放疗后的 2 周内肺不张好转，另外 23% 的患者在放疗 2 周后才出现类似效果[197]。

综合治疗

前文讨论的有一点我们不能忽视，即单一气管镜下治疗不能满足每一位恶性中央气道阻塞的患者。一份综合治疗计划对于多数想要获得相对满意治疗效果的患者是必需的。最近的多个病例研究已经证实了多种模式的治疗，即气管镜介入联合外照射、化疗和手术，能更好地缓解症状和治疗晚期中央气道阻塞患者[5,75,96,198-200]。95% 的中央气道阻塞患者接受综合治疗后气管腔重新开放[96,199]。这些研究中的多数患者，联合机械减瘤和激光消融或电烙术治疗腔内气道肿瘤；同时气管支架用于外源性气管压迫的患者。这也提示了综合治疗比单一模式治疗更具有优势。比如有报道显示，非小细胞肺癌中央气道阻塞的患者接受综合治疗后其生存期比仅仅接受 Nd:YAG 治疗的生存期延长了 4.9 个月。另一项研究中，接受单一模式治疗的患者 3 年存活率仅为 2.3%，而接受综合治疗的有 22%[198]。尽管我们清楚既往数据用来进行生存分析的局限性，但这些结果进一步强调了需要一位专门从事卫生保健的专家提供不同的治疗模式，来为恶性中央气道阻塞患者获取理想的治疗效果。

结 论

中央气道阻塞患者有多种治疗方式可供选择。每一例患者对相关技术的选择依赖于中央气道阻塞的严重程度及类型，快速解除其症状是必需的，同时专业技术、患者个人喜好及费用也需要考虑。不管怎么样，有一点需要认识到，即气管镜下介入治疗的首要原则是解除严重的症状如呼吸困难和咯血，以改善患者的生存质量，而不是仅仅延长生存期。但是对患者有获益的很多气管镜技术费用相对较高，有时候难以进行治疗。因此，因晚期和转移瘤或者严重终末期系统性疾病而预期寿命 <3 个月的患者在接受这些操作时需要格外慎重。能通过非气管镜下诊疗手段缓解患者的症状的方法是更好的。此外，我们应充分

认识到多数患者心肺储备功能的严重损害。因此，为避免会引起相关并发症的操作所进行的任何努力都是必要的。很多气管镜治疗都是昂贵的，需要时刻将医疗保健成本记在心里。我们对患者不能夸大这些方法，而是应该慎重、保守，选用性价比高的方法。

参考文献

1. Lee P, Kupeli E, Mehta AC. Therapeutic bronchoscopy in lung cancer. Laser therapy, electrocautery, brachytherapy, stents and photodynamic therapy. Clin Chest Med. 2002;23:241–56.
2. Ernst A, Feller-Kopman D, Becker HD, Mehta AC. Central airway obstruction. Am J Respir Crit Care Med. 2004;169:1278–97.
3. Freitag L. Interventional endoscopic treatment. Lung Cancer. 2004;45 Suppl 2:S235–8.
4. Williamson JP, Phillips MJ, Hillman DR, Eastwood PR. Managing obstruction of the central airways. Intern Med J. 2010;40:399–410.
5. Stephens KE, Wood DE. Bronchoscopic management of central airway obstruction. J Thorac Cardiovasc Surg. 2000;119:289–96.
6. Theodore PR. Emergent management of malignancy related acute airway obstruction. Emerg Med Clin North Am. 2009;27:231–41.
7. Folch E, Mehta AC. Airway interventions in the tracheobronchial tree. Semin Respir Crit Care Med. 2008;29:441–52.
8. Brodsky JB. Bronchoscopic procedures for central airway obstruction. J Cardiothorac Vasc Anesth. 2003;17:638–46.
9. Gorden JA, Ernst A. Endoscopic management of central airway obstruction. Semin Thorac Cardiovasc Surg. 2009;21:263–73.
10. Dela Cruz CS, Tanoue LT, Matthay RA. Lung cancer: epidemiology, etiology, and prevention. Clin Chest Med. 2011;32:605–44.
11. Sorensen JB. Endobronchial metastases from extrapulmonary solid tumors. Acta Oncol. 2004;43:73–9.
12. Braman SS, Whitcomb ME. Endobronchial metastasis. Arch Intern Med. 1975;135:543–7.
13. Kiryu T, Hoshi H, Matsui E, et al. Endotracheal/endobronchial metastasis. Chest. 2001;119:768–75.
14. Shepherd MP. Endobronchial metastatic disease. Thorax. 1982;37:362–5.
15. Ognibene FP, Shelhamer JH. Kaposi's sarcoma. Clin Chest Med. 1988;9:459–65.
16. Garay SM, Belenko M, Fazzini E, Schinella R. Pulmonary manifestations of Kaposi's sarcoma. Chest. 1987;91:39–43.
17. Zibrak JD, Silvestri RC, Costello P, Marlink R, Jensen WA, Robins A, et al. Bronchoscopic and radiologic features of Kaposi's sarcoma involving the respiratory system. Chest. 1986;90:476–9.
18. Webb BD, Walsh GL, Roberts DB, Sturgis EM. Primary tracheal malignant neoplasms: the University of Texas MD Anderson Cancer Center experience. J Am Coll Surg. 2006;202:237–46.
19. Honings J, Gaissert HA, Van Der Heijden HFM, et al. Clinical aspects and treatment of tracheal malignancies. Acta Otolaryngol. 2010;130:763–72.
20. Zimmer W, DeLuca SA. Primary tracheal neoplasms: recognition, diagnosis and evaluation. Am Fam Physician. 1992;45:2651–7.
21. Gaissert HA, Grillo HC, Shadmehr MB, et al. Long term survival after resection of primary adenoid cystic and squamous cell carcinoma of trachea and carina. Ann Thorac Surg. 2004;78:1889–97.
22. Murgu SD, Colt HG. Tracheobronchomalacia and excessive dynamic airway collapse. Respirology. 2006;11:388–406.
23. Marel M, Pekarek Z, Spasova I, et al. Management of benign stenosis of the large airways in the University hospital in Prague, Czech Republic, in 1998–2003. Respiration. 2005;72:622–8.
24. Perotin JM, Jeanfaivre T, Thibout Y, et al. Endoscopic management of idiopathic tracheal stenosis. Ann Thorac Surg. 2011;92:297–302.
25. Brichet A, Verkindre C, Dupont J, et al. Multidisciplinary approach to management of post intubation tracheal stenosis. Eur Respir J. 1999;13:888–93.
26. Hollingsworth HM. Wheezing and stridor. Clin Chest Med. 1987;8:231–40.
27. Geffin B, Grillo HC, Cooper JD, Pantoppidan H. Stenosis following tracheostomy for respiratory care. JAMA. 1971;216:1984–8.
28. Jabbardarjani H, Kiani A, Karimi S, Kharabian S, Masjedi MR. Role of endoscopic treatments in patients with adenoid cystic carcinoma. J Bronchol. 2007;14:251–4.
29. Stoller JK. Spirometry: a key diagnostic test in pulmonary medicine. Cleve Clin J Med. 1992;59:75–8.
30. Acres JC. Clinical significance of pulmonary function tests: upper airway obstruction. Chest. 1981;80:207–11.
31. Boiselle PM, Ernst A. Recent advances in central airway imaging. Chest. 2002;121:1651–60.
32. Boiselle PM, Reynolds KF, Ernst A. Multiplanar and three-dimensional imaging of the central airways with multidetector CT. Am J Roentgenol. 2002;179:301–8.
33. Boiselle PM. Multislice helical CT of the central airways. Radiol Clin North Am. 2003;41:561–74.
34. Lee KS, Lunn W, Feller-Kopman D, Ernst A, Hatabu H, Boiselle PM. Multislice CT evaluation of airway stents. J Thorac Imaging. 2005;20:81–8.
35. Fettetti GR, Kocier M, Calaque O, et al. Follow up after stent insertion in the tracheobronchial tree: role of helical computed tomography in comparison with flexible bromchoscopy. Eur Radiol. 2003;13:1172–8.
36. Dialani V, Ernst A, Sun M, et al. MDCT detection of airway stent complications: comparison with bronchoscopy. Am J Roentgenol. 2008;191:1576–80.
37. LoCicero III J, Costello P, Campos CT, et al. Spiral CT with multiplanar and three-dimensional reconstructions accurately predicts tracheobronchial pathology. Ann Thorac Surg. 1996;62:811–7.
38. Remy-Jardin M, Remy J, Artaud D, Fribourg M, Duhamel A. Volume rendering of the tracheobronchial tree: clinical evaluation of bronchographic images. Radiology. 1998;208:761–70.
39. Haponik EF, Aquino SL, Vining DJ. Virtual bronchoscopy. Clin Chest Med. 1999;20:201–17.
40. Fleiter T, Merkle EM, Aschoff AJ, et al. Comparison of real time virtual and fiberoptic bronchoscopy in patients with bronchial carcinoma: opportunities and limitations. Am J Roentgenol. 1997;169:1591–5.
41. Finkelstein SE, Schrump DS, Nguyen DM, Hewitt SM, Kunst TF, Summers RM. Comparative evaluation of super high-

resolution CT scan and virtual bronchoscopy for the detection of tracheobronchial malignancies. Chest. 2003;124:1834–40.
42. Allah MF, Hussein SRA, Al-Asmar ABH, et al. Role of virtual bronchoscopy in the evaluation of bronchial lesions. J Comput Assist Tomogr. 2012;36:94–9.
43. De wever W, Vendecaveye V, Lanciotti S, Verschakelen JA. Multidetector CT-generated virtual bronchoscopy: an illustrated review of the potential clinical indications. Eur Respir J. 2004;23:776–82.
44. Hoppe H, Dinkel HP, Walder B, von Allmen G, Gugger M, Vock P. Grading airway stenosis down to the segmental level using virtual bronchoscopy. Chest. 2004;125:704–11.
45. Whiteman SC, Yang Y, Gey van Pittius D, et al. Optical coherence tomography: real time imaging of bronchial airways microstructures and detection of inflammatory/neoplastic morphologic changes. Clin Cancer Res. 2006;12:813–8.
46. Williamson JP, Armstrong JJ, McLaughlin RA, et al. Measuring the airway dimensions during bronchoscopy using anatomical optical coherence tomography. Eur Respir J. 2010;35:34–41.
47. Williamson JP, McLaughlin RA, Phillips MJ, Armstrong JJ, Becker S, Walsh JH, et al. Using optical coherence tomography to improve diagnostic and therapeutic bronchoscopy. Chest. 2009;136:272–6.
48. Colt HG. Functional evaluation before and after interventional bronchoscopy. In: Bollinger CT, Mathur PN, editors. Interventional bronchoscopy. Basel, Switzeland: S. Krager; 2000. p. 55–64.
49. Schuurmans MM, Michaud GC, Diacon AH, Bolliger CT. Use of ultrathin bronchoscope in the assessment of central airway obstruction. Chest. 2003;124:735–9.
50. Oki M, Saka H. Thin bronchoscope for evaluating stenotic airways during stenting procedure. Respiration. 2011;82:509–14.
51. Helmers RA, Sanderson DR. Rigid bronchoscopy. the forgotten art. Clin Chest Med. 1995;16:393–9.
52. Ayers ML, Beamis Jr JF. Rigid bronchoscopy in the twenty-first century. Clin Chest Med. 2001;22:355–64.
53. Colt HG, Harrell JH. Therapeutic rigid bronchoscopy allows level of care changes in patients with acute respiratory failure from central airways obstruction. Chest. 1997;112:202–6.
54. Kurimoto N, Murayama M, Yoshioka S, Nishisaka T, Inai K, Dohi K. Assessment of usefulness of endobronchial ultrasonography in determination of depth of tracheobronchial tumor invasion. Chest. 1999; 115:1500–6.
55. Miyazu Y, Miyazawa T, Kurimoto N, Iwamoto Y, Kanoh K, Kohno N. Endobronchial ultrasonography in the assessment of centrally located early-stage lung cancer before photodynamic therapy. Am J Respir Crit Care Med. 2002;165:832–7.
56. Miyazawa T, Miyazu Y, Iwamoto Y, Ishida A, Kanoh K, Sumiyoshi H, et al. Stenting at the flow-limiting segment in tracheobronchial stenosis due to lung cancer. Am J Respir Crit Care Med. 2004;169:1096–102.
57. Herth F, Becker HD, LoCicero 3rd J, Ernst A. Endobronchial ultrasound in therapeutic bronchoscopy. Eur Respir J. 2002;20:118–21.
58. Sarkiss M. Anesthesia for bronchoscopy and interventional pulmonology: from moderate sedation to jet ventilation. Curr Opin Pulm Med. 2011;17:274–8.
59. Conacher ID, Paes LL, McMohan CC, Morritt GN. Anesthetic management of laser surgery for central obstruction: a 12-year case series. J Cardiothorac Vasc Anesth. 1998;12:153–6.
60. Milner QJW, Abdy S, Allen JG. Management of severe tracheal obstruction with helium/oxygen and a laryngeal mask airway. Anesthesia. 1997;52:1087–9.
61. Brodsky JB. Anesthetic considerations for bronchoscopic procedures in patients with central-airway obstruction. J Bronchol. 2001;8:36–43.
62. McMahon CC, Rainey L, Fulton B, Conacher ID. Central airway compression. Anaesthetic and intensive care consequences. Anaesthesia. 1997;52:158–62.
63. Mathisen DJ, Grillo HC. Endoscopic relief of malignant airway obstruction. Ann Thorac Surg. 1989;48:469–75.
64. Watters MP, McKenzie JM. Inhalational induction with sevoflurane in an adult with severe complex central airways obstruction. Anaesth Intensive Care. 1997;25:704–6.
65. Purugganan R. Intravenous anesthesia for thoracic procedures. Curr Opin Anaesthesiol. 2008;21:1–7.
66. Choudhury M, Saxena N. Total intravenous anaesthesia for tracheobronchial stenting in children. Anaesth Intensive Care. 2002;30:376–9.
67. El-Baz N, Jensik R, Faber LP, Faro RS. One-lung high-frequency ventilation for tracheoplasty and bronchoplasty: a new technique. Ann Thorac Surg. 1982;34:564–71.
68. Biro P, Layer M, Becker HD, Herth F, Wiedemann K, Seifert B, et al. Influence of airway-occluding instruments on airway pressure during jet ventilation for rigid bronchoscopy. Br J Anaesth. 2000;85:462–5.
69. Plummer S, Hartley M, Vaughan RS. Anaesthesia for telescopic procedures in the thorax. Br J Anaesth. 1998;80:223–34.
70. Macdonald AG. A brief historical review of nonanaesthetic causes of fires and explosions in the operating room. Br J Anaesth. 1994;73:847–56.
71. Denton RA, Dedhia HV, Abrons HL, Jain PR, Lapp NL, Teba L. Long-term survival after endobronchial fire during treatment of severe malignant airway obstruction with the Nd:YAG laser. Chest. 1988;94:1086–8.
72. Ernst A, Simoff M, Ost D, Goldman Y, Herth FJF. Prospective risk-adjusted morbidity and mortality outcome analysis after therapeutic bronchoscopy procedures. Results of a multi-institutional outcomes database. Chest. 2008;134:514–9.
73. Amjadi K, Voduc N, Cruysberghs Y, et al. Impact of interventional bronchoscopy on quality of life in malignant airway obstruction. Respiration. 2008;76:421–8.
74. Oviatt PL, Stather DR, Michaud G, MacEachern P, Tremblay A. Exercise capacity, lung function, and quality of life after interventional bronchoscopy. J Thorac Oncol. 2011;6:38–42.
75. Hans CC, Prasetyo D, Wright GM. Endobronchial palliation using Nd:YAG laser is associated with improved survival when combined with multimodal adjuvant treatments. J Thorac Oncol. 2007;2:59–64.
76. Razi SS, Levovics RS, Schwartz G, et al. Timely airway stenting improves survival in patients with malignant central airway obstruction. Ann Thorac Surg. 2010;90:1088–93.
77. Venuta F, Rendina EA, Dr Giacomo T, et al. Endoscopic treatment of lung cancer invading the airway before induction chemotherapy and surgical resection. Eur J Cardiothorac Surg. 2001;20:464–7.
78. Chhajed PN, Baty F, Pless M, Somandin S, Tamm M, Brutsche MH. Outcome of treated advanced nonsmall cell lung cancer with and without central airway obstruction. Chest. 2006;130:1803–7.
79. Daddi G, Puma F, Avenia N, Santoprete S, Casadei S, Urbani M. Resection with curative intent after endoscopic treatment of airway obstruction. Ann Thorac Surg. 1998;65:203–7.
80. Venuta F, Rendina EA, De Giacomo T, et al. Nd:YAG laser resection of lung cancer invading the airway as a bridge to surgery and palliative treatment. Ann Thorac Surg. 2002;74:995–8.
81. Bolliger CT, Suteja TG, Strausz J, Freitag L. Therapeutic bronchoscopy with immediate effects:laser, electrocautery, argon plasma coagulation, and stents. Eur Respir J. 2006;27:1258–71.
82. Vergnon JM, Huber RM, Moghissi K. Place of cryotherapy, brachytherapy, and photodynamic therapy in therapeutic bronchoscopy of lung cancers. Eur Respir J. 2006;28:200–18.

83. Lunn W, Garland R, Ashiku S, Thurer RL, Feller-Kopman D, Ernst A. Microdebrider bronchoscopy: a new tool for the interventional bronchoscopist. Ann Thorac Surg. 2005;80: 1485–8.
84. Lunn W, Bagherzadegan N, Munjampappi SK, Feller-Kopman D, Ernst A. Initial experience with a rotating airway microdebrider. J Bronchol. 2008;15:91–4.
85. Hautmann H, Gamarra F, Jurgen K, Huber RM. Fiberoptic bronchoscopic balloon dilatation in malignant tracheobronchial stenosis. Chest. 2001;120:43–9.
86. Noppen M, Schlesser M, Meysman M, Peche R, Vincken W. Bronchoscopic balloon dilatation in the combined management of postintubation stenosis of trachea in adults. Chest. 1997;112:1136–40.
87. Lee KH, Ko GY, Song HY, Shim TS, Kim WS. Benign tracheobronchial stenosis: long term clinical experience with balloon dilation. J Vasc Interv Radiol. 2002;13(9 pt 1):909–14.
88. Sheski FD, Mathur PN. Long-term results of fiberoptic bronchoscopic balloon dilation in the management of benign tracheobronchial stenosis. Chest. 1998;114:796–800.
89. DeGarcia J, Culebras M, Alverez A, et al. Bronchoscopic balloon dilatation in the management of bronchial stenosis following lung transplantation. Respir Med. 2007;101:27–33.
90. Mayse ML, Greenheck J, Friedman M, Kovitz KL. Successful bronchoscopic balloon dilation on nonmalignant tracheobronchial obstruction without fluoroscopy. Chest. 2004;126:634–7.
91. Shitrit D, Kuchuk M, Zismanov V, et al. Bronchoscopic balloon dilation of tracheobronchial stenosis: long-term follow-up. Eur J Cardiothorac Surg. 2010;38:198–210.
92. Kim JH, Shin JH, Song HY, et al. Tracheobronchial laceration after balloon dilation for benign strictures. Incidence and clinical significance. Chest. 2007;131:1114–7.
93. van Boxem TJ, Westerga J, Venmans BJ, Postmus PE, Suteja G. Tissue effects of bronchoscopic electrocautery: bronchoscopic appearance and histologic changes of bronchial wall after electrocautery. Chest. 2000;117:887–91.
94. Sutedja K, van Kralingen, Schramel FMNH, Postmus PE. Fiberoptic bronchoscopic electrosurgery under local anesthesia for rapid palliation in patients with central airway malignancies: a preliminary report. Thorax. 1994;49:1243–6.
95. Coulter TD, Mehta AC. The heat is on. Impact of endobronchial electrosurgery on the need for Nd-YAG laser photoresection. Chest. 2000;118:516–21.
96. Wahidi MM, Unroe MA, Adlakha N, Beyea M, Shofer SL. The use of electrosurgery as the primary ablation modality for malignant and benign airway obstruction. J Thorac Oncol. 2011;6:1516–20.
97. van Boxem TJ, Venmans BJ, Schramel FM, et al. Radiographically occult lung cancer treated with fiberoptic eloectrocautery: a pilot study of simple and inexpensive technique. Eur Respir J. 1998;11:169–72.
98. Sutedja T, van Boxem TJ, Schramel FM, et al. Endobronchial electrocautery is an excellent alternative for Nd:YAG laser to treat airway tumors. J Bronchol. 1997;4:101–5.
99. Horinouchi H, Miyazawa T, Takada K, et al. Safety study of endobronchial electrosurgery for tracheobronchial lesions. Multicenter prospective study. J Bronchol. 2008;15:228–32.
100. Reichle G, Freitag L, Kullman HJ, Prenzel R, Macha HN, Farin G. Argon plasma coagulation in bronchology: a new method-alternative or complimentary? J Bronchol. 2000;7:109–17.
101. Morice RC, Ece T, Keus L. Endobronchial argon plasma coagulation for treatment of hemoptysis and neoplastic airway obstruction. Chest. 2001;119:781–7.
102. Okada S, Yamauchi H, Ishimori S, satoh S, Sugawara H, Tanaba Y. Endoscopic surgery with a flexible bronchoscope and argon plasma coagulation for tracheobronchial tumors. J Thorac Cardiovasc Surg. 2001;121:180–3.
103. Crosta C, Spaggiari L, De Stefano A, et al. Endoscopic argon plasma coagulation for palliative treatment of malignant airway obstruction: early results in 47 cases. Lung Cancer. 2001;33:75–80.
104. Keller CA, Hinerman R, Singh A, Alverez F. The use of endoscopic argon plasma coagulation in airway complications after solid organ transplantation. Chest. 2001;119:1968–75.
105. Reddy C, Majid A, Michaud G, et al. Gas embolism following bronchoscopic argon plasma coagulation. A case series. Chest. 2008;134:1066–9.
106. Chan AL, Tharratt RS, Siefkin AD, Albertson TE, Volz EG, Allen RP. Nd:YAG laser bronchoscopy. Rigid or fiberoptic mode? Chest. 1990;98:271–5.
107. Brutinel WM, Cortese DA, Edell DA, McDougall JC, Prakash UB. Complications of Nd:YAG laser therapy. Chest. 1989;94:902–3.
108. Cavaliere S, Venuta F, Foccoli P, Toninelli C, La Face B. Endoscopic treatment of malignant airway obstructions in 2,008 patients. Chest. 1996;110:1536–42.
109. Dumon JF, Shapshay S, Bourcereau J, et al. Principles of safety in application of neodymium-YAG laser in bronchology. Chest. 1984;86:163–8.
110. Dumon JF, Reboud E, Garbe L, Aucomte F, Meric B. Treatment of tracheobronchial lesions by laser photoresection. Chest. 1982;81:278–84.
111. Cavaliere S, Foccoli P, Farina PL. Nd:YAG loaser bronchoscopy. A five year experience with 1396 applications in 1000 patients. Chest. 1988;94:15–21.
112. Kvale PA, Eichenhorn MS, Radke JR, Miks V. YAG laser photoresection of lesions obstructing the central airways. Chest. 1985;87:283–8.
113. Brutinel WM, Cortese DA, McDougall JC, Gillio RG, Bergstralh EJ. A two-year experience with the neodymium-YAG laser in endobronchial obstruction. Chest. 1987;91:159–65.
114. Hujala K, Sipila J, Grenman R. Endotracheal and bronchial laser surgery in the treatment of malignant and benign lower airway obstruction. Eur Arch Otorhinolaryngol. 2003;260:219–22.
115. Hermes A, Heigener D, Gatzemeier U, Schatz J, Reck M. Efficacy and safety of bronchoscopic laser therapy in patients with tracheal and bronchial obstruction: a retrospective single institution report. Clin Respir J. 2012;6:67–71.
116. Toty L, Personne C, Colchen A, Vourch G. Bronchoscopic management of tracheal lesions using the neodymium yttrium aluminum garnet laser. Thorax. 1981;36:175–8.
117. George PJM, Garrett CPO, Hetzel MR. Role of neodymium YAG laser in the management of tracheal tumors. Thorax. 1987;42:440–4.
118. Stanopoulos IT, Beamis JF, Martinez FJ, Vergos K, Shapshay SM. Laser bronchoscopy in respiratory failure from malignant airway obstruction. Crit Care Med. 1993;21:386–91.
119. Hetzel MR, Nixon C, Edmondstone WM, et al. Laser therapy in 100 tracheobronchial tumors. Thorax. 1985;40:341–5.
120. Gilmartin JJ, Veale D, Cooper BG, Keavey PM, Gibson GJ, Morritt GN. Effects of laser treatment on respiratory function in malignant narrowing of central airways. Thorax. 1987;42:578–82.
121. George PMJ, Clarke G, Tolfree S, Garrett CPO, Hetzel MR. Changes in regional ventilation and perfusion of lung after endoscopic laser treatment. Thorax. 1990;45:248–53.
122. Venuta F, Rendina EA, De Giacomo T, et al. Nd:YAG laser resection of lung cancer invading the airway as bridge to surgery and palliative treatment. Ann Thorac Surg. 2002;74:995–8.
123. Eichenhorn MS, Kvale PA, Miks VM, et al. Initial combination therapy with YAG laser photoresection and irradiation for

123. inoperable non-small cell carcinoma of lung. A preliminary report. Chest. 1986;89:782–5.
124. Gelb AF, Epstein JD. Neodymium-yttrium aluminum garnet laser in lung cancer. Ann Thorac Surg. 1987;43:164–7.
125. Desai SJ, Mehta AC, VanderBurg MS, Golish JA, Ahmad M. Survival experience following Nd:YAG laser photoresection for primary bronchogenic carcinoma. Chest. 1988;94:939–44.
126. Shea JM, Allen RP, Tharratt RS, Chan AL, Seifkin AD. Survival of patients undergoing Nd:YAG laser therapy compared with Nd:YAG laser therapy and brachytherapy for malignant airway disease. Chest. 1993;103:1023–31.
127. Moghissi K, Dixon K. Bronchoscopic Nd:YAG laser treatment in lung cancer, 30 year on: an institutional review. Lasers Med Sci. 2006;21:186–91.
128. Casey KR, Fairfax WR, Smith SJ, Dixon JA. Intratracheal fire ignited by the Nd:YAG laser during treatment of tracheal stenosis. Chest. 1983;84:295–6.
129. Krawtz S, Mehta AC, Wiedemann HP, et al. Nd:YAG laser induced endobronchial burn. Management and long term follow-up. Chest. 1989;95:916–8.
130. Ilgner J, Falter F, Westhofen M. Long-term follow up after laser induced endotracheal fire. J Laryngol Otol. 2002;116:213–5.
131. van Boxem T, Muller M, Venmans B, Postmus B, Suteja T. Nd:YAG laser vs. bronchoscopic electrocautery for palliation of symptomatic airway obstruction: a cost-effectiveness study. Chest. 1999;116:1108–12.
132. Walsh D, Maiwand MO, Nath A, Lockwood P, Lloyd M, Saab M. Bronchoscopic cryotherapy for advanced bronchial carcinoma. Thorax. 1990;45:509–13.
133. Mathur PN, Wolfe KM, Busk MF, Briet M, Datzman M. Fiberoptic bronchoscopic cryotherapy in the management of tracheobronchial obstruction. Chest. 1996;110:718–23.
134. Lee SH, Choi WJ, Sung SW, et al. Endoscopic cryotherapy of lung and bronchial tumors: a systemic review. Korean J Intern Med. 2011;26:137–44.
135. Marasso A, Gallo E, Massaglia GM, Onoscuri M, Bernardi V. Cryosurgery in bronchoscopic treatment of tracheobronchial stenosis. Indications, limits, personal experience. Chest. 1993;103:472–4.
136. Maiwand MO. Cryotherapy for advanced carcinoma of the trachea and bronchi. Br Med J. 1986;293:181–2.
137. Asimakopoulos G, Beeson J, Evan J, Maiwand MO. Cryosurgery for malignant endobronchial tumors. Analysis of outcome. Chest. 2005;127:2007–14.
138. Maiwand MO. The role of cryosurgery in palliation of tracheobronchial carcinoma. Eur J Cardiothorac Surg. 1999;15:764–8.
139. Bertoletti L, Elleuch R, Kaczmarek D, Jean-Francois R, Vergnon JM. Bronchoscopic cryotherapy treatment of isolated endoluminal typical carcinoid tumors. Chest. 2006;130:1405–11.
140. Deygas N, Froudarakis M, Ozenne G, Vergnon JM. Cryotherapy in early superficial bronchogenic carcinoma. Chest. 2001;120:26–31.
141. Vergnon JM, Schmitt T, Alamartine E, Barthelemy JC, Fournel P, Emonot A. Initial combined cryotherapy and irradiation for unresectable non-small cell lung cancer. Preliminary results. Chest. 1992;102:1436–40.
142. Forest V, Hadjeres R, Bertrand R, Jean-Francois R. Optimization and molecular signaling of apoptosis in sequential cryotherapy and chemotherapy combination in human A549 lung cancer xenografts in SCID mice. Br J Cancer. 2009;100:1896–902.
143. Forest V, Peoch M, Campos L, Guyotat D, Vergnon JM. Benefits of a combined treatment of cryotherapy and chemotherapy on tumor growth and late cryoinduced angiogenesis in a non-small cell lung cancer model. Lung Cancer. 2006;54:79–86.
144. Hetzel M, Hetzel J, Schumann C, Marx N, Babiak A. Cryorecanalization: a new approach for the immediate management of acute airway obstruction. J Thorac Cardiovasc Surg. 2004;127:1427–31.
145. Schumann C, Hetzel M, Babiak A, et al. Endobronchial tumor debulking with a flexible cryoprobe for immediate treatment of malignant stenosis. J Thorac Cardiovasc Surg. 2010;1309:997–1000.
146. Edell ES, Cortese DA. Photodynamic therapy: its uses in management of bronchogenic carcinoma. Clin Chest Med. 1995;16:455–63.
147. Cecic I, Minchinton AI, Korbelik M. The impact of complement activation on tumor oxygenation during photodynamic therapy. Photochem Photobiol. 2007;83:1049–55.
148. Dougherty TJ, Marcus SL. Photodynamic therapy. Eur J Cancer. 1992;28A:1734–42.
149. Moghissi K, Dixon K, Stringer M, Freeman T, Thorpe A, Brown S. The place of bronchoscopic photodynamic therapy in advanced unresectable lung cancer: experience on 100 cases. Eur J Cardiothorac Surg. 1999;15:1–6.
150. Ernst A, Garland R, Beamis JF. Photodynamic treatment in lung cancer. J Bronchol. 1996;6:285–8.
151. Mehrishi S, Ost D. Photodynamic therapy. J Bronchol. 2002;9:218–22.
152. McCaughan JS, Williams TS. Photodynamic therapy for endobronchial malignant disease: a prospective fourteen year study. J Thorac Cardiovasc Surg. 1997;114:940–7.
153. Ernst A, Freitag L, Feller-Koppman D, LoCicero J, Ost D. Photodynamic therapy for endobronchial obstruction is safely performed with flexible bronchoscopy. J Bronchol. 2003;10:260–3.
154. Moghissi K, Dixon K, Hudson E, Stringer M, Brown S. Endoscopic laser therapy in malignant tracheobronchial obstruction using sequential Nd:YAG laser and photodynamic therapy. Thorax. 1997;52:281–3.
155. Freitag L, Ernst A, Thomas M, Prenzel R, Wahlers B, Macha HN. Sequential photodynamic therapy (PDT) and high dose brachytherapy for endobronchial tumor control in patients with limited bronchogenic carcinoma. Thorax. 2004;59:790–3.
156. Moghissi K, Dixon K, Parsons RJ. A controlled trial of Nd:YAG laser versus photodynamic therapy for advanced malignant bronchial obstruction. Laser in Med Sci. 1993;8:269–73.
157. Diaz-Jimenez JP, Martinez-Bellarin JE, Llunell A, Farrero E, Rodriguez A, Castro MJ. Efficacy and safety of photodynamic therapy versus Nd:YAG laser resection in NSCLC with airway obstruction. Eur Respir J. 1999;14:800–5.
158. Moghissi K, Dixon K, Andrew J, Thorpe C, Stringer M, Oxtoby C. Photodynamic therapy in early central lung cancer: a treatment option for patients ineligible for surgical resection. Thorax. 2007;62:391–5.
159. Corti L, Toniolo L, Boso C, et al. Long-term survival of patients treated with photodynamic therapy for carcinoma in situ and early non-small cell lung carcinoma. Lasers Surg Med. 2007;39:394–402.
160. Mathur PN, Edell E, Sutedja T, Vergnon JM. Treatment of early non-small cell lung cancer. Chest. 2003;123:176–80.
161. Moghissi K, Dixon K. Is bronchoscopic photodynamic therapy a therapeutic option in lung cancer? Eur Respir J. 2003;22:535–41.
162. Nag S, Kelly JF, Horton JL, et al. Brachytherapy for carcinoma of the lung. Oncology (Winston Park). 2001;15:371–81.
163. Ozkok S, Karakoyun-Celik O, Goksel T, et al. High dose rate endobronchial brachytherapy in the management of lung cancer: response and toxicity evaluation in 158 patients. Lung Cancer. 2008;62:326–33.
164. Kelly JF, Delclos ME, Morice RC, et al. High dose rate brachytherapy effectively palliates symptoms due to airway

tumors: the 10-year M.D. Anderson cancer center experience. Int J Radiat Oncol Biol Phys. 2000;48:697–702.
165. Anacak Y, Mogulcok N, Ozkok S, et al. High dose rate endobronchial brachytherapy in combination with external beam radiation therapy for Stage III non-small cell lung cancer. Lung Cancer. 2011;34:253–9.
166. Hernandez P, Gursahaney A, Roman T, et al. High dose rate brachytherapy for the local control of endobronchial carcinoma following external radiation. Thorax. 1996;51:354–8.
167. DuRand IA, Barber PV, Goldring J, et al. British Thoracic Society guidelines for advanced diagnostic and therapeutic flexible bronchoscopy in adults. Thorax. 2011;66:iii1–21.
168. Guarnaschelli JN, Jose BO. Palliative high dose rate endobronchial brachytherapy for recurrent carcinoma: The University of Louisville experience. J Palliat Med. 2010;13:981–9.
169. Goldman JM, Bulman AS, Rathemell AJ, Carey BM, Muers MF, Joslin CA. Physiological effect of endobronchial radiotherapy in patients with major airway occlusion by carcinoma. Thorax. 1993;48:110–4.
170. Mallick I, Sharma SC, Behera D. Endobronchial brachytherapy for symptom palliation in non-small cell lung cancer- analysis of symptom response, endoscopic improvement and quality of life. Lung Cancer. 2007;55:313–8.
171. Chella A, Ambrogi MC, Ribechini A, et al. Combined Nd:YAG laser/HDR brachytherapy versus Nd:YAG laser only in malignant central airway involvement: a prospective randomized study. Lung Cancer. 2000;27:169–75.
172. Stout R, Barber P, Burt P, et al. Clinical and quality of life outcomes in the first United Kingdom randomized trial of endobronchial brachytherapy (intraluminal radiotherapy) vs external beam radiotherapy in palliative treatment of inoperable nonsmall cell lung cancer. Radiother Oncol. 2000;56:323–7.
173. Langendijk H, de Jong J, Tjwa M, et al. External irradiation versus external irradiation plus endobronchial brachytherapy in inoperable non-small cell lung cancer: a prospective randomized study. Radiother Oncol. 2001;58:257–68.
174. Bastin KT, Mehta MP, Kinsella TJ. Thoracic volume radiation sparing following endobronchial brachytherapy: a quantitative analysis. Int J Radiat Oncol Biol Phys. 1993;25:703–7.
175. Fuwa N, Matsumoto A, Kamata M, et al. External irradiation and intraluminal irradiation using middle dose rate iridium in patients with roentgenographically occult lung cancer. Int J Radiat Oncol Biol Phys. 2001;49:965–71.
176. Marsiglia H, Baldeyrou P, Lartigau E, et al. High dose rate brachytherapy as sole modality for early stage endobronchial carcinoma. Int J Radiat Oncol Biol Phys. 2000;47:665–72.
177. Hennequin C, Bleichner O, Tredaniel J, et al. Longterm results of endobronchial brachytherapy: a curative treatment? Int J Radiat Oncol Biol Phys. 2007;67:425–30.
178. Guilcher MA, Prevost B, Sunyach MP, et al. High dose rate brachytherapy for non-small cell carcinoma: a retrospective study of 226 patients. Int J Radiat Oncol Biol Phys. 2011;79:1112–6.
179. Halkos ME, Godette KD, Lawrence EC, Miller JI. High dose rate brachytherapy in the management of lung transplant airway stenosis. Ann Thorac Surg. 2003;76:381–4.
180. Brenner B, Kramer MR, Katz A, et al. High dose rate brachytherapy for non-malignant airway obstruction: new treatment option. Chest. 2003;124:1605–10.
181. Madu CN, Machuzak MS, Sterman DH, et al. High dose rate brachytherapy for the treatment of benign obstructive endobronchial granulation tissue. Int J Radiat Oncol Biol Phys. 2006;66:1450–6.
182. Tendulkar RD, Fleming PA, Reddy CA, Gildea TA, Machuzak M, Mehta AC. High dose rate endobronchial brachytherapy for recurrent airway obstruction from hyperplastic granulation tissue. Int J Radiat Oncol Biol Phys. 2008;70:701–6.
183. Hara R, Itami J, Aruga T, et al. Risk factors for massive hemoptysis after endobronchial brachytherapy in patients with tracheobronchial malignancies. Cancer. 2001;92:2623–7.
184. Gollis SW, Ryder WD, Burt PA, et al. Massive hemoptysis, death and other morbidity associated with high dose rate intraluminal radiotherapy for carcinoma of bronchus. Radiother Oncol. 1996;39:105–16.
185. Langendijk JA, Tjwa MK, de Jong JM, et al. Massive hemoptysis after radiotherapy in inoperable nonsmall cell lung carcinoma: is endobronchial radiotherapy really a risk factor? Radiother Oncol. 1998;49:175–83.
186. Bedwinek J, Petty A, Bruton C, et al. The use of high dose rate endobronchial brachytherapy to palliate symptomatic endobronchial recurrence of previously irradiated bronchogenic carcinoma. Int J Radiat Oncol Biol Phys. 1991;22:23–30.
187. Speiser B, Spratling I. Remote afterloading brachytherapy for local control of endobronchial carcinoma. Int J Radiat Oncol Biol Phys. 1993;25:579–89.
188. Speiser B, Spratling I. Intermediate dose rate remote afterloading brachytherapy for intraluminal control of bronchogenic carcinoma. Int J Radiat Oncol Biol Phys. 1990;18:1443–8.
189. Saad CP, Murthy S, Krizmaniach G, Mehta AC. Self-expandable metallic airway stents and flexible bronchoscopy. Long-term outcome analysis Chest. 2003;124:1993–9.
190. Husain SA, Finch D, Ahmad M, Morgan A, Hetzel MR. Long term follow up of Ultraflex metallic stents in benign and malignant airway obstruction. Ann Thorac Surg. 2007;83:1251–6.
191. Wood DE, Liu YH, Vallieres E, Karmey-Jones R, Mulligan MS. Airway stenting for malignant and benign tracheobronchial stenosis. Ann Thorac Surg. 2003;76:167–74.
192. Noppen M, Stratakos G, Amjadi K, et al. Stenting allows weaning and extubation in ventilator or tracheostomy dependency secondary to benign airway disease. Respir Med. 2007;101:139–45.
193. Breitenbucher A, Chhajed PN, Brtusche MH, Mordasini C, Schilter D, Tamm M. Long term follow up and survival after ultraflex stent insertion in the management of complex malignant airway stenosis. Respiration. 2008;75:443–9.
194. Reinfuss M, Mucha-Malecka A, Walasek T, et al. Palliative thoracic radiotherapy in non-small cell lung cancer. An analysis of 1250 patients. Palliation of symptoms, tolerance and toxicity. Lung Cancer. 2011;71:344–9.
195. Majid OA, Lee S, Khushalani S, Seydel HG. The response of atelectasis from lung cancer to radiation therapy. Int J Radiat Oncol Biol Phys. 1986;12:231–2.
196. Chetty KG, Moran EM, Sassoon CS, Viravathana T, Light RW. Effect of radiation therapy on bronchial obstruction due to bronchogenic carcinoma. Chest. 1989;95:582–4.
197. Reddy SP, Marks JE. Total atelectasis of the lung secondary to malignant airway obstruction. Response to radiation therapy. Am J Clin Oncol. 1990;13:394–400.
198. Santos RS, Raftopoulos Y, Keenan RJ, Hala A, Maley RH, Landreneau RJ. Bronchoscopic palliation of primary lung cancer. Single or multimodality therapy? Surg Endoscopy. 2004;18:931–6.
199. Jeon K, Kim H, Yu CM, et al. Rigid bronchoscopic intervention in patients with respiratory failure caused by malignant central airway obstruction. J Thorac Oncol. 2006;1:319–23.
200. Neyman K, Sundest A, Espinoza A, Kongerud J, Fosse E. Survival and complications after interventional bronchoscopy in malignant central airway obstruction. A single center experience. J Bronchol Intervent Pulmonol. 2011;18:233–8.

第 9 章

气道支架

Pyng Lee and Atul C. Mehta

本章提要　支架置入是减轻恶性肿瘤中央气道阻塞的常用方法，也用于炎性及感染性气道狭窄的扩张、肺移植术后气道开裂和气管支气管软化。覆膜支架可用于封堵（支）气管食管瘘、开裂的肺切除术后残端。根据患者情况、气道狭窄的特点、医师的专业知识和设备决定使用何种支架。管状支架的放置需要先用硬质支气管镜扩张狭窄，而金属支架可以应用支气管镜灵活使用。本章就常用气道支架的优缺点、技术以及与支架放置相关的并发症进行讨论。

关键词　气道支架，覆膜支架，中央气道狭窄，硬质支气管镜。

引　言

支架是一个能够保持管腔通畅的中空、圆柱形的假腔。它最早由 19 世纪的牙医查尔斯（同时发明了牙科夹板）发明，又称查尔斯支架。气道支架置入术发明至今已有 1 个多世纪，其作用包括限制气道内肿瘤或肉芽组织内生性生长，平衡气道内外的压力[1]。覆膜支架兼有屏障作用，动静态性能决定其支撑效果[2]。第一例治疗气道狭窄的气道支架置入手术由 Trendelenburg[3] 和 Bond[4] 完成，并很快由 Brunings 和 Albrecht 在 1915 年发展为内镜下应用[5]。1965 年，Montgomery 设计了 T 形支架，外侧支由硅酮和橡胶构成，用来治疗声门下狭窄。目前硅酮已成为最常用的支架材料[6]。然而，当时的硅酮支架会破坏气道纤毛清除分泌物的能力，直到 Dumon 提出一种专门用于（支）气管的支架这一问题才有突破。Dumon 支架的制作材料为硅酮，外壁有一些钉状突起，对纤毛运动的影响较小，价格相对低廉，容易移除和替换。限制其广泛应用的一个重要因素是支架置入需要硬质支气管镜[7]。据美国胸科医师学会的调查，美国北部的肺科医师只有 5% 接受过硬质支气管镜培训[8]。此外，声门下的硅酮支架耐受性较差，在面对复杂性气管狭窄时容易移位。针对上述缺点，原本为气管支气管树的血管系统开发的金属支架应运而生[9,10]。金属支架易用纤维支气管镜操作，但会引起支架结点处肉芽组织的明显内生，并嵌入气管壁，增加了移除的难度[10]。金属支架和管状支架可用于恶性狭窄，而在良性疾病中则推荐使用硅酮及混合支架，这样可避免金属支架相关的远期并发症。因此，理想的支架应该是容易置入和移除，能根据狭窄形状调整尺寸，重建管腔抵抗压力，有足够的弹性贴合气道形态，不引起缺血，不侵蚀相邻结构，不容易移位，不诱发感染，不干扰气道内纤毛运动，不诱发肉芽组织，生物相容性好，无刺激性，价格易接受。选择理想的支架已经成为介入肺科医师、放射科医师、胸外科医师、耳鼻喉科医师参与中央气道狭窄患者管理的一部分。

支架置入的适应证（表9.1）

大约30%的肺癌患者会出现中央气道阻塞，其中的35%会死于窒息、咯血、阻塞性肺炎[11]。气道支架置入术是一种有价值的气管镜辅助技术，目的是重建挤压或狭窄的气道，支撑软化的气管支气管以及封闭支气管食管瘘[11,12]。虽然切除原发肿瘤和重建气道能提供最为可靠的治疗，但大部分恶性中央气道狭窄诊断时已是晚期。因此，气管镜治疗加上气道支架置入不仅能快速缓解症状和改善生存质量，还能作为化疗的辅助治疗并可能延长生存时间[1,11-14]。与先前的观点相反，现在的观点认为，如果治疗恰当，恶性气道狭窄并不预示预后不佳。Chhajed团队证明恶性中央气道狭窄在激光、支架治疗后化疗的预后（8.2个月）和那些无气道梗阻的姑息性化疗的预后（8.4个月）相似[15]。

继发于气管插管后的损伤、炎症和感染性疾病的良性气道狭窄，如果患者有基础疾病或相关的合并症不宜手术修复，可能需要放置支架。肺移植后短时间内出现气道开裂的患者置入支架可能获得收益。克利夫兰诊所使用非覆膜金属支架作为肺移植术后重度吻合口开裂的替代治疗，不仅气道愈合良好，而且容易移除（8周内）[16]。

支架类型

支架的种类繁多，根据所用材料及制作工艺分为3大类：①管状（高分子聚合物）：Montgomery T形管, Dumon, Polyflex, Noppen, Hood；②金属（覆膜或非覆膜）：

表9.1 支架的适应证

恶性肿瘤
1. 外来气管压迫或黏膜下病变所致的气道阻塞
2. 气管内肿瘤经激光治疗后堵塞50%以上
3. 侵袭性支气管肿瘤生长，重复激光治疗后复发
4. 肿瘤所致骨性支架破损
5. 支气管食管瘘，依次放置气道和食管支架

良性气道疾病
1. 纤维化瘢痕或瓶颈以下狭窄
   (1) 外伤：气管插管、气管切开、激光、球囊成形术
   (2) 感染：支气管内膜结核、组织胞浆菌病-纤维性纵隔炎、疱疹病毒、白喉、鼻硬结克雷伯菌
   (3) 炎症：Wegener肉芽肿、结节病、炎性肠病、异物吸入
   (4) 肺移植术后吻合口并发症
2. 气管支气管软化症
   (1) 弥漫性：特发性、复发性多软骨炎、气管支气管肥大（Mounier-Kuhn syndrome）
   (2) 局限性：气管切开术、化疗后肺移植
3. 良性肿瘤
   (1) 乳头状瘤病
   (2) 淀粉样变性

Gianturco，Palmaz，Ultraflex；③混合式（金属环加固的硅胶）：Orlowski，Dynamic（图 9.1 和 9.2）。管状支架价格低廉，易于再放置和移除。缺点包括支架移位，肉芽肿形成，黏液堵塞，支架厚度与气道内径比例不佳；无法贴合非规则气道；难以放置在远端气道；干扰纤毛清除功能；需要硬质支气管镜放置。硬质支气管镜操作是一大障碍，全球范围内相关技术的培训量正在骤减[8]。

金属支架由于置入方便、普及较广，可在门诊使用。根据使用方法进行分类：球囊扩张支架（被动膨胀式支架）依赖于适合靶点直径的球囊，而自膨胀式支架具有形状记忆能力，在移出工作孔道后能恢复至预定形状（图 9.4）。其他优点包括能够放射显影，有更大的通气面积，有贴合气道的生理弯曲，保留了纤毛的清除功能，架在叶段支气管开口处而不影响通气。主要缺点是支架内肉芽组织形成、感染，6~8 周嵌入气管后难以移除和再放置（图 9.5 A，B）。

支架选择

除了放置位置，狭窄的形状和长度，有无气管软化或瘘管也是支架选择时需要考虑的因素。针对气管支气管的内径选择合适尺寸的支架是至关重要的。合适的支架能减少并发症的发生，如支架移位，黏液堵塞，肉芽肿形成和肿瘤生长。管状支架的放置需要硬质支气管镜，而金属支架则可通过纤维支气管镜放置，在门诊就能使用。支架的选择应具体情况具体分析。内镜医师选择支架的类型和内径时需考虑到患者的收益和预后、气道的病理改变、后续的治疗以及技术、设备和团队。管状支架最适于良性狭窄，因为它容易更换和移除，对黏膜的损伤也较小。复发性多软骨炎或气管肥大综合征则首选非覆膜金属支架，因为它们对纤毛清除功能的干扰及移位的概率较小[19,20]。慢性阻塞性肺病引起的呼气性气道塌陷，在标准化治疗包括无创通气失败[21]后，可考虑使用容易移除

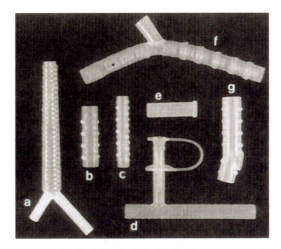

图 9.1 管状和混合支架的类型。A. Rusch 支架；B. Dumon 气管支架；C. Dumon 支气管支架；D. Montgomery T 管；E. Hood 支气管支架；F. Orlowski 支架；G. Hood 可定制气管支气管支架

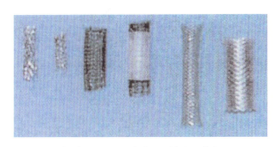

图 9.2 各类型金属支架，从左到右：Palmaz 支架、Strecker 支架，非覆膜 UltraFlex 支架，覆膜 UltraFlex 支架，非覆膜 Wall 支架，覆膜 Wall 支架

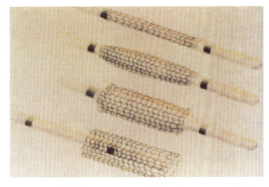

图 9.3 球囊扩张 Palmaz 支架和 Strecker 支架。球囊扩张支架由球囊支撑起合适的内径

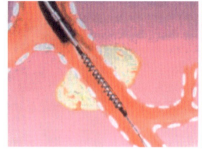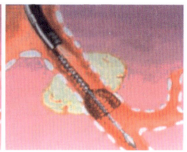

图 9.4 自膨胀 Ultraflex 支架放置系统：Ultraflex 支架由工作孔道内的拉钩送至目标位置后释放

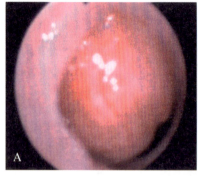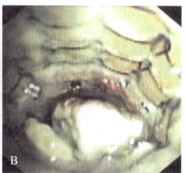

图 9.5 支架相关并发症。A. 硅酮 Dumon 支架致远端阻塞性肉芽肿形成；B.Ultraflex 支架致远端肉芽肿形成伴铜绿假单胞菌感染。

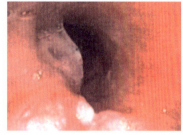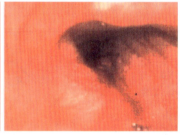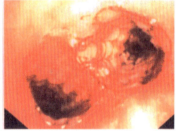

图 9.6 左主支气管食管瘘伴食管癌所致的右主支气管浸润。由纤维支气管镜放置的 2 个覆膜自膨胀金属支架

的支架。覆膜金属支架和管状支架都能应用于恶性狭窄[11,14,15,17,18]和气管食管瘘（图 9.6）[22,23]。

支架置入技术

支架放置前最好使用硬质支气管镜、导管或球囊确定狭窄气道的最佳扩张直径。肿瘤组织可以用激光或电烧灼去除，经球囊或钳夹处理后再放置支架。管状支架通常用硬质支气管镜放置，而金属支架则用纤维支气管镜放置。

管状支架

Montgomery 支架

Montgomery 支架至今只做了些许修改，一直用于声门下气管狭窄的治疗[6]。制作材料由硅酮取代了早期的丙烯酸，3 条管腔都有不同的内径和长度。该支架一般用于气管切开术后，可在气管切开时放置或经硬质支气管镜放置。突出在气管造口外的部分是为环状软骨或声门狭窄设计的，开放时可清洁气道，关闭支架通常在激光切除气道恢复通畅后放置（图 9.7）。在一项多中心试验中，对 1 574 例患者放置了该支架，其中 698 例为恶性气道梗阻。结果 9.5% 发生支架移位，8% 有肉芽肿形成，4% 出现管腔再次狭窄（恶性狭窄随访 4 个月，良性病变随访 14 个月）[24]。Diaz-Jimenez 和 Cavaliere 的研究得到类似的结果[11]。Dumon 支架自推出以来，已成为应用最广的支架，许多专家视其为"金标准"。成人和儿童均能使用，视气管狭窄情况选用合适的内径和长度。还有一种分叉支架，称为 Dumon Y 支架，可缓解下段气管和 / 或气管分叉处狭窄（图 9.8）。然而 Dumon 支架并不适用于气管支气管软化或封堵气管 - 食管瘘，因为该支架的固定依赖于气道壁与突起之间的压力和摩擦阻力。

Noppen 支架

Noppen 支架的材料是聚乙烯，外侧壁有类似夹板螺钉的结构，需要特殊设备放置。有研究表明 Noppen 支架治疗良性气道狭窄时较少发生移位[26]。

Polyflex 支架

Polyflex 支架是自膨胀式支架，由交叉的聚酯涤纶线嵌入硅酮制成，由硬质支气管镜放置。交叉点由钨制成，可以显影。与上两种支架相比，它有更薄的管壁。可选择不同的长度和内径，适用于良恶性气道狭窄和气管食管瘘。锥形部分可用来封闭残端瘘。但是，它表面光滑，较易移位。在一组研究中，12 例患者共使用了 16 个 Polyflex 支架，用于肺移植后的吻合口狭窄、气管狭窄、气管支气管软化、骨软骨质沉着性气管支气管病、复发性多软骨炎、支气管胸膜瘘。该支架的移位率高达 75%，多发生在支架放置后 24 小时至 7 个月[27]。

Dynamic 支架

Dynamic 支架为分叉的硅酮支架，马蹄形的金属环结构模拟了气管软骨和无软骨的后壁，

表 9.2　Dumon 支架和覆膜 Ultraflex 支架比较

特性	Dumon 支架	覆膜 Ultraflex 支架
机械因素		
高内外径比值	−	+++
耐压缩	+	++
径向力	+	++
移位	−	+
适用变形气道	−	+++
可移除	+++	−
膨胀	−	++
定制	+++	−
兼容性		
生物惰性	++	++
肉芽组织	+	−
肿瘤内生	+	−
简便性		
能由纤维支气管镜放置	−	+++
意识清晰下局部麻醉	−	++
X 线透视定位	−	+++
是否易再放置	++	−
价格		
价廉	+	−

注：−. 否；+. 轻；++. 中；+++. 重

时可以说话。因为管腔的一端固定在气管造口处，所以极少发生移位；因为不靠紧贴气道来固定位置，所以对上段气管血液和淋巴回流的影响较少。故此管对高度气管狭窄是比较安全的。

Dumon 支架

Dumon 是由硅酮制成的圆管状支架，外周布满突起，由硬质支气管镜放置[7]。Dumon

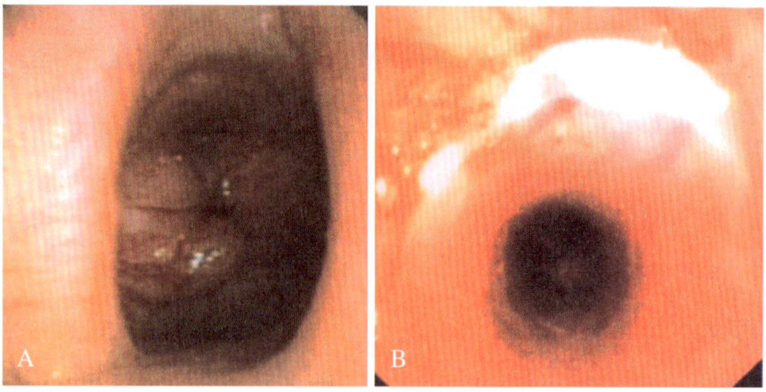

图 9.7 A. 气管腺样囊性癌引起气道几乎完全阻塞；B. 激光切除肿瘤和经硬质支气管镜放置硅酮支架

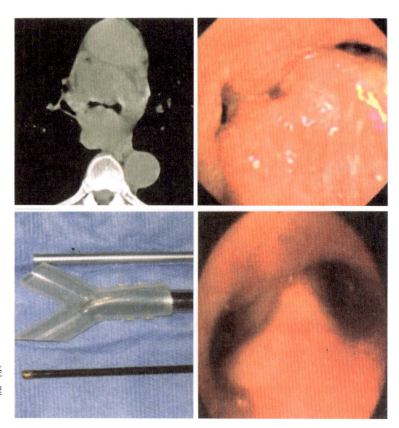

图 9.8 Y 形 Dumon 支架经硬质支气管镜放置，缓解淋巴结转移所致隆突受压

咳嗽时就由气管膜部向内部突出。此类支架一般用于气管、隆突、主支气管处的狭窄，也用于气管支气管软化、气管支气管肥大症和支气管食管瘘，用专用钳或硬质支气管镜放置较为方便（图 9.9），支架断裂、分泌物滞留等情况少见。

金属支架

球囊扩张支架

Palmaz 支架和 Strecker 支架可以扩张到 11~12 mm，限用于儿童。Palmaz 支架不适用于成人，因其可塑性好但弹性差，剧烈咳嗽、肿

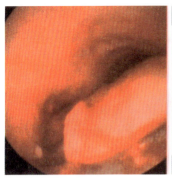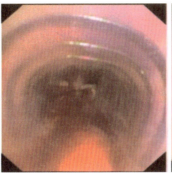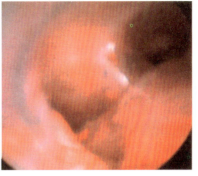

图 9.9 Y 型 Rusch 支架模拟气道结构：前部有金属环加固，后部较柔软

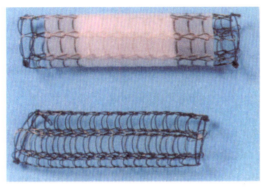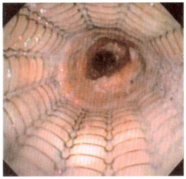

图 9.10 覆膜及非覆膜 Ultraflex 支架

瘤或血管结构的压迫会造成其塌陷、阻塞和移位[28]。Strecker 支架可扩张至 20~40 mm，用于成人的指征仅限于短段狭窄，因为不需调度上的调节[29]。Palmaz 支架和 Strecker 支架无覆膜，在放化疗后可能松动，故不适合恶性狭窄。

自膨胀支架

Ultraflex 支架是最常用的自膨胀式支架，有覆膜和非覆膜两种。Ultraflex 支架通过均匀的径向力固定支架，降低了黏膜穿孔的风险。它采用 1 根具有形状记忆功能的镍钛合金，因而在低温时具有良好的可塑性，而温度较高时，支架立刻恢复至设计形状。Miyazawa 等共放置了 54 根 Ultraflex 支架治疗 34 例无法手术治疗的恶性气道狭窄患者。82% 患者的呼吸困难立刻得到缓解。未发现痰液潴留及支架移位；支架能够移除和再放置，放置在声门下也较安全[30]。它不需 X 线透视辅助即可放置，减少了辐射暴露[31]。常见的并发症包括传染性支气管炎（15.9%），阻塞性肉芽肿（14.6%，需要多次介入治疗再通），肿瘤内生（6.1%），此外，4 例患者支架发生移位，1 例 2 年后支架软化[32]。

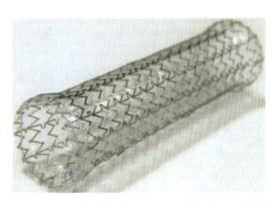

图 9.11 混合支架（Alveolus 支架），可由纤维支气管镜或硬质支气管镜放置，X 线显影

Alveolus 支架

Alveolus 支架是一种聚氨酯覆膜金属支架，因其可以很容易地被移除而用于非肿瘤性气道狭窄，可用硬质支气管镜或纤维支气管镜放置。由特有的装置通过纤维支气管镜通道确定合适的大小。此装置的末端带有测量工具，测量范围是 6~12 mm，另一端有手柄。当内部导线从手柄上收回时，测量装置的外圈张开。一旦释放了可通过气管镜观察到的由颜色条编码的管腔直径来选择合适尺寸的支架。Alveolus 支架是一个钛镍合金网固定的同心环经激光雕刻而成的支架。因其结构特征，它的长度容易更改，放置前无须压缩[33]。已有由该支架塌陷引起咯血和呼吸困难的相关报道[34]。

参考文献

1. Bolliger CT, Sutedja TG, Strausz J, Freitag L. Therapeutic bronchoscopy with immediate effect: laser, electrocautery, argon plasma coagulation and stents. Eur Respir J. 2006;27:1258–71.
2. Freitag L. Tracheobronchial stents. In: Bolliger CT, Mathur PN, editors. Interventional bronchoscopy, Progress in respiratory research, vol. 30. Basel, Switzerland: Karger; 2000. p. 171–86.
3. Trendelenburg F. Beitrage zu den Operationen an den Luftwegen. Langenbecks Arch Chir. 1872;13:335.
4. Bond CJ. Note on the treatment of tracheal stenosis by a new T-shaped tracheostomy tube. Lancet. 1891;I:539–40.
5. Brunings W, Albrecht W. Direkte Endoskopie der Luft und Speisewege. Stuttgart: Enke; 1915. p. 134–8.
6. Montgomery WW. T-tube tracheal stent. Arch Otolaryngol. 1965;82:320–1.
7. Dumon JF. A dedicated tracheobronchial stent. Chest. 1990;97:328–32.
8. Colt HG, Prakash UB, Offord KP. Bronchoscopy in North America: survey by the American Association for Bronchology. J Bronchol. 2000;7:8–25.
9. Dasgupta A, Dolmatch BC, Abi-Saleh WJ, et al. Selfexpandable metallic airway stent insertion employing flexible bronchoscopy: preliminary results. Chest. 1998;114:106–9.
10. Lemaire A, Burfeind WR, Toloza E, et al. Outcomes of tracheobronchial stents in patients with malignant airway disease. Ann Thorac Surg. 2005;80:434–8.
11. Cavaliere S, Venuta F, Foccoli P, et al. Endoscopic treatment of malignant airway obstruction in 2008 patients. Chest. 1996;110:1536–42.
12. Colt HG, Harrell JH. Therapeutic rigid bronchoscopy allows level of care changes in patients with acute respiratory failure from central airways obstruction. Chest. 1997;112:202–6.
13. Bolliger CT, Probst R, Tschopp K, Soler M, Perruchoud AP. Silicone stents in the management of inoperable tracheobronchial stenoses. Indications and limitations. Chest. 1993;104:1653–9.
14. Lee P, Kupeli E, Mehta AC. Therapeutic bronchoscopy in lung cancer. Laser therapy, electrocautery, brachytherapy, stents, and photodynamic therapy. Clin Chest Med. 2002;23:241–56.
15. Chhajed PN, Baty F, Pless M, et al. Outcome of treated advanced non-small cell lung cancer with and without airway obstruction. Chest. 2006;130:1803–7.
16. Mughal MM, Gildea TR, Murthy S, et al. Short-term deployment of self-expanding metallic stents facilitates healing of bronchial dehiscence. Am J Respir Crit Care Med. 2005;172:768–71.
17. Mehta AC, Dasgupta A. Airway stents. Clin Chest Med. 1999;20:139–51.
18. Rafanan AL, Mehta AC. Stenting of the tracheobronchial tree. Radiol Clin North Am. 2000;38:395–408.
19. Dunne JA, Sabanathan S. Use of metallic stents in relapsing polychondritis. Chest. 1994;105:864–7.
20. Collard PH, Freitag L, Reynaert MS, et al. Terminal respiratory failure from tracheobronchomalacia. Thorax. 1996;51:224–6.
21. Murgu SD, Colt HG. Complications of silicone stent insertion in patients with expiratory central airway collapse. Ann Thorac Surg. 2007;84:1870–7.
22. Colt HG, Meric B, Dumon JF. Double stents for carcinoma of the esophagus invading the tracheobronhial tree. Gastrointest Endosc. 1992;38:485–9.
23. Freitag L, Tekolf E, Steveling H, et al. Management of malignant esophago-tracheal fistulas with airway stenting and double stenting. Chest. 1996;110:1155–60.
24. Dumon J, Cavaliere S, Diaz-Jimenez JP, et al. Sevenyear experience with the Dumon prosthesis. J Bronchol. 1996;3:6–10.
25. Diaz-Jimenez JP, Farrero Munoz E, et al. Silicone stents in the management of obstructive tracheobronchial lesions:2 year experience. J Bronchol. 1994;1:15–8.
26. Noppen M, Meysman M, Claes I, et al. Screw-thread vs. Dumon endoprosthesis in the management of tracheal stenosis. Chest. 1999;115:532–5.
27. Gildea TR, Murthy SC, Sahoo D, et al. Performance of a self-expanding silicone stent in palliation of benign airway conditions. Chest. 2006;130:1419–23.
28. Slonim SM, Razavi M, Kee S, et al. Transbronchial Palmaz stent placement for tracheo-bronchial stenosis. J Vasc Interv Radiol. 1998;9:153–60.
29. Strecker EP, Liermann D, Barth KH, et al. Expandable tubular stents for treatment of arterial occlusive diseases: experimental and clinical results. Radiology. 1990;175:87–102.
30. Miyazawa T, Yamakido M, Ikeda S, et al. Implantation of Ultraflex nitinol stents in malignant tracheobronchial stenoses. Chest. 2000;118:959–65.
31. Herth F, Becker HD, LoCicero J, Thurer R, Ernst A. Successful bronchoscopic placement of tracheobronchial stents without fluoroscopy. Chest. 2001;119:1910–2.
32. Saad CP, Murthy S, Krizmanich G, et al. Selfexpandable metallic airway stents and flexible bronchoscopy. Chest. 2003;124:1993–9.
33. Hoag JB, Juhas W, Morrow K, Standiford SB, Lund ME. Predeployment length modification of a selfexpanding metallic stent. J Bronchol. 2008;15:185–90.
34. Trisolini R, Paioli D, Fornario V, Agli LL, Grosso D, Patelli M. Collapse of a new type of self-expanding metallic tracheal stent. Monaldi Arch Chest Dis. 2006;65:56–8.

第 10 章
支气管热成形术治疗重症哮喘
Sumita B. Khatri and Thomas R. Gildea

本章提要 支气管热成形术（BT）是药物治疗效果不佳的难治性重症哮喘患者的一种新的治疗方法。高剂量吸入糖皮质激素和长效支气管舒张剂后无法控制症状的人群可用本方法。BT 使用射频能量减少哮喘中反应过度的气道平滑肌。由于气道平滑肌关系到气道高反应性和气道收缩，BT 可以辅助抗炎治疗。热能由主支气管远端传输至直径 3~10 mm 的可见气道，右肺中叶除外。BT 包括 3 个不同的部分，最常见的并发症为哮喘急性发作，因此操作前后均需密切监测。临床试验已经证明 BT 较为安全，且能提高哮喘患者的生存质量，改善其症状，提高卫生资源利用率。故 FDA 在 2010 年批准 BT 治疗哮喘。最近有证据表明 BT 能使患者受益 2 年之久。选择合适的患者，优化复杂的条件，以及持续的哮喘管理是改善预后的关键因素，能够减少不良事件的发生。随着相关经验的积累，将会有更多的哮喘患者从中受益。

关键词 重症哮喘，顽固性哮喘，支气管热成形术，射频消融术。

引　言

支气管热成形术（BT）是药物治疗效果不佳的难治性重度持续性哮喘患者的一种新的治疗方法。BT 是在可视条件下控制射频能量对气道平滑肌进行热处理，在 2010 年经 FDA 批准用于重症哮喘的治疗[1,2]。完整的 BT 治疗通常在门诊完成，它包括 3 个不同的部分，每个部分至少持续 3 周。治疗时通过在支气管镜工作通道引入导管将热能引导至直径 3~10 mm 的可见气道内。治疗的顺序由远及近。最先处理右下叶，然后左下叶，最后双侧上叶。由于可能引起肺不张和右肺中叶综合征，故右肺中叶一般不治疗。临床试验证明，对于药物治疗控制不佳的重症哮喘患者，BT 是安全的，并能改善症状、提高生存质量和医疗资源利用率。BT 最常见的不良反应是呼吸系统并发症，如哮喘发作[2-5]。选择合适的患者和哮喘的优化管理对 BT 的成功开展是至关重要的。BT 最适合那些药物治疗无效但对 BT 耐受性较好的患者。在这一章节中，我们将讨论 BT 的科学依据，临床应用，步骤，并发症等。

科学依据：哮喘的病理生理及治疗效果的潜在机制

哮喘与慢性气道炎症、气道高反应和气流阻塞有关。包括嗜酸性粒细胞、肥大细胞、淋巴细胞、巨噬细胞、中性粒细胞和上皮细胞在内的多种细胞[6]在哮喘的发病机制中发挥作用。呼吸急促和支气管痉挛在哮喘中较为常见，与组胺、白三烯、前列腺素、过敏或非过敏性因素有关。持续的炎症可引起气道重塑，基底膜增厚，胶原纤维沉积，杯状细胞增生伴黏液分泌增加，血管增生，平滑肌肥厚等[6,7]。这些变化可能导致不可逆的气道狭窄和阻塞，即使药物治疗也难以控制[6]。在慢性难治性哮喘患者中，气道平滑肌出现的过度增生和肥厚，在某些情况下导致异常的支气管痉挛和气道关闭。虽然气道高反应性可以暂时用支气管舒张剂和抗炎治疗控制，但控制进行性加重的平滑肌肥大颇具难度。BT正是着眼于此。

气道平滑肌在哮喘中的作用尚未完全阐明。早期针对气道阻塞和气流受限机制的研究表明，75%的鼻后气流受限发生在前6~8级气道，暗示较大的气道也参与其中[8]。正常气道中，平滑肌在结构支持、通气、促进黏液清除、咳嗽和促进淋巴回流中发挥作用。然而在哮喘患者中，气道平滑肌参与支气管痉挛，并通过炎症介质促进气道高反应。此外，气道平滑肌细胞通过合成细胞因子和肥大细胞浸润介导气道炎症和重塑[9-11]。气道平滑肌细胞因其非必需的作用被称为"肺的附件"[12]。没有证据表明，去除气道平滑肌会明显抑制正常的气道功能，但是异常的气道平滑肌会加重哮喘的严重程度。因此，针对肥大平滑肌的治疗可能是重症持续性哮喘的干预靶点[13]。

临床应用：重症难治性哮喘和支气管热成形术的适用人群

哮喘是一种伴有发作性呼吸困难、咳嗽、喘息的慢性气道炎症，人群中的发病率约为8%[6]。大多数哮喘患者能够通过抗炎治疗、行为改变和疾病管理控制症状。自从国家哮喘教育和预防计划（NAEPP）临床实践指南发布以来（1991、1997、2002年），我们对哮喘的病理生理机制和治疗有了更深刻的认识[14-16]。2007版最新指南强调了对哮喘严重程度分类的重要性。然而哮喘控制评估（包括损害和风险评估）同样重要。目前，重症哮喘占所有哮喘的10%，因发作频繁，往往需要紧急救治，占用了较多的医疗资源。哮喘的住院负担沉重，据估计，每年超过456 000人住院，140万患者因此耽误了工作[6,17]。多数情况下，抗炎治疗和远离过敏原是能够控制哮喘发作的。但有些重症哮喘的患者，即使经过充分的药物治疗后症状仍难以控制。为了更好地发现和管理重症难治性哮喘患者，美国胸科学会（ATS）将重度难治性哮喘定义为需持续或间歇（超过半年）口服或高剂量吸入糖皮质激素方能控制的哮喘（图10.1）[18]。此外，需满足下述次要标准中的至少两个：持续气道阻塞和最大呼气流量（PEF）的变化，每日需额外药物控制，吸入/口服类固醇激素减量致哮喘加重，每年多于3次口服糖皮质激素冲击治疗，急救治疗，最近发生过致命性哮喘[19]。这些重症哮喘患者较适合BT。

临床试验：哮喘支气管热成形术的发展和评估

射频消融术已用于肺癌和心律失常的治疗[20,21]。动物（狗）试验中，针对气道平滑肌使用射频消融术能够减少平滑肌数量[1]。之后，通过对非哮喘、轻中度哮喘和中重度哮喘患者的临床研究和试验，确定了BT的适应证、不良反应和预期结果[2-5]。

前期的动物试验证实，对狗的气道应用热能（65℃和75℃）能够持续抑制气道高反应长达3年[1]。热能治疗1周后即可发现气道平滑肌退化或消失，且这些变化的程度与气道高反应的程度成反比。试验动物的不良反应包括咳嗽、气道壁炎性水肿、黏液潴留、热能接触部位的灼伤等。这项超过3年的研究尚未发现平滑肌再生的证据。

随后的临床研究将纳入人群定为将行肺癌切除术的患者[2]。8例患者[平均年龄（58±8.3）岁]在术前5~20天对需切除的直径1 cm气道进行BT治疗（55℃和65℃）。每例患者治疗3~9个点。术中内镜下可见除部分气道狭窄或线性灼伤外，其余肺组织无明显变化。组织学检查显示，65℃热处理后的气道平滑肌与未

难治性哮喘：典型临床特征的会议共识 *, †

主要特征：为控制轻-中度持续性哮喘：
1. 半年或以上持续或间歇口服糖皮质激素
2. 需高剂量 ICS 治疗

药 物	剂量（μg/d）	剂 量
a. 丙酸倍氯米松	> 1 260	> 40 puffs（42 μg/ 吸入） > 20 puffs（84 μg/ 吸入）
b. 布地奈德	> 1 200	> 6 puffs
c. 氟尼缩松	> 2 000	> 8 puffs
d. 丙酸氟替卡松	> 880	> 8 puffs（110 μg） > 4 puffs（220 μg）
e. 曲安奈德	> 2 000	> 20 puffs

次要特征：
1. 每日除 ICS 外，还需 LABA、茶碱或白三烯拮抗剂等药物治疗
2. 每日或几乎每日需 SABA 控制哮喘症状
3. 持续性气流受限（FEV1 < 80% 预计值；PEF 昼夜变异 > 20%）
4. 每年至少 1 次哮喘的急救处理
5. 每年至少 3 种口服类固醇激素冲击治疗
6. 口服或吸入糖皮质激素减量 < 25% 后症状急剧恶化
7. 过去有致命性哮喘发作

注：*. 需排除诱发加重的因素存在，以及患者感觉普遍粘连
†. 难治性哮喘的定义需至少 1 项主要标准和 2 项次要标准

图 10.1 重症难治性哮喘美国胸科协会共识。[引自 2012 American Thoracic Society. Proceedings of the ATS workshop on refractory asthma: current understanding, recommendations, and unanswered questions. American Thoracic Society. Am J Respir Crit Care Med Dec 2000;162（6）:2341–2351. Official journal of the American Thoracic Society]

处理组相比数量减少了 50%，且无明显咯血、呼吸道感染和支气管过度刺激等表现。一项前瞻性研究观察了 BT 治疗 16 例轻度至中度哮喘患者的效果[22]。参与者在 BT 治疗当天及前一天服用 30~50 mg 的泼尼松。3 次 BT 治疗之间相隔 3 周（不治疗右肺中叶）。BT 治疗后使用支气管舒张剂可改善 12 周和 1 年时的 FEV1，但与 2 年后相比无显著差异。无症状天数在治疗后 12 周增加了 50%~73%（P=0.015），2 年后的气道高反应显著降低（乙酰胆碱法）。最常见的副作用为咳嗽、呼吸困难、喘息、支气管痉挛，多出现在治疗后的 2~5 天内，通常不严重，也不需住院治疗。1~2 年后行胸部 CT 检查未发现有肺实质或支气管壁结构的变化。此项研究证实，BT 治疗轻中度哮喘是安全可行的。

第一个围绕 BT 的大型多中心研究采用前瞻性随机非盲法，观察了吸入糖皮质激素（ICS）和长效 β 受体激动剂（LABA）的中重度哮喘患者[3]。入选者为每日需要 200 mg 或更多与丙酸倍氯米松等效 ICS 且无法停用 LABA 的哮喘患者，随机接受 BT+ICS+LABA 或 ICS+LABA 治疗。112 例患者（18~65 岁）在参加试验前哮喘持续 6 周，FEV1 占预计值 60%~85%，乙酰甲胆碱诱导气道高反应后 FEV1 减少 20%（< 8 mg/ml）。在持续至少 9 周的 3 部分治疗后的 3、6、9 月尝试停用 LABA，治疗组 3 月和 12 月的轻度发

作次数和抢救药物使用数量明显降低，3、6、12月时的晨起峰流速有所改善。无症状天数及哮喘生活质量评分（AQLQ 和 ACQ）较对照组明显增加。然而，治疗组也在 BT 期间出现了更多的呼吸道不良事件，因哮喘发作、肺下叶不张、胸膜炎住院的人数也较多[3]。此外，BT 组 FEV1 或气道高反应无明显变化。此试验中治疗组哮喘症状和轻度发作次数有改观，但仍需要增设随机试验组与安慰剂组[3]。

为评价 BT 在重症哮喘患者中的安全性，Pavord 团队进行了重症哮喘试验（Research in Severe Asthma, RISA）[4]。此项研究中，高剂量吸入激素（>750 mg 氟替卡松/日），泼尼松 30 mg/d，FEV1 占预测值 50%，乙酰甲胆碱试验阳性的哮喘患者（n=17）随机接受 BT 或药物治疗（n=17）。16 周的 BT 治疗期中，吸入和口服类固醇的剂量没有改变，之后进入为期 14 周的类固醇减量期（2~4 周减量 20%~25%）。不良事件包括 7 例住院患者，其中哮喘加重 4 例，

肺不张 2 例。尽管 BT 治疗后短期内哮喘相关的发病率有所增加，但 BT 组急救吸入装置的使用率明显减少，FEV1 得到改善，AQLQ 和 ACQ 评分也有所增加。安慰剂效应虽然存在，但 BT 疗效更确切[4]。

随后的临床研究解决了安慰剂效应[5]。部分参与者被随机分为纤维支气管镜对照组（无射频治疗）。此试验对除纤维支气管镜检查人员外的所有患者及调查人员双盲。主要比较的是治疗组与对照组在 6，9，12 月时的 AQLQ 评分，同时还比较了哮喘控制评分、症状评分、峰流速、急救药物使用和 FEV1。两组的特征基线基本相同（BT 组 196 例，对照组 101 例）。超过 80% 的参与者符合重症难治性哮喘的 ATS 标准[19]。但最近 1 年内曾因哮喘急性发作至少住院 3 次、至少 3 次下呼吸道感染、至少 4 次增加糖皮质激素用量的患者除外。结果显示，BT 组 6，9，12 月时的 AQLQ 基线水平较对照组明显提高（图 10.2）。但两组的 AQLQ 评分只

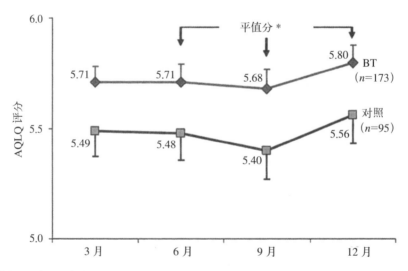

图 10.2　治疗组生活质量变化。BT 组和对照组治疗 12 月后 AQLQ 评分变化。* 后验概率 = 97.9%。[引自 2012 American Thoracic Society. Castro M, Rubin AS, Laviolette M, et al. Effectiveness and safety of bronchial thermoplasty in the treatment of severe asthma: a multicenter, randomized, double-blind, sham-controlled clinical trial. Am J Respir Crit Care Med. Jan 15 2010;181（2）:116–124. Official Journal of the American Thoracic Society]

相差 0.5。与对照组相比，BT 组急性加重次数有所减少 [0.48:0.70，平均加重次数 = 加重次数 /（人·年）；后验概率 =96%]，急诊数量也减少了 84%（图 10.3）。两组均有不良事件发生。在治疗阶段，BT 组有 16 例患者需要住院治疗，呼吸道症状包括哮喘加重、肺不张、下呼吸道感染、FEV1 下降、哮喘引起的蛀牙。其中 1 例咯血患者行支气管动脉栓塞治疗。相比之下，对照组只有 2 例需要住院治疗。有趣的是，对照组中 64% 的病例提示了安慰剂的作用[23]。BT 组则有 79% 的患者 AQLQ 评分增加，且增幅 > 0.5。因此，此项大型多中心随机双盲对照临床研究表明，BT 能长期改善哮喘患者的生存质量，降低医疗费用[5]，但早期并发症较多，且费用昂贵。

FDA 的许可和长期跟踪

2010 年 FDA 批准 Alair® 系统用于治疗 18 岁以上的重症持续性哮喘患者和 ICS 及 LABA 控制不佳的哮喘患者[24]。大多数机构根据已发表的研究来确定适应人群。ICS 和 LABA 控制不佳的重症持续性哮喘患者可考虑 BT 治疗。作为批准条件的一部分，FDA 还需要一项 AIR2 长期随访研究，进而确定可以预测 BT 的远期疗效的因素。一项为期 2 年的 AIR2 研究证实，接受 BT 治疗的患者哮喘急性发作次数、不良事件次数、急诊需求和住院次数均下降，遗憾的是无法与对照组比较，因对照组的大部分患者在治疗后 1 年失访，且未收集哮喘生存质量方面的信息[25]。此外，FDA 还需一项前瞻性开放单组多中心的研究来评估治疗效果、短期和长期的安全性。

BT 器械和步骤说明

BT 在 Alair® 系统中进行，通过纤维支气管镜内径 2 mm 的工作管道提供的射频热能改变气道平滑肌（图 10.4）[26]。导丝远端的电极可逐级治疗

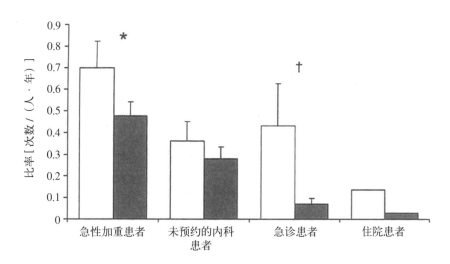

图 10.3　BT 治疗后医疗事件发生情况。严重恶化（需全身应用糖皮质激素或加倍 ICS），急诊治疗，住院治疗。白色：对照组。黑色：BT 组。数值用"平均值 ± 标准误"表示。* 后验概率 = 95.5%；† 后验概率 = 99.9%。[引自 2012 American Thoracic Society. Castro M, Rubin AS, Laviolette M, et al. Effectiveness and safety of bronchial thermoplasty in the treatment of severe asthma: a multicenter, randomized, double-blind, sham-controlled clinical trial. Am J Respir Crit Care Med. Jan 15 2010;181（2）:116–124. Official Journal of the American Thoracic Society]

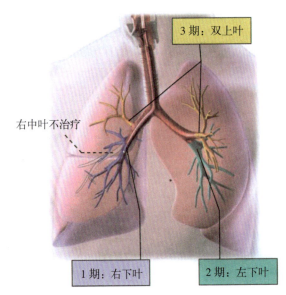
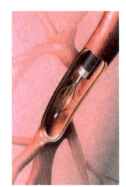

图 10.4　BT 传送射频热灼烧平滑肌，减少支气管痉挛，改善症状。治疗分 3 期进行，定位精细。首先是右下叶，其次是左下叶，最后双肺上叶。右中叶一般不处理（经允许引自 Gildea TR, Khatri SB, Castro M. Bronchial thermoplasty: A new treatment for severe refractory asthma. Cleve Clin J Med 2011; 78:477–485。印刷自 2011 Cleveland Clinic Foundation.）

到最小直径 3 mm 的叶段支气管。电极可自由撑开，撑开后的 4 个点接触气道壁，每个点都有 5 mm 的治疗区域。控制单元可检测热能，避免过热。

BT 治疗前需全面评估患者。治疗前后的护理重点总结在表 10.1 内。符合下列条件的患者可考虑 BT：①最大剂量药物治疗下仍难以控制的哮喘。②至少 1 年未抽烟。③无射频消融相关的禁忌证。④能暂停抗凝治疗。⑤得到控制的胃食管反流病、鼻窦疾病、阻塞性睡眠呼吸暂停低通气综合征、声带功能紊乱。装有起搏器或除颤器的患者禁用，育龄妇女需行孕检。

为减轻炎症反应，患者在术前 3 天至术后 1 天应每天预防性服用 50 mg 泼尼松。过去 6 周有需全身性糖皮质激素治疗的哮喘，6 周内有下呼吸道感染史，或 1~2 周内有上呼吸道感染者，需推迟 BT 治疗。BT 前 1 天及当天需进行评估，确保哮喘稳定。术前常规雾化吸入沙丁胺醇（2.5~5.0 mg）可稳定肺功能。BT 当天的 FEV1 变异率需控制在 10%~15%。完整的疗程分为相对独立的 3 期，每期间隔 2~3 周。一般首先处理右下叶，然后为左下叶，最后是双上叶（图 10.5）。治疗通过纤维支气管镜内直径 ≥ 2 mm 的通道进行。治疗过程通常需要镇静（如芬太尼，咪达唑仑，局部使用利多卡因）。在长期咳嗽或感到不适时，可以使用全身麻醉。治疗时吸入的氧气浓度需严格控制在 40% 以下，患者躯干部位需放置接地胶垫。

BT 治疗需要专业的解剖知识和能力，以确保治疗不重复，不遗漏。每期操作需要重复 50~75 次，治疗时间为 40~60 分钟。患者治疗后至少休息 3~4 小时，确保术后肺功能高于基线的 80%。术后 1 天需服用 50 mg 泼尼松[27]。

并发症

最常见的并发症是哮喘，通常在术后 1~7 天发作。不良事件在积极治疗组更常见，包括需住院治疗的哮喘加重、肺不张、下呼吸道感染和胸膜炎[3,6]。为确保安全，严格把控适应证、术中及术后积极监测、术后随访是必要的（表10.1）。

限 制

BT 并非适用于所有重症哮喘患者。大多数情况下，服用抗炎药物和远离过敏原可较好地控制哮喘。对那些大剂量药物无法控制的持续性哮喘患者，需要考虑是否存在其他影响因素。肺功能较差、症状不稳定的患者不宜 BT 治疗。

BT 价格昂贵，无法进行成本 - 效益分析，限制了其普及。

应当注意，BT 只适用于哮喘，治疗经验不能推广至 COPD 和支气管扩张。目前吸烟者不包括在临床试验中。吸烟患者多数情况下不考虑 BT 治疗。其他注意事项包括：能够耐受纤维支气管镜检测，暂停抗凝治疗，间质性肺病、肺气肿或囊性纤维化等呼吸系统疾病的存在。控制不佳的高血压、临床症状明显的心血管疾病、安装起搏器或除颤器的患者不适合 BT 治疗。

展 望

由于 BT 是治疗哮喘的新方法，不断积累的临床经验将有助于确定可能获得最大收益的患者。BT 虽不能治愈哮喘，但能改善气道痉挛和气道高反应。BT 治疗需要细心且经验丰富的操作人员及术后的密切随访。此外，通过观察性研究确定患者特征和由生物标志物预测成功率也是必要的。

结 论

一些临床试验证实了 BT 的安全性和可行性，提高了药物控制不佳哮喘的临床疗效。同时表明，哮喘是（小）气道的疾病，治疗直径 3 mm 或更大的气道有助于改善症状及生存质量、降低医疗费用[5]。

表 10.1　BT 患者护理概述

患者选择
- 哮喘确诊
- 大量药物治疗仍未控制的难治性哮喘
- 支气管舒张剂使用前 FEV1 > 60%
- 得到控制的胃食管反流病、阻塞性睡眠呼吸暂停低通气综合征、鼻窦疾病
- 无严重的冠状动脉疾病或心律失常
- 耐受停抗凝治疗
- 至少 1 年未吸烟
- 未埋入心脏起搏器或除颤器
- 耐受纤维支气管镜检查

预处理
- 最大化哮喘治疗
- BT 治疗前 3 天及治疗当天口服泼尼松 50 mg/d
- 排除妊娠。育龄妇女行妊娠检测
- 气管镜检查前雾化吸入沙丁胺醇

推迟 BT 治疗
- 无法控制的支气管痉挛
- SpO_2 < 90%（非吸氧）
- 近 6 周有需要增加类固醇剂量才能控制的哮喘急性加重
- 先前有过持续性气道炎症、红斑或感染
- 过去 2 周内有上呼吸道感染
- 过去 6 周内有下呼吸道感染

治疗过程中
- 放置接地垫
- 吸入氧分压 < 40%
- 至少准备 2 根导管
- 气管镜检查时控制咳嗽

治疗后护理
- 留观 3~4 小时
- FEV1 稳定在术前值的 80% 以上时可出院
- 术后 1 天服用 50 mg 泼尼松
- 24~48 小时内电话联系患者
- 2~3 周时正式评估疗效，安排后期 BT 治疗

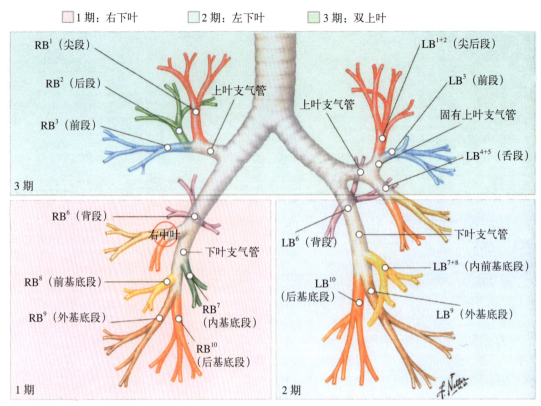

图 10.5 BT 治疗分 3 期进行。右肺中叶通常不治疗。治疗需谨慎，避免遗漏或重复。RB：右主支气管；LB：左主支气管

参考文献

1. Danek CJ, Lombard CM, Dungworth DL, et al. Reduction in airway hyperresponsiveness to methacholine by the application of RF energy in dogs. J Appl Physiol. 2004;97:1946–53.
2. Miller JD, Cox G, Vinic L, Lombard CM, Loomas BE, Danek CJ. A prospective feasibility study of bronchial thermoplasty in the human airway. Chest. 2005;127:1999–2006.
3. Cox G, Thomson NC, Rubin AS, et al. Asthma control during the year after bronchial thermoplasty. N Engl J Med. 2007;356:1327–37.
4. Pavord ID, Cox G, Thomson NC, et al. Safety and efficacy of bronchial thermoplasty in symptomatic, severe asthma. Am J Respir Crit Care Med. 2007;176:1185–91.
5. Castro M, Rubin AS, Laviolette M, et al. Effectiveness and safety of bronchial thermoplasty in the treatment of severe asthma: a multicenter, randomized, doubleblind, sham-controlled clinical trial. Am J Respir Crit Care Med. 2010;181:116–24.
6. National Asthma Education and Prevention Program, National Heart Lung and Blood Institute. Expert Panel Report 3:Guidelines for the Diagnosis and Management of Asthma, summary report 2007. J Allergy Clin Immunol. 2007;120:S94–138.
7. Akinbami L, Moorman J, Liu X. Asthma prevalence, health care use, and mortality: United States, 2005–2009. National health statistics reports, No. 32. Hyattsville, MD: National Center for Health Statistics; 2011.
8. Ingram RH, McFadden ER. Localization and mechanisms of airway responses. N Engl J Med. 1977;297:596–600.
9. Solway J, Irvin CG. Airway smooth muscle as a target for asthma therapy. N Engl J Med. 2007;356:1367–9.
10. Berger P et al. Tryptase-stimulated human airway smooth muscle cells induce cytokine synthesis and mast cell chemotaxis. FASEB J. 2003;17:2139–41.
11. Carroll NG, Mutavdzic S, James AL. Distribution and degranulation of airway mast cells in normal and asthmatic subjects. Eur Respir J. 2002;19:879–85.
12. Mitzner W. Airway smooth muscle: the appendix of the lung. Am J Respir Crit Care Med. 2004;169:787–90.
13. Cox PG et al. Radiofrequency ablation of airway smooth muscle for sustained treatment of asthma: preliminary investigations. Eur Respir J. 2004;24(4):659–63.
14. NHLBI, EPR. Expert panel report: guidelines for the diagnosis and management of asthma (EPR 1991). NIH Publication No. 91-3642. Bethesda, MD: US Department of Health and Human Services; National Institutes of Health; National Heart, Lung, and Blood Institute; National Asthma Education and Prevention Program, 1991; 1991.

15. NHLBI, EPR-2. Expert panel report 2: guidelines for the diagnosis and management of asthma (EPR-2 1997). NIH Publication No. 97-4051. Bethesda, MD: US Department of Health and Human Services; National Institutes of Health; National Heart, Lung, and Blood Institute; National Asthma Education and Prevention Program, 1997; 1997.
16. NHLBI, EPR-Update 2002. Expert panel report: guidelines for the diagnosis and management of asthma. Update on selected topics 2002 (EPR–Update 2002). NIH Publication No. 02-5074. Bethesda, MD: US Department of Health and Human Services; National Institutes of Health; National Heart, Lung, and Blood Institute; National Asthma Education and Prevention Program, June 2003; 2002.
17. National Center for Health Statistics (NCHS), Centers for Disease Control and Prevention, National health interview survey (NHIS 2005). 2005.
18. American Thoracic Society. Proceedings of the ATS workshop on refractory asthma: current understanding, recommendations, and unanswered questions. Am J Respir Crit Care Med, 2000;162:2341–51.
19. Moore WC, Bleecker ER, Curran-Everett D, et al. Characterization of the severe asthma phenotype by the National Heart, Lung, and Blood Institute's Severe Asthma Research Program. J Allergy Clin Immunol. 2007;119:405–13.
20. Ambrogi MC, Fanucchi O, Lencioni R, Cioni R, Mussi A. Pulmonary radiofrequency ablation in a single lung patient. Thorax. 2006;61:828–9.
21. Benussi S, Cini R, Gaynor SL, Alfieri O, Calafiore AM. Bipolar radiofrequency maze procedure through a transseptal approach. Ann Thorac Surg. 2010;90:1025–7.
22. Cox G, Miller JD, McWilliams A, Fitzgerald JM, Lam S. Bronchial thermoplasty for asthma. Am J Respir Crit Care Med. 2006;173:965–9.
23. Wise RA, Bartlett SJ, Brown ED, et al. Randomized trial of the effect of drug presentation on asthma outcomes: the American Lung Association Asthma Clinical Research Centers. J Allergy Clin Immunol. 2009;124:436–44. 444e1-8.
24. FDA. Approval of Alair bronchial thermoplasty system: Alair catheter and Alair RF controller. 2010.
25. Castro M, Rubin A, Laviolette M, et al. Persistence of effectiveness of bronchial thermoplasty in patients with severe asthma. Ann Allergy Asthma Immunol. 2011;107:65–70.
26. Gildea TR, Khatri SB, Castro M. Bronchial thermoplasty: a new treatment for severe refractory asthma. Cleve Clin J Med. 2011;78:477–85.
27. Mayse M, Laviolette M, Rubin AS, et al. Clinical pearls for bronchial thermoplasty. J Bronchol. 2007; 14:115–23.

第 11 章
经支气管镜肺减容术
Cheng He and Cliff K. C. Choong

本章提要 慢性阻塞性肺病（COPD）是世界范围内导致呼吸系统发病和死亡的主要病因之一。肺减容术已经被证实对以上叶肺为优势肺和低运动耐量的 COPD 患者有效，但是它也伴随着许多不足：严重的并发症、住院时间长和高费用。近几年，许多支气管镜技术尝试在取得相似效果的同时，减少并发症的发生和相关费用的产生。有研究报道，在非均质性肺气肿患者的气道放置单向支气管瓣膜会有一定的临床收益。对于肺大叶完全阻塞和缺少侧支通气的患者，肺减容术后的功能恢复更好。虽然目前已经开始尝试对均质性肺气肿患者使用特别设计的支架作为气道旁路，但是支架阻塞仍然是主要问题。还有一些新的研究表明，使用支气管肺减容线圈、支气管内密封胶和经支气管镜热蒸汽消融术能取得相似结果。经支气管镜肺减容术领域正在快速发展，因此需要更多临床研究来确定理想患者和最有效的技术。

关键词 经支气管镜肺减容术，慢性阻塞性肺病，支气管瓣膜，气道旁路，经支气管镜热蒸汽消融术，肺减容线圈。

引 言

肺气肿是一种以肺组织缺失为特点的不可逆性、进展性和衰弱性疾病。现有的治疗严重肺气肿的方法包括内科治疗和手术治疗。尽管包括吸入疗法和肺康复疗法在内的内科治疗有效，但是许多患者还是会出现明显的肺功能缺失。手术治疗为肺减容术和肺移植。肺移植只在高选择性的患者中进行，并且存在供体缺乏、需要终身接受免疫抑制治疗的限制，以及永久性排斥反应、闭塞性细支气管炎和感染的风险。美国国家肺气肿治疗试验证明对于合理选择的、双上肺为主和低运动耐量的非均质性肺气肿患者，肺减容术能显著改善肺功能、运动耐量、生存质量和生存率[1]。但是，由于肺减容术的高筛选标准和手术相关的发病和死亡风险，我们已经在寻找更新、更安全的肺减容方法。

对严重肺气肿的支气管内治疗方法在过去的 10 年中已经出现。各式各样的方法被报道，包括支气管瓣膜和线圈、支气管镜下放置气道旁路支架和通过生物学试剂诱导反应性瘢痕形成[2-9]。这些新方法的目的是提供治疗严重肺气肿的微创方法，避免传统手术方法的致病率、死亡率和高费用的问题。同时，由于肺减容术或肺移植可以考虑的患者较少，相比之下，这些不同的治疗方法有希望被应用到更广大的患者群体中。技术选择依赖于 CT 影像形态学下肺气肿亚型的区分，可以是均质性的或非均质性的。我们将会对各种支气管镜技术和现有的数据进行综述。

观念一：用于非均质性肺气肿患者的支气管气道内放置单向活瓣

第一个观念是将单向活瓣放置于气道内，使得气流只能朝气道外流动（如呼气方向气流），而不能通过活瓣向气道内流动。这样做是为了通过一些支气管活瓣阻断肺段和亚段气道对所有过度膨胀节段或肺叶的气流供应，以产生有效的肺减容作用。支气管活瓣的不同大小使它可以放置在不同大小的支气管内，它通过纤维支气管镜的工作通道放置，必要时可以移除[10,11]。

这种治疗方法针对非均质性肺气肿的患者，适用人群和肺减容术类似。Pulmonx 和 Spiration 两个公司分别生产 Zephyr 支气管活瓣（图11.1）和螺旋伞状支架（图 11.2）[12,13]。尽管两种活瓣的设计不同，但是它们都具备上面描述的特点。两种活瓣具体的设计和特色可以在两个公司的网站上找到[12,13]。

Pulmonx 的 Zephry 单向活瓣

Zephyr® 支气管活瓣是一种由覆盖硅胶膜的镍钛合金自膨式固定器连接的单向鸭嘴活瓣[12]。它可以通过 2.8 mm 的纤维支气管镜放置。这个装置的目的是将患病肺的部分（过度膨胀）隔离开，只让患病肺呼出的气体和分泌物通过，避免气体进入阻断部分。诱导隔离的肺气肿节段出现肺不张能获得理想的肺减容效果，从而让肺活动更有生理学价值。

在多个独立试验和一个多中心试验取得有利结果后，又进行了两个随机试验[3,14-17]。支气管内瓣膜减轻肺气肿试验（VENT）是一个随机的、前瞻性的和多中心试验，它对比了对重度非均质性肺气肿使用 Zephyr 支气管活瓣（Pulmonx）和最佳内科治疗的安全性和有效性。共同主要疗效终点是采用多属性、意向性治疗分析方法检测第一秒用力呼气容积和 6 分钟行走测试的百分比改变（从基线到 6 个月）。在美国支气管内瓣膜减轻肺气肿试验中入组了 321 例患者，其中的 220 例被随机分配到使用支气管活瓣治疗组，101 位被分配到对照组（标准内科治疗）。试验中观察到支气管活瓣组的一秒用力呼气容积（组间中位数差异 6.8%，$P=0.002$）和 6 分钟行走测试（中位数差异 5.8%，$P=0.019$）比起对照组有适度改善[3]。这些肺功能、运动耐量和症状上的适度改善同时伴随 COPD、肺炎和咯血频数加重等代价。观察到的整体结果和欧洲支气管内瓣膜减轻肺气肿试验的研究结果类似[14]。

来自美国和欧洲两方面的支气管内瓣膜减轻肺气肿试验为理解影响生理学和临床预后的重要的患者因素提供了有价值的见解。在亚组分析中区别出两个影响获得最佳肺减容效果和临床反应的因素：①肺叶完全阻塞；②非均质

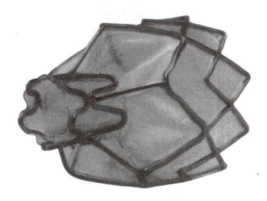

图 11.1　Zephyr 支气管活瓣（来自 Pulmonx 有限公司，加利福尼亚）

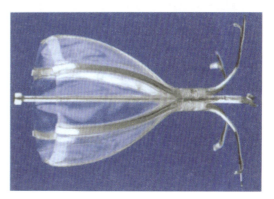

图 11.2　螺旋伞状支架

性更强，且治疗肺叶和邻近肺叶之间有完整的肺裂。

高分辨率 CT 被用来定量靶治疗肺叶的体积改变、判断肺裂的完整性和识别支气管活瓣治疗后的肺叶阻塞。在两项支气管内瓣膜减轻肺气肿试验中，伴有完整肺裂的患者接受支气管活瓣治疗后第一秒用力呼气容积比肺裂不完整的患者有显著改善（美国支气管内瓣膜减轻肺气肿试验：6 个月内 16.2% vs. 2%）。通过支气管活瓣将靶肺叶从节段气道中完全隔离，在理论上可以获得期望的肺减容效果。确实，对于CT 上肺裂完整、存在肺叶阻塞的患者（如最理想活瓣放置治疗患者）使用支气管活瓣比不存在肺叶阻塞的患者预后更好：靶肺叶容积平均减少 80% vs. 29%、在 6 个月内增加 26% vs. 6%（欧洲支气管内瓣膜减轻肺气肿试验）。并且，对欧洲支气管内瓣膜减轻肺气肿试验队列的进一步分析发现，临床反应和肺减容程度直接相关[18]。

一些患者在进行了支气管活瓣放置后，仍然无法取得显著的肺减容效果。这个结果被认为是称作侧支通气（CV）的现象造成的[18,19]。对切除的人肺叶研究发现，21%~30% 的斜裂和近 88% 的右水平裂存在严重缺失，并且这些肺裂不完整的区域会出现 CV[20,21]。在正常肺中，这些侧支通道的阻力比较高，导致了 CV 最小。而肺气肿时这些通道的阻力比气道阻力低，使得肺叶间出现 CV。将支气管活瓣放置于存在 CV 的地方不太可能会出现肺不张，因为气体会通过侧支通道进入靶肺叶。因此，能识别这些"后门"通道，并能够只针对 CV 低或缺失的肺叶优化肺叶隔离效果，使得借助支气管活瓣可显著改善预后[18]。

在支气管内瓣膜减轻肺气肿试验中发现，胸部 CT 上肺裂完整度与支气管活瓣放置后肺叶体积改变和第一秒用力呼气容积改善程度有联系。基于这个发现，可以推测在选择支气管镜肺减容患者时，CT 上肺裂的完整度可以当作 CV 缺乏的指标。高分辨率 CT 上非均质性肺气肿的表现更明显，也能作为低 CV 或没有 CV 的影像学生物指标。

与此同时也发展出了检测 CV 的支气管镜系统（Chartis），它是由装有远端顺应性球囊组件的一次性使用导管组成的，通过球囊的膨胀阻断气道[12]。气体只能通过导管的内腔从目标间隔流出进入外界。连接到控制台后，气道流量和压力能直接显示（图 11.3）。气道阻力可以计算，并且随后可以测定在隔离的肺间隔中是否存在 CV。测定气流的逐渐减少提示球囊阻塞远端气道的 CV 缺乏，而持续的气流读数提示在靶肺叶存在 CV。在最近一项入组 80 例患者的研究中，评估了这个系统用来识别能够受益于支气管活瓣治疗患者的有效性[18]。高分辨率 CT 被用来识别存在最严重肺气肿破坏的肺叶，即认为是支气管活瓣放置的靶肺叶，并且使用 Chartis 评估这一肺叶。虽然 Chartis 在活瓣放置前进行，但是它并不影响靶肺叶的选择。主要的终点结果是靶肺叶容积减少 > 350 ml，这个结果标准来自支气管内瓣膜减轻肺气肿试验，研究观察到对照组（只进行内科治疗）的最大靶肺叶容积减少量很少有超过这一水平的[3,18]。Chartis 在预测活瓣放置后的显著肺减容作用上达到了 75% 的精确度：对 51

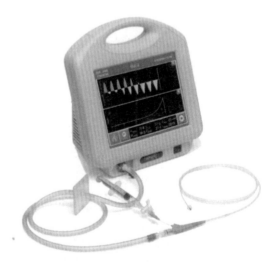

图 11.3 Chartis 系统（来自 Pulmonx 有限公司，加利福尼亚）

例患者中 36 例被分类为 CV 阴性的患者实现了靶肺体积减小 ≥ 350 ml。这个结果等同于单独进行高分辨率 CT 肺裂完整性分析，后者的精确度为 77%[22]。Chartis 存在的技术问题是会导致一些患者不显示测量结果[23]。存在最小 CV 时，Chartis 系统在识别合适的靶肺叶上是对高分辨率 CT 的有价值的补充，能确保对支气管活瓣治疗的最佳反应。但是，对它的潜力的预测还需要进一步更高功效的随机研究评估。

螺旋伞状支架

类似于 Zephyr 活瓣，螺旋伞状支架也是一个留置支气管内装置，被设计用来阻塞气流进入肺气肿的靶肺段。这个单向活瓣位于 6 个聚氨酯覆盖的镍钛合金支架上，形状像一把雨伞，允许活瓣变构并密封气道，同时对黏膜施加最小压力（图 11.4）[13]。螺旋伞状支架能够通过胸片可见（图 11.5），并且在许多病例中，随访胸片可以发现气体潴留显著减少（图 11.6）。

螺旋伞状支架预试验研究团队在 2009 年发表了一份报道，该研究入组了 98 例双上肺为主的非均质性肺气肿患者。在 3 年的单组病例系列、开放性队列研究中，他们在 13 个国际医学中心进行治疗，将支气管活瓣放置在双侧肺上叶[10]。虽然 56% 的患者在健康相关的生存质量上出现临床上有意义的改善，但是这和标准肺

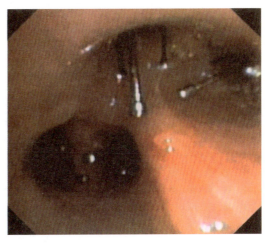

图 11.4 放置在节段支气管的螺旋伞状支架在支气管镜下的外观

功能与运动研究的改善没有关联。通过 CT 证明了 > 85% 的患者出现靶肺叶容积减少。一定比例的患者非靶肺叶（如非肺上叶）容积也有所增加，而总肺容积保持不变。吸入气体的重新导向，包括吸入气体转向健康肺组织，并且通过灌注扫描的改变证实，非上叶（非治疗）肺实质通气/灌注匹配的改善可以作为临床预后改善的机制。

最常见的器械相关副作用是气胸（n=8），推测是邻近组织的张力导致的，抑或是肺叶或肺段容积减小时，肺小泡、大泡或粘连出现过

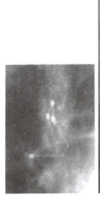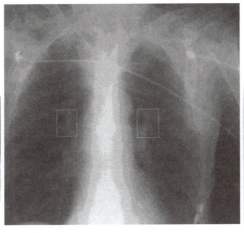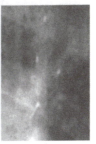

图 11.5 胸片显示了两上肺放置的螺旋伞状支架

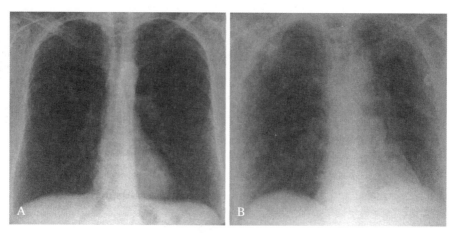

图 11.6　螺旋伞状支架放置前（A）和放置后（B）的胸片。在术后的胸片中观察到肺过度通气和气体潴留显著减少

度膨胀。同时治疗肺舌段和肺上叶时，肺叶不张和产生气胸之间的相关性最明显，导致18例患者中的6例出现左侧气胸。停止舌段治疗后没有发现左侧气胸的进一步发作。螺旋伞状支架没有手术相关死亡的报道，30天死亡率是1.1%，相比肺减容术更佳（美国国家肺气肿治疗试验中30天死亡率为16%）[24]。鉴于支架放置技术的成功率为99.7%，并且不发生支架移位或支架侵蚀，相关感染概率<2.5%，因此作者总结，主要的安全性预后目标成功达成[10]。

美国多中心数据在2010年发表，该数据囊括了上述研究中98例患者中的91例，并得出相似的结果和结论[4]。

2012年Ninane等发表了第一个对支气管活瓣治疗的双盲、对照评估研究[25]。这项随机研究使用了螺旋伞状支架进行双侧不完全阻塞靶肺叶治疗。37例患者置入活瓣，而36例进行假手术支气管镜检查。阳性反应者的标准基于圣乔治呼吸问卷（SGRQ）的分数改变，≥4分时与CT下测得肺容积改变（双上肺容积减小，伴非治疗肺叶容积代偿增加≥7.5%）的复合终点作为标准。在3个月后，24%的治疗组患者被鉴定为阳性反应者，而对照组没有。治疗组的容积存在显著的由双上肺（均数±标准差，−7.3%±9.0%）向非治疗肺叶（6.7%±14.5%）的转移，而对照组没有显著改变（$P<0.05$）。然而，两组间不存在肺功能、呼吸困难和圣乔治呼吸问卷（SGRQ）分数的统计学显著差异。另外，对照组的存在证明了明显的安慰剂作用，两组的圣乔治呼吸问卷分数（SGRQ）都有0~4分的改善。因此，在缺乏功能改变的情况下，临床治疗结果的可信度成了问题[10]。重要的是，这项随机对照研究表明，肺叶不完全阻塞的治疗方法虽然是安全的，但是对大多数接受支气管活瓣治疗的非均质性肺气肿患者没有效果。最新的一项小型随机研究支持这一结论，这项研究表明当采取单肺叶完全阻塞方法时，螺旋伞状支架在提供临床上和生理学上的显著改善方面确实比双侧部分肺叶治疗更有优势[26]。

观念二：均质性肺气肿患者使用气道旁路

第二个观念是使用气道旁路支架。之前提到过，气体通过非解剖通道从肺的一部分移动到另一部分（肺内）的能力被称为"CV"，并且由Van Allen等在1930年观察到[27]。正常肺中侧支通道的高阻力消除了CV，与之相反，肺气肿患者肺的CV往往存在并提供气体分布的重要通道。虽然 CV 会妨碍支气管活瓣治疗肺气肿，但是从某种程度上说，也是一种有利因素。实验和临床工作已经证明了在肺气肿的肺实质和支气管气道（如气道旁路）间创造的直接通道能利用肺气肿中广泛存在的 CV，进而改善呼气的气流和容积，否则呼气的气流和容积会被呼气时周围小的气道塌陷所限制[6,8]。

气道旁路涉及经支气管开窗以及随后的气道旁路支架置入[6,9,28,29]。支架由不锈钢嵌入硅胶制作而成，并用紫杉醇浸泡来改善支架通畅性[9]。支架被装在一个传输装置上，并通过纤维支气管镜上 2 mm 的工作通道在检查时放置。支架放置要通过肺段或亚段，为潴留气体离开提供额外解剖气道，因此可减少过度充气。

气道旁路支架针对严重均质性肺气肿患者，不像单向支气管活瓣（Zephry 单向活瓣和螺旋伞状支架）针对非均质性肺气肿患者。气道旁路支架（Exhale 肺气肿治疗系统）由 Broncus 科技有限公司（山景城，加利福尼亚，美国）制造。它的设计和特色在公司网站上能够找到[30]。

EASE 试验：呼气气道支架治疗肺气肿试验

呼气气道支架治疗肺气肿随机试验的研究结果在 2012 年发表，它旨在评估对严重均质性肺气肿患者进行的支气管镜气道旁路的安全性和临床疗效[5]。315 例由均质性肺气肿引起过度充气（余气量和肺总量比例 ≥ 0.65）的患者被随机分配到气道旁路组和假手术对照组。6 个月主要终点结果是基于肺功能和临床疗效测量的复合终点：用力肺活量 ≥ 12%，修改版医学研究委员会呼吸困难程度（mMRC）计分减少 ≥ 1 分。

在支气管镜检查后 1 天观察到气道旁路组患者比起对照组肺功能出现显著改善。但是，这些短期作用在 1 个月时消失，并且直到试验结束和 12 个月的随访时仍然如此。在随访过程中，支架组 mMRC 计分的均值比对照组更好，但是在缺乏肺功能参数改善的情况下，这些临床测量的意义受到限制。

除了 mMRC 计分外，所有主要和次要检测结果都在 6 个月时回到基线，失去最初效果。这被认为是多因素的综合结果，包括在没有放置支架部位出现旁路、支架被咳出和支架不通畅。CT 分析了支架放置的无组织密度肺叶（即支架通畅），结果表明 6 个月时残气量有所减少（− 8.4%），结果和第 1 天时接近（− 10%）。以紫杉醇硅胶聚合物为基础的药物释放支架不能保持支架通畅性，6 个月时只有 21% 的支架被 CT 分析认定为通畅，而第 1 天时是 66%。

分配到气道旁路组患者的气胸、咯血和 COPD 急性加重的概率更高。但是，12 个月时两组 COPD 急性加重和肺部感染的概率相似。气道旁路组 12 个月时死亡率为 6.7%，而假手术对照组为 6.5%，表现出相似的 Kaplan-Meier 生存曲线。

紫杉醇维持支架通透性的效果不像动物研究结果显示得那么好[9]。尽管操作安全性可以接受，但是呼气气道支架治疗肺气肿试验结果不能说明严重均质性肺气肿患者接受气道旁路支架治疗后有持续的远期效果。

其他观念

下面我们描述一些其他的支气管镜肺减容方法。

支气管肺减容线圈

支气管肺减容线圈（RePneu® LVRC）由镍钛合金丝制成，通过支气管镜放置后能造成肺实质压缩（图 11.7）。肺减容线圈法起作用不像单向支气管活瓣那样，不要求 CV 缺失。一项可行性研究评估了 11 例使用肺减容线圈法的患者，观察到术后 3 个月时没有严重副作用。这项研究入组了非均质性和均质性肺气肿患者。尽管样本队列较小，但是非均质性肺气肿患者术后的临床疗效比均质性肺气肿患者更好[2]。

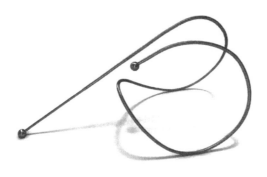

图 11.7　RePneu 肺减容线圈（来自 PneumRx 有限公司，加利福尼亚）

密封胶

已经有支气管镜肺减容术直接应用密封胶（肺气肿密封胶，ELS，Aeriseal）使肺气肿区域塌陷的报道。ELS 在 25 例严重（全球 COPD 倡议组织，GOLD Ⅲ 期和Ⅳ期）非均质性肺气肿患者上进行初步测试[7]。ELS 治疗与肺功能、运动耐量和生存质量评定的改善有关。CT 分析提示在治疗部位诱导局部肺不张。有意思的是，GOLD 分期Ⅲ期患者比Ⅳ期表现出更好的生理获益。这个结果体现Ⅳ期患者组织破坏程度更强，推测需要额外肺减容才能产生和Ⅲ期患者类似的效果。尽管 ELS 治疗的早期结果激励人心，但是必须记得比起支气管活瓣，这个疗法的过程是不可逆的。

支气管镜热蒸汽消融术

支气管镜热蒸汽消融术（BTVA）通过特殊的导管将精确数量的蒸汽直接送到靶肺段。热反应通过引起局部炎症反应、永久性纤维化和肺不张来获得对非均质性肺气肿患者靶向、完整和永久的肺减容效果。支气管镜热蒸汽消融术的潜在优势是它的成功不依赖于 CV。Snell 等[31]报道了 44 例双上肺为主的非均质性肺气肿患者单侧支气管镜热蒸汽消融术的预后。19 例患者报道出现副作用，其中 COPD 急性加重最常见。副作用最易发（62%）于支气管镜热蒸汽消融术后第一个 30 天内。在 3 个月时，平均 48% 的患者实现靶肺叶减容，17% 的患者第一秒用力呼气容积得到改善，两个作用均持续到随访 6 个月后。大多数患者在 6 个月时功能检查结果（圣乔治呼吸问卷）也得到显著改善。

结　论

根据疾病类型区分肺气肿患者逐渐变得恰当。最新证据表明非均质性肺气肿患者通过使用支气管瓣膜能获得显著的生理学和临床益处。重要的是，这一作用在活瓣放置造成完全肺叶阻塞时最明显，并且和 CV 缺乏息息相关，CT 上完整肺裂的存在是 CV 的间接指标。实际上，这强调了常规应用高分辨率 CT 的必要性，不仅为了选择适用不同支气管镜技术的患者，也为了更加准确地识别有积极反应的患者。后者通过靶向选择存在完整肺裂的肺叶来确保完全阻塞肺叶，进一步引起有效的靶肺叶减容。两项最新报道也提示对支气管活瓣治疗反应良好的患者存在存活优势[15,16]。另外，伴随着一些新的发展，例如 Chartis 系统的改进，我们会有一些工具能用来测定是否存在 CV，因此能促进患者选择的改善。令人失望的是，EASE 试验报道气道旁路对均质性肺气肿患者没有持续作用。但是，不应该就此否定该方法在急性期的积极作用。这种作用提示如果能缓解支架阻塞的问题，那么这就是一个有价值的方法。

随着对支气管镜肺减容技术在不同类型肺气肿患者中的作用的更深入的认识和对治疗指征更清晰的定义，该技术的作用将会持续演变。更新的方法带来希望，如支气管镜线圈、生物制剂和热疗，但是需要进一步的研究，包括随机对照研究。关于终点的临床相关且生理学可行的重要问题将会达成共识，以期能够提供一个对比不同内镜治疗方法的研究平台。

参考文献

1. Fishman A, Martinez F, Naunheim K, Piantadosi S, Wise R, Ries A, et al. A randomized trial comparing lung-volume-reduction surgery with medical therapy for severe emphysema. N Engl J Med. 2003;348:2059–73.
2. Herth FJ, Eberhard R, Gompelmann D, Slebos DJ, Ernst A. Bronchoscopic lung volume reduction with a dedicated coil: a clinical pilot study. Ther Adv Respir Dis. 2010;4:225–31.
3. Sciurba FC, Ernst A, Herth FJ, Strange C, Criner GJ, Marquette CH, et al. A randomized study of endobronchial valves for advanced emphysema. N Engl J Med. 2010;363:1233–44.
4. Sterman DH, Mehta AC, Wood DE, Mathur PN, McKenna Jr RJ, Ost DE, et al. A multicenter pilot study of a bronchial valve for the treatment of severe emphysema. Respiration. 2010;79:222–33.
5. Shah PL, Slebos DJ, Cardoso PF, Cetti E, Voelker K, Levine B, et al. group Ets. Bronchoscopic lung-volume reduction with Exhale airway stents for emphysema (EASE trial): randomised, sham-controlled, multicentre trial. Lancet. 2011;378:997–1005.
6. Choong CK, Cardoso PF, Sybrecht GW, Cooper JD. Airway bypass treatment of severe homogeneous emphysema: taking advantage of collateral ventilation. Thorac Surg Clin. 2009;19:239–45.
7. Herth FJ, Gompelmann D, Stanzel F, Bonnet R, Behr J, Schmidt B, et al. Treatment of advanced emphysema with emphysematous lung sealant [AeriSeal(R)]. Respiration. 2011;82:36–45.
8. Choong CK, Macklem PT, Pierce JA, Das N, Lutey BA, Martinez CO, et al. Airway bypass improves the mechanical properties of explanted emphysematous lungs. Am J Respir Crit Care Med. 2008;178:902–5.
9. Choong CK, Phan L, Massetti P, Haddad FJ, Martinez C, Roschak E, et al. Prolongation of patency of airway bypass stents with use of drug-eluting stents. J Thorac Cardiovasc Surg. 2006;131:60–4.
10. Springmeyer SC, Bolliger CT, Waddell TK, Gonzalez X, Wood DE, Teams IBVVPTR. Treatment of heterogeneous emphysema using the spiration IBV valves. Thorac Surg Clin. 2009;19:247–53. ix–x.
11. Venuta F, Rendina EA, Coloni GF. Endobronchial treatment of emphysema with one-way valves. Thorac Surg Clin. 2009;19:255–60. x.
12. Pulmonx Inc. 2012. http://www.pulmonx.com. Accessed 19 Sept 2012.
13. Spiration Inc. 2012. http://www.spiration.com . Accessed 19 Sept 2012.
14. Herth FJ, Noppen M, Valipour A, Leroy S, Vergnon JM, Ficker JH, et al. Efficacy predictors of lung volume reduction with Zephyr valves in a European cohort. Eur Respir J. 2012;39:1334–42.
15. Hopkinson NS, Kemp SV, Toma TP, Hansell DM, Geddes DM, Shah PL, et al. Atelectasis and survival after bronchoscopic lung volume reduction for COPD. Eur Respir J. 2011;37:1346–51.
16. Venuta F, Anile M, Diso D, Carillo C, De Giacomo T, D'Andrilli A, et al. Long-term follow-up after bronchoscopic lung volume reduction in patients with emphysema. Eur Respir J. 2012;39:1084–9.
17. Kotecha S, Westall GP, Holsworth L, Pham A, Williams TJ, Snell GI. Long-term outcomes from bronchoscopic lung volume reduction using a bronchial prosthesis. Respirology. 2011;16:167–73.
18. Herth FJ, Eberhardt R, Gompelmann D, Ficker JH, Wagner M, Ek L, Schmidt B, Slebos DJ. Radiological and clinical outcomes of using chartis to plan endobronchial valve treatment. Eur Respir J 2013;41:302–8
19. Shah PL, Geddes DM. Collateral ventilation and selection of techniques for bronchoscopic lung volume reduction. Thorax. 2012;67:285–6.
20. Kent EM, Blades B. The Anatomic Approach to Pulmonary Resection. Ann Surg. 1942;116:782–94.
21. Herth FJ, Gompelmann D, Ernst A, Eberhardt R. Endo scopic lung volume reduction. Respiration. 2010;79:5–13.
22. Gompelmann D ER, Slebos DJ, et al. Study of the Use of Chartis® Pulmonary Assessment System as a Predictor of Collateral Ventilation as Compared to Computed Tomography. Pulmonx Inc.: http://www.zephyrelvr 2012.com/media/28872/ers_poster_chartis_and_ct_final_14_sept_2011pdf . Accessed 19 Sept 2012.
23. Gompelmann D, Eberhardt R, Michaud G, Ernst A, Herth FJ. Predicting atelectasis by assessment of collateral ventilation prior to endobronchial lung volume reduction: a feasibility study. Respiration. 2010;80:419–25.
24. Criner GJ, Sternberg AL. National Emphysema Treatment Trial: the major outcomes of lung volume reduction surgery in severe emphysema. Proc Am Thorac Soc. 2008;5:393–405.
25. Ninane V, Geltner C, Bezzi M, Foccoli P, Gottlieb J, Welte T, et al. Multicentre European study for the treatment of advanced emphysema with bronchial valves. Eur Respir J. 2012;39:1319–25.
26. Eberhardt R, Gompelmann D, Schuhmann M, Reinhardt H, Ernst A, Heussel CP. Herth FJ. Chest: Complete unilateral versus partial bilateral endoscopic lung volume reduction in patients with bilateral lung emphysema; 2012.
27. Van Allen CLG, Richter HG. Gaseous interchange between adjacent lung lobules. Yale J Biol Med. 1930;2:297.
28. Choong CK, Haddad FJ, Gee EY, Cooper JD. Feasibility and safety of airway bypass stent placement and influence of topical mitomycin C on stent patency. J Thorac Cardiovasc Surg. 2005;129:632–8.
29. Lausberg HF, Chino K, Patterson GA, Meyers BF, Toeniskoetter PD, Cooper JD. Bronchial fenestration improves expiratory flow in emphysematous human lungs. Ann Thorac Surg. 2003;75:393–7. discussion 398.
30. Broncus Technologies Inc. 2012. http://www.broncus.com . Acessed 19 Sept 2012.
31. Snell G, Herth FJ, Hopkins P, Baker KM, Witt C, Gotfried MH, et al. Bronchoscopic thermal vapour ablation therapy in the management of heterogeneous emphysema. Eur Respir J. 2012;39:1326–33.

第 12 章
支气管镜用于治疗支气管胸膜瘘

Yaser Abu El-Sameed

本章提要 支气管胸膜瘘指支气管树和胸膜腔之间存在直接通道。肺切除术是最常见的支气管胸膜瘘病因。其他常见病因包括肺部感染、肺结核、自发性气胸和创伤。支气管胸膜瘘是最严重的肺部手术并发症之一,伴随着高发病率和死亡率。胸部 CT 和支气管镜常用于明确诊断、识别瘘道的病因和位置。支气管胸膜瘘治疗困难,并且其治疗依赖潜在的心肺储备、营养状态、能够适应一次重大手术、可用专家情况和瘘道的大小与部位。直径 > 5 mm、位于中心的瘘道最有可能受益于手术。许多支气管镜技术也被描述用于治疗支气管胸膜瘘。直径 ≤ 5 mm 的外周支气管胸膜瘘也可以考虑进行支气管镜干预,特别是对体弱和高手术风险的患者。近些年支气管内活瓣成功治疗了许多此类患者的支气管胸膜瘘。

关键词 支气管胸膜瘘,持续漏气,气胸,支气管活瓣。

引 言

支气管胸膜瘘被定义为气管支气管树和胸膜腔之间的通道[1,2]。自从采用有效的抗微生物和抗结核治疗后,随着手术技术的进步,支气管胸膜瘘的发生率显著降低。肺切除后支气管胸膜瘘的发生率是 1.5%~28%[3-7]。肺叶切除术后的发生率更低(0.5%)[6]。它的发生也受到支气管吻合方式和需要进行手术的潜在疾病进程的影响[8-10]。这一章讨论了支气管胸膜瘘的病因、危险因素、诊断和治疗。焦点在于支气管镜在治疗支气管胸膜瘘中的新兴作用。对手术选择和技术的详细讨论不在这篇综述的讨论范围。

病因和危险因素

超过 2/3 的支气管胸膜瘘作为肺切除术的术后并发症出现,包括全肺切除术[7,11]。其他病因包括肺部感染、自发性气胸、胸部创伤、肺癌放疗或化疗、肺结核以及机械通气并发症[2,7,11]。在肺癌手术中,右肺切除术与支气管胸膜瘘风险显著增加有关,特别当进行纵隔淋巴结清扫并且在支气管残端阳性时[12]。有报道很好地描述了由于有肺部炎症,特别是活跃肺结核时进行肺切除术后发生的支气管胸膜瘘[13]。其他危险因素包括急性呼吸窘迫综合征(ARDS)、营养不良和气胸[4,14-18]。射频消融术用于治疗肺部恶性肿瘤时也会并发瘘道形成[19]。支气管胸膜瘘也会自发出现。

肺癌患者肺切除术后发生支气管胸膜瘘的最常见部位是手术残端[20]。一些特定因素会增加这些患者发生支气管胸膜瘘的风险。这些因素包括发烧、类固醇使用、血沉增高、白细胞增多、贫血和支气管镜吸痰[20]。一项研究入组了 221 例进行了肺切除术的非小细胞肺癌(NSCLC)患者,其中 5 例出现支气管胸膜瘘[21]。单变量分析发现手术期输血、手术前呼吸道感染、新辅助疗法、右肺切除术、手工吻合支气管、术后住院天数和机械通气都是支气管胸膜瘘发生的重要危险因素。在多变量分析中，只有术前呼吸道感染和右肺切除术是独立危险因素[21]。局部因素被认为是肺切除术后发生支气管胸膜瘘的危险因素，包括支气管残端阳性、长支气管残端、支气管血供紊乱、残端吻合技术不合格、存在脓胸、扩大切除和术前放疗[22-24]。

肺结核和支气管胸膜瘘发生的关联是显著的[16,25,26]。瘘道能在肺结核患者肺切除术后出现，或由空洞自发产生[16,26,27]。Pomerantz 等提到 85 例存在耐药结核杆菌感染的患者肺切除术后支气管胸膜瘘发生率为 10.5%[28]。几乎所有多重耐药肺结核患者在右肺切除术后发生支气管胸膜瘘。

最好的防止支气管胸膜瘘的支气管吻合技术已经讨论过。一项报道评估了 625 位病例的支气管吻合情况[29]。支气管胸膜瘘发生率为 3.8%，比起手工吻合支气管残端的患者，它更常见于使用吻合器吻合的患者。在一系列 209 例由于恶性疾病进行肺切除术的患者中，Hubaut 等[30]发现手工吻合残端的支气管胸膜瘘发生率为 2.4%。其他人也报道了手工吻合时支气管胸膜瘘发生率低[12,23,31]。由于一些专家仍选择常规吻合器吻合，而另一些建议手工吻合，所以对吻合方式的争议仍然存在[32]。在肺切除术中使用吻合器的好处包括最大限度地减少手术区域感染、减少吻合所需时间以及增加分离血管的安全性[32-34]。出于这些考虑，一些学者提倡在这些患者中继续常规使用吻合器吻合[32-35]。

发病率和死亡率

支气管胸膜瘘是小细胞肺癌患者肺切除术后最害怕的并发症。它也跟高死亡率有关，范围在 25%~71.2%，其中最常见的死因是吸入性肺炎和后续的急性呼吸窘迫综合征[12,16,23,36-38]。肺炎也可能来自脓胸的物质通过瘘道对正常肺的污染[36,39,40]。支气管胸膜瘘也跟高发病率有关[6]。支气管胸膜瘘的吻合延迟会导致脓胸、需要手术引流和延长抗生素治疗[41]。意料之中的是，许多患者发生明显的营养不良和低白蛋白水平。导致预后恶化的因素包括呼吸动力受损、对侧肺污染和慢性胸膜感染[42]。除了住院时间延长外，其他综合征包括肺不张、医院获得性肺炎和血栓栓塞疾病[19,39]。

机械通气是发生支气管胸膜瘘较为明确的危险因素。一项研究回顾了 4 年间所有机械通气的病例，发现 1 700 例患者中有 39 例出现支气管胸膜瘘[17]。这 39 例患者的死亡率为 67%，当支气管胸膜瘘发生在疾病晚期时，死亡率更高。所有 8 例每次呼吸最大漏气量超过 500 ml 的患者均死于该疾病[17]。治疗呼吸机依赖患者的支气管胸膜瘘特别有挑战性，因为气道正压会妨碍气道和胸膜间瘘道的闭合。据一项报道，借助网膜固定术和肌肉移位术及时干预慢性脓胸和支气管胸膜瘘与降低发病率、死亡率相关[43]。

就 诊

支气管胸膜瘘患者可能因为早期急性发作前来就诊，也可能因为潜伏发作延迟就诊。急性支气管胸膜瘘是次于张力性气胸和肺部溢流的致死原因[2]。支气管胸膜瘘会导致能引起感染的物质突然从胸膜腔进入气道和肺实质[1,44]。渗出物可能溢到两肺气道引起急性呼吸恶化。支气管胸膜瘘的其他急性表现包括皮下气肿和术后胸片上胸腔积液的减少或消失。术后胸导管持续漏气也提示支气管胸膜瘘。在术后和胸导管移除后出现发热、咳嗽伴化脓性痰和胸膜腔气液平面出现或升高都提示支气管胸膜瘘的可能[3]。

另外，支气管胸膜瘘患者会因为发热、体重降低和咳嗽的慢性恶化前来就诊。这些患者的胸膜腔通常有纤维化和慢性感染存在[1,15,16]。

支气管胸膜瘘的诊断和定位

胸部CT扫描能用于检测支气管胸膜瘘的病因。Ricci等[45]报道CT扫描能用于鉴别和定位55%的需要手术治疗支气管胸膜瘘的病因。亚甲蓝已经被用于定位带有胸导管患者的支气管胸膜瘘的位置[46]。方法是将亚甲蓝注射到支气管残端中，然后观察胸导管中是否可见[47]，但是这种定位支气管胸膜瘘的方法不再受欢迎。

支气管镜不仅能够对中央型支气管胸膜瘘进行直接成像，也能对许多外周型病例进行充分定位[48-50]。对远端支气管胸膜瘘的定位，需要借助球囊导管阻塞，方法是将一个球囊导管传递到通向瘘道的支气管段[51-54]。在这项技术中，将球囊有条不紊地穿过支气管镜的工作通道，进入每个有问题的支气管段，然后持续膨胀30~120秒。集液瓶中漏气的减少提示该部位就是与支气管胸膜瘘连接的支气管段[51-54]。可以使用5F的Fogarty导管，一些其他导管也有报道描述[55]。如果中央型支气管胸膜瘘无法直接成像，或是阻塞远端支气管胸膜瘘不能显著减少或停止漏气，那么支气管镜方法就不再适合。

治 疗

支气管胸膜瘘的治疗方案除了各种支气管镜干预外，还包括手术治疗和内科治疗。治疗支气管胸膜瘘的患者首先要解决紧急情况，比如张力性气胸[56,57]。治疗的其他重要部分是胸膜腔合理引流、充分抗生素治疗、营养支持和治疗导致支气管胸膜瘘的潜在疾病[58-61]。

各种针对闭合支气管胸膜瘘的手术方法成功率在80%~95%之间，但是，它们常伴随高发病率和死亡率[43,62,63]。手术方法包括脓胸引流和用不同皮瓣加强支气管残端。慢性脓胸可能需要胸廓成形术取出部分胸壁[64,65]。当肺叶切除术合并支气管胸膜瘘时[66]，通常需要完全支气管切除。视频辅助胸腔镜手术（VATS）被越来越多地用于治疗持续很久的支气管胸膜瘘，并且成功率高[67]。一项最新的手术技术包括胸腔清创，随后缝合支气管残端，并且使用大网膜或肌瓣包盖加固[68,69]。如果无法鉴别支气管胸膜瘘，那么进行开窗手术并每日换药会有帮助。

在过去，支气管镜在支气管胸膜瘘中的作用仅限于评估支气管残端和排除各种感染。近年来，支气管镜在治疗支气管胸膜瘘患者中的作用更加突出。如今，对于那些不适合手术和无法耐受胸部大手术的支气管胸膜瘘患者，支气管镜干预为它们提供了一种治疗选择[37,70]。支气管镜也能用于一些危重患者的过渡治疗，直到他们的情况得到改善，能承受对瘘道的手术治疗[71]。在一项报道中，光纤支气管镜也已经被用来经皮显像和检查支气管胸膜瘘[72]。不幸的是，关于支气管镜干预的绝大多数数据仅限于个案报道或小样本研究。目前的文献无法对各种可用的支气管镜干预方法进行充分对比。介入科医师需要进行临床判断选择患者及特定的干预方法进行支气管镜治疗。

Hartmann and Rausch[73]在1977年第一次报道了用甲基氰基丙烯酸酯闭合术后外周型支气管胸膜瘘。在同一年，Ratliff等[54]报道了通过在支气管镜下放置铅丸控制一例支气管胸膜瘘的患者。自此，出现许多借助支气管镜使用各种装置治疗支气管胸膜瘘的报道。支气管镜干预通常用于小瘘道或一般状况差的患者[2,7]。支气管镜技术控制支气管胸膜瘘的疗效随着瘘道直径的增大而降低[12,74]。

一项收录96个病例的综述描述了全肺切除术后支气管胸膜瘘的自然进程[36]，并且21例经手术治疗的患者，成功闭合支气管胸膜瘘，而11例接受支气管镜干预的患者也治疗成功。然而，总的术后死亡率是31%。另一个重要的综述对比了在肺切除术后支气管胸膜瘘中使用支气管镜闭合支气管胸膜瘘和传统开胸方法的差别[42]。这个研究确定了6个病例系列，每个系列都有超过2例肺切除术后支气管胸膜瘘的患者。85例肺切除术后支气管胸膜瘘患者接受支气管镜方法来治疗支气管胸膜瘘。各种支气管镜干预的成功率为30%。死亡率为40%，再次反映了该患者群体的高死亡率。

尚无研究比较不同支气管镜干预用于治疗支气管胸膜瘘的作用。由于支气管镜治疗通常在直径>5 mm的瘘道中成功率不高，因此支气管胸膜瘘的大小是一项评估支气管镜干预预后的重要因素[75-77]。使用支气管镜技术成功治疗的报道通常在≤5 mm的支气管胸膜瘘患者中[75-78]。总之，使用支气管镜方法闭合支气管胸膜瘘的适应证包括高手术风险、瘘道<5 mm[79]。对于大的支气管胸膜瘘病例，通常需要行开胸手术[80]。

支气管镜治疗支气管胸膜瘘基于将不同材料和小装置送到支气管胸膜瘘的部位。包括使用不同封闭胶、明胶海绵、抗生素、无水乙醇注射、硅胶填料、线圈、气道支架、Amplatzer封堵器、支气管内单向活瓣和其他装置等[50-55,81-100]。

合成胶水

氰基丙烯酸酯胶是常用的治疗支气管胸膜瘘的密封胶。一旦这种胶水和组织接触，它就形成一个多聚体并凝固。通过这种方式，胶水起到屏障作用，并诱导炎症和随后的纤维组织形成。在支气管镜检查时，使用前面提到的技术定位支气管胸膜瘘后，将一根导管穿过工作通道靠近支气管胸膜瘘部位。下一步注射0.5~1 ml的胶水到瘘道中[37,50,101-105]。胶水治疗被认为是一种费用低的干预方法，并且能在门诊进行[103]。有一项在支气管镜下使用甲基-2-氰基丙烯酸酯闭合肺切除术后支气管胸膜瘘的报道[106]。在入组的12例患者中，成功率为83%。另一个病例系列研究中，9例患者借助支气管镜注射正丁基氰基丙烯酸酯胶关闭支气管胸膜瘘[103]。在8例患者中，胶水成功封住瘘道。由于在这项研究中没有出现并发症，所以作者建议将这个方法用于高手术风险的患者。Histo-acryl组织胶水也通过黏膜下注射的方式用来治疗支气管胸膜瘘[107]。在这项报道中，非小细胞肺癌患者在右肺切除术后出现支气管胸膜瘘。黏膜下注射胶水通过减小瘘道直径帮助闭合瘘道。胶水也会加快肉芽组织的形成。尽管有这些成功的报道，Belda-Sanchís等[108]发表了一篇Cochrane综述，不建议将手术密封剂用于治疗肺癌患者肺切除后的漏气。这篇2010年的综述收录了16个试验，结果表明术后漏气虽然减少了，但是住院时间没有明显减少[108]。

纤维蛋白胶

纤维蛋白胶已经被成功地用于支气管镜下闭合小的肺切除术后支气管胸膜瘘[70,96,109-112]。它被用于中央型[70,96,109]和外周型[51]支气管胸膜瘘的治疗。手术过程包括借助导管在目标部位注射1 ml纤维蛋白原，随后快速注射1 ml凝血酶（1 000 U/ml）。混合物形成一个纤维蛋白凝块并封住瘘道。一项动物研究评估了纤维蛋白胶减少实验性肺漏气的作用[113]。胶水被用在支气管胸膜瘘的胸膜侧。术后评估显示胶水治疗组动物没有出现粘连增加，并在3个月时完全吸收。

组织黏合剂

一项报道收录了38例接受胸部手术的患者，检验了基于人血清白蛋白与明胶的医用软组织黏合剂治疗支气管胸膜瘘的作用[114]。黏合剂能够闭合肺部瘘道，并预防来自手术残端的漏气。另一篇文章报道了在2例患者中通过相同的材料成功闭合复杂支气管胸膜瘘[115]。

明胶海绵

Jones等描述了使用明胶海绵作为短暂性支气管堵塞器阻塞外周型支气管胸膜瘘的技术[97]。明胶海绵容易得到和使用，在1个月内能完全吸收[3]。

组织扩张器

通过黏膜下注射组织扩张器进行支气管镜

阻塞支气管胸膜瘘，这项技术被报道过。该方法可以单独使用，也可以联合支气管镜注射正丁基氰基丙烯酸酯胶使用[74]。一项报道描述了2例支气管胸膜瘘患者获得了成功治疗[74]。使用的组织扩张器是一种生物兼容制剂，由热解碳涂层珠悬浮在包含β-葡聚糖的水基载体胶中制备而成。热解碳涂层珠作为物理填料能闭合瘘道。另一项关于组织扩张器治疗肺叶切除术后持续性肺瘘的报道提示其预后良好[116]。在该研究中，肺癌患者在右侧双肺叶切除术后出现胸腔积脓。引流积脓后使用肌瓣来闭合瘘道，但仍存在残腔和持续漏气，植入组织扩张器能够紧密固定肌瓣并解决漏气。

抗生素

多西环素作为胸膜硬化剂被成功地使用，通过胸导管给药治疗持续的支气管胸膜瘘[117]。在一个病例报道中，多西环素被用于治疗严重肺炎造成慢性瘘道形成和呼吸衰竭的患者[90]。支气管内滴注四环素能使瘘道闭合、患者情况改善。相似的病例报道已经发表[52]。

无水乙醇

最初，酒精通过直视下壁内注射治疗胃隆起性病变[118]。有报道称借助支气管镜壁内注射无水乙醇可治疗恶性气管支气管病变[95]。局部注射无水乙醇也被用作支气管镜下闭合支气管胸膜瘘。注射引起的黏膜肿胀最初能控制支气管胸膜瘘，随后肉芽组织形成使得瘘道闭合[118,119]。一项报道收录了5例中央型支气管胸膜瘘的患者，他们通过支气管镜下瘘道黏膜下注射无水乙醇获得成功治疗[89]。治疗后没有出现并发症。该方法能减少住院费用和持续时间，并改善患者的生活质量。

氩离子凝固术和Nd:YAG激光

有报道介绍了一例使用氩离子凝固术治疗气管支气管吻合失败发生支气管胸膜瘘的病例[120]。这种方法旨在为肺切除术后小的非复杂性瘘提供替代治疗。该报道中，一例56岁的非小细胞肺癌患者接受袖式肺切除术。患者在术后3个月出现咳嗽咳痰。在它的吻合接口处发现两条小的瘘道，但没有证据支持肿瘤复发。在局麻下通过支气管镜应用氩离子凝固术，术后无并发症。术后对患者随访到18个月，没有出现任何症状。瘘道的愈合可以归因于机械创伤和伤口愈合引起的纤维化。Kiriyama等报道了使用支气管Nd:YAG激光对肺切除术后小的中央型支气管胸膜瘘进行无创闭合[121]。

硅胶填料

硅胶填料已经被成功地用于治疗顽固性气胸引起的支气管胸膜瘘。Watanabe等[93]报道了他们通过支气管栓（图12.1）阻塞迁延性支气管胸

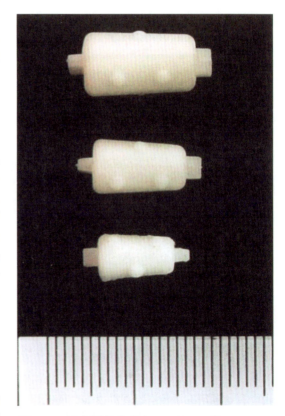

图12.1　支气管栓（来自Sukagawa和Watanabe医师）

膜瘘的经验。77.6% 的患者漏气停止或显著减少（图 12.2）。还有报道借助硅胶栓塞材料在内镜下阻塞支气管来控制射频消融引起的顽固性支气管胸膜瘘[122]。该报道中，一例 58 岁的非小细胞肺癌男性患者接受射频消融后并发气胸。尽管延长了胸部引流时间，但是漏气仍然持续。后借助硅胶栓子阻塞支气管，使得漏气停止。

线圈

关于使用线圈控制支气管胸膜瘘已经有许多报道[99,100,123]。在其中一个报道中，支气管镜被用来将血管造影栓塞线圈放在大的支气管胸膜瘘上，以便更好地控制漏气[99]。另一个病例系列报道了一种永久堵塞小的外周气道的方法，它借助改良血管造影技术将血管栓塞线圈放置于支气管内[100]。这个方法被应用于 5 例复杂肺实质漏气患者。所有没有并发症的患者都实现了完全或大部分控制。支气管镜下通过金属线圈和胶水阻塞支气管治疗支气管胸膜瘘的技术已经有过报道[91]。该技术是将血管栓塞线圈固定在支气管胸膜瘘区域后，在上面喷洒氰基丙烯酸酯胶水。喷洒的胶水消除了线圈间隔，并使线圈稳定。所有使用该方法的患者都成功了，除了 1 例伴有大瘘道的患者[91]。Uchida 等报道了 1 例支气管胸膜瘘的妇女，通过放置血管栓塞线圈治疗[124]，患者在脓胸手术治疗后出现多发性支气管胸膜瘘，这些瘘道可以通过支气管内放置血管栓塞线圈阻塞。操作后不久，来自瘘道的漏气停止，引流管在 2 天后拔除。

气道支架

气道支架通常被用于治疗和食管连通的气管或支气管瘘道[125-128]。它的作用已经延伸到了治疗肺切除术后的支气管胸膜瘘[129-133]。Watanabe 等描述了通过支气管支架放置合并脓腔冲洗成功治疗支气管胸膜瘘[129]。一例 67 岁男性肺癌患者在肺叶切除术后出现支气管胸膜瘘。重新缝合支气管残端和使用不同的皮瓣没有作用。而将 Dumon 支架放在支气管闭合残端能够控制瘘道。Tayama 等[130] 描述了另一个相似的病例，该肺癌患者在全肺切除术后出现支气管胸膜瘘。通过放置改良版 Dumon 支架来有效闭合残端。硅胶支架移动的高发生率会导致支气管胸膜瘘复发，因此可以使用全覆盖自膨胀金属支架（SEMSs）提供对瘘道更好的控制。Takahashi 等[134] 报道了使用 Ultraflex 膨胀支架治疗大的全肺切除术后支气管胸膜瘘[134]。这例患者出现术后脓胸和曲霉菌病。一个 Ultraflex 膨胀支架被置入以堵塞支气管胸膜瘘的严重漏气。这例患者的总体状况得到改善，并且在放置支架后 1 个月出院。最近一项研究评估了在大的全肺切除术后瘘患者的多学科管理中，使用定制锥形气管支气管自膨胀金属支架的疗效和预后[132]。这些支架被用于 7 例全肺切除术后的支气管胸膜瘘患者，他们的瘘道直径 > 6 mm。术后所有患者的漏气均停止，但是死亡率仍然高达 67%，主要死因是败血症。另一项关于锥形气管支气管自膨胀金属支架的最新研究得到了阳性结果，它评估了该支架用于治疗全肺切除术后的支气管胸膜瘘患者的可行性、疗效和安全性[80]。为了让支气管裂开部位不出现漏气，6

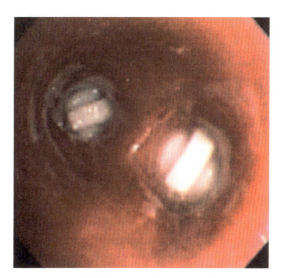

图 12.2 支气管栓通过纤维支气管镜放置（来自 Sukagawa 和 Watanabe 医师）

例患者接受该手术，5例患者全肺切除术后出现的支气管胸膜瘘直径＞5 mm，1例患者在气管袖式全肺切除术后出现吻合口裂开。支架借助钛螺旋大头钉固定在气管黏膜。所有患者的支气管漏气都立刻消失。成功移除支架后没有出现并发症，并且所有患者都实现了支气管裂开的永久性吻合。

Amplatzer封堵器

Amplatzer封堵器（AD）通常被用于治疗充血性心力衰竭[135-138]。一项报道描述了3例接受支气管镜治疗的患者，通过置入房间隔缺损封堵器控制瘘道[139]。其中两个瘘道直径＞10 mm。操作为微创，并能缓解支气管胸膜瘘。另一个病例报道描述了如何通过支气管镜下置入Amplatzer封堵器成功闭合支气管胸膜瘘，该患者在全肺切除术后出现了右主支气管的支气管胸膜瘘[140]。相似地，一个房间隔缺损封堵器被用于闭合曲菌球患者肺叶切除术后的支气管瘘道，能使漏气立刻减少[141]。在随访支气管镜检查时，这个装置几乎都被肉芽组织覆盖。这项支气管内技术似乎能安全有效地治疗大的支气管胸膜瘘。Passera等[142]提供了一个病例，患者在双下肺叶切除术后并发大的支气管胸膜瘘，并在初次手术后1个月时出现脓胸。对患者立刻通过开窗胸廓造口术进行治疗。手术清创后放置一个Amplatzer封堵器闭合瘘道。随后胸廓造口术通过真空辅助闭合疗法快速结束。该联合治疗获得了成功的预后。

Fruchter等最近描述了一个病例报道，通过Amplatzer封堵器治疗了10例患者的11处支气管胸膜瘘[86]。操作在清醒镇静下完成。镍钛合金双盘封堵器直接在支气管镜引导下借助导丝放置，阻塞瘘道。操作在9例患者中获得成功，并且支气管胸膜瘘相关的症状消失。该操作没有副作用或并发症，能够被患者很好地耐受。该结果平均持续到随访后9个月。对比自膨胀金属支架，Amplatzer封堵器能让气道免于外源性材料的影响，这就避免了黏液嵌塞的问题。Amplatzer封堵器不像常见的金属支架那样需要被移除。

支气管内单向活瓣

支气管内单向活瓣是支气管胸膜瘘不同治疗装置的最新补充。它最初被设计用来对部分肺气肿患者进行支气管镜肺减张术[143]。支气管内单向活瓣作为一种单向活瓣，能够让呼出的气体和分泌物流动，但是停止气体吸入。它被固定在气道内，和支气管壁紧密相连，能阻止任何装置附近的漏气。早期的病例报道描述了支气管内单向活瓣用于控制顽固性肺胸膜瘘[55,66,144]。这些报道收录了手术治疗无法闭合支气管胸膜瘘的脓胸患者。其余患者由于太虚弱无法经受手术[19,145-150]。Travaline发表了一组大规模病例，入组了40例持续漏气的患者[151]。这些患者接受支气管内单向活瓣作为支气管胸膜瘘的主要治疗方法。漏气的完全和部分缓解率分别为47.5%和45%。胸导管在支气管内单向活瓣置入后平均持续时间为21天（中位数7.5天；四分位距3~29天）。活瓣置入和出院间的平均时间为（19±28）天（中位数11；四分位距4~27天）。另一个报道描述了7例连续性复杂性支气管胸膜瘘患者，他们通过支气管内单向活瓣获得成功治疗[152]。El-Sameed等[153]报道了治疗持续性支气管胸膜瘘的成功经验，包括对文献的回顾。他们治疗了4例存在不同类型持续漏气的患者（图12.3和图12.4）。其中2例支气管胸膜瘘的病因是肺结核。所有患者都在术后得到改善，所有患者的活瓣都成功移除，没有出现并发症。这些报道表明支气管内单向活瓣能够通过纤维支气管镜在清醒镇静下轻松放置。目前Emphasys单向活瓣（EBV）和螺旋伞状支架（IBV）可供使用。自从2006年美国食品药物管理局（FDA）的人道主义器械豁免项目赋予螺旋伞状支架人道主义用途称号后，它能被用于任何接受肺切除术或肺减张术，包括术后持续漏气7天或更久的患者[154]。尽管该方法对一些类似的患者有吸引力，但是

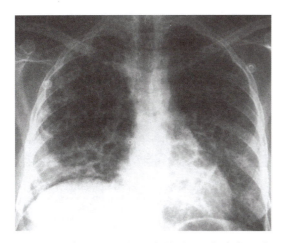

图 12.3　胸片显示在患者的右上肺叶有 3 个支气管内单向活瓣，该患者的迁延性支气管胸膜瘘是晚期支气管扩张症引起的（获得了 Springer Science 和 Business Media 的允许）

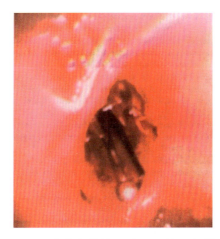

图 12.4　一张支气管镜图片显示放置在断裂支气管残端的支气管内单向活瓣

需要更大型的研究明确支气管内单向活瓣在支气管胸膜瘘治疗中的作用。

总　结

能用于治疗支气管胸膜瘘的支气管镜干预方法有很多。但是，大多数文献是病例系列或有限的病例报道，治疗复杂的支气管胸膜瘘的最佳方法没有明确指南。支气管镜方法看起来有利于高手术风险的患者。瘘道的大小和定位瘘道的能力有助于选择进行手术还是支气管镜干预治疗。目前没有任何的对比研究支持某个特定支气管镜干预方法胜过其他治疗方法。患者的状况、支气管胸膜瘘的评估、资源的获取以及支气管镜专科医师的经验仍然是选择特定技术的重要因素。该领域显然需要未来的研究指导处理这些具有挑战性的棘手情况。

参考文献

1. Baumann MH, Sahn SA. Medical management and therapy of bronchopleural fistulas in the mechanically ventilated patient. Chest. 1990;97:721–8.
2. Lois M, Noppen M. Bronchopleural fistulas: an overview of the problem with special focus on endoscopic management. Chest. 2005;128:3955–65.
3. McManigle JE, Fletcher GL, Tenholder MF. Bronchoscopy in the management of bronchopleural fistula. Chest. 1990;97:1235–8.
4. Sonobe M, Nakagawa M, Ichinose M, et al. Analysis of risk factors in bronchopleural fistula after pulmonary resection for primary lung cancer. Eur J Cardiothorac Surg. 2000;18:519–23.
5. Turk AE, Karanas YL, Cannon W, Chang J. Staged closure of complicated bronchopleural fistulas. Ann Plast Surg. 2000;45:560–4.
6. Cerfolio RJ. The incidence, etiology, and prevention of postresectional bronchopleural fistula. Semin Thorac Cardiovasc Surg. 2001;13:3–7.
7. Sirbu H, Busch T, Aleksic I, et al. Bronchopleural fistula in the surgery of non-small cell lung cancer: incidence, risk factors, and management. Ann Thorac Cardiovasc Surg. 2001;7:330–6.
8. Sato M, Saito Y, Nagamoto N, et al. An improved method of bronchial stump closure for prevention of bronchopleural fistula in pulmonary resection. Tohoku J Exp Med. 1992;168(3):507–13.
9. Al-Kattan K, Cattelani L, Goldstraw P. Bronchopleural fistula after pneumonectomy for lung cancer. Eur J Cardiothorac Surg. 1995;9:479–82.
10. Conlan AA, Lukanich JM, Shutz J, Hurwitz SS. Elective pneumonectomy for benign lung disease: modern-day mortality and morbidity. J Thorac Cardiovasc Surg. 1995;110(4 Pt 1):1118–24.
11. Algar FJ, Alvarez A, Aranda JL, et al. Prediction of early bronchopleural fistula after pneumonectomy: a multivariate

analysis. Ann Thorac Surg. 2001;72:1662–7.
12. Asamura H, Naruke T, Tsuchiya R, et al. Bronchopleural fistulas associated with lung cancer operations. Univariate and multivariate analysis of risk factors, management, and outcome. J Thorac Cardiovasc Surg. 1992;104:1456–64.
13. Shields TW, Ponn RB. Complications of pulmonary resection. In: Shields TW, LoCicero J, Ponn RB, editors. General thoracic surgery. 5th ed. Philadelphia: Williams and Wilkins; 2000. p. 1113–22.
14. Malave G, Foster ED, Wilson JA, Munro DD. Bronchopleural fistula—present-day study of an old problem. A review of 52 cases. Ann Thorac Surg. 1971;11:1–10.
15. Hankins JR, Miller JE, Attar S, Satterfield JR, McLaughlin JS. Bronchopleural fistula. Thirteenyear experience with 77 cases. J Thorac Cardiovasc Surg. 1978;76:755–62.
16. Steiger Z, Wilson RF. Management of bronchopleural fistulas. Surg Gynecol Obstet. 1984;158:267–71.
17. Pierson DJ, Horton CA, Bates PW. Persistent bronchopleural air leak during mechanical ventilation. A review of 39 cases. Chest. 1986;90:321–3.
18. Frytak S, Lee RE, Pairolero PC, Arnold PG, Shaw JN. Necrotic lung and bronchopleural fistula as complications of therapy in lung cancer. Cancer Invest. 1988;6:139–43.
19. Abu-Hijleh M, Blundin M. Emergency use of an endobronchial one-way valve in the management of severe air leak and massive subcutaneous emphysema. Lung. 2010;188:253–7.
20. Sato M, Saito Y, Fujimura S, et al. Study of postoperative bronchopleural fistulas—analysis of factors related to bronchopleural fistulas. Nihon Kyobu Geka Gakkai Zasshi. 1989;37:498–503.
21. Panagopoulos ND, Apostolakis E, Koletsis E, et al. Low incidence of bronchopleural fistula after pneumonectomy for lung cancer. Interact Cardiovasc Thorac Surg. 2009;9:571–5.
22. Ferguson MK. Assessment of operative risk for pneumonectomy. Chest Surg Clin N Am. 1999;9:339–51.
23. Wright CD, Wain JC, Mathisen DJ, Grillo HC. Postpneumonectomy bronchopleural fistula after sutured bronchial closure: incidence, risk factors, and management. J Thorac Cardiovasc Surg. 1996;112:1367–71.
24. Klepetko W, Taghavi S, Pereszlenyi A, et al. Impact of different coverage techniques on incidence of postpneumonectomy stump fistula. Eur J Cardiothorac Surg. 1999;15:758–63.
25. Ellis JH, Sequeira FW, Weber TR, Eigen H, Fitzgerald JF. Balloon catheter occlusion of bronchopleural fistulae. AJR Am J Roentgenol. 1982; 138:157–9.
26. Donath J, Khan FA. Tuberculous and posttuberculous bronchopleural fistula. Ten year clinical experience. Chest. 1984;86:697–703.
27. Johnson TM, McCann W, Davey WN. Tuberculous bronchopleural fistula. Am Rev Respir Dis. 1973; 107:30–41.
28. Pomerantz M, Madsen L, Goble M, Iseman M. Surgical management of resistant mycobacterial tuberculosis and other mycobacterial pulmonary infections. Ann Thorac Surg. 1991;52:1108–11; discussion 1112.
29. Uçvet A, Gursoy S, Sirzai S, et al. Bronchial closure methods and risks for bronchopleural fistula in pulmonary resections: how a surgeon may choose the optimum method? Interact Cardiovasc Thorac Surg. 2011;12:558–62.
30. Hubaut JJ, Baron O, Al Habash O, et al. Closure of the bronchial stump by manual suture and incidence of bronchopleural fistula in a series of 209 pneumonectomies for lung cancer. Eur J Cardiothorac Surg. 1999;16:418–23.
31. Péterffy A, Calabrese E. Mechanical and conventional manual sutures of the bronchial stump. A comparative study of 298 surgical patients. Scand J Thorac Cardiovasc Surg. 1979;13:87–91.
32. Asamura H, Kondo H, Tsuchiya R. Management of the bronchial stump in pulmonary resections: a review of 533 consecutive recent bronchial closures. Eur J Cardiothorac Surg. 2000;17:106–10.
33. Weissberg D, Kaufman M. Suture closure versus stapling of bronchial stump in 304 lung cancer operations. Scand J Thorac Cardiovasc Surg. 1992;26:125–7.
34. Vester SR, Faber LP, Kittle CF, Warren WH, Jensik RJ. Bronchopleural fistula after stapled closure of bronchus. Ann Thorac Surg. 1991;52:1253–7; discussion 1257-8.
35. Takaro T. Use of staplers in bronchial closure. In: Grillo HC, Eschapasse H, editors. International trends in general thoracic surgery. Philadelphia: W.B. Saunders; 1987. p. 452–7.
36. Hollaus PH, Lax F, El-Nashef BB, et al. Natural history of bronchopleural fistula after pneumonectomy: a review of 96 cases. Ann Thorac Surg. 1997;63:1391–6; discussion 1396-7.
37. Torre M, Chiesa G, Ravini M, Vercelloni M, Belloni PA. Endoscopic gluing of bronchopleural fistula. Ann Thorac Surg. 1987;43:295–7.
38. Uramoto H, Hanagiri T. The development of bronchopleural fistula in lung cancer patients after major surgery:31 years of experience with 19 cases. Anticancer Res. 2011;31:619–24.
39. Sarkar P, Chandak T, Shah R, Talwar A. Diagnosis and management bronchopleural fistula. Indian J Chest Dis Allied Sci. 2010;52:97–104.
40. Darling GE, Abdurahman A, Yi Q-L, et al. Risk of a right pneumonectomy: role of bronchopleural fistula. Ann Thorac Surg. 2005;79:433–7.
41. Fernández-Díaz JA, García-Gallo C, Goicolea-Ruigómez J, Varela-de UA. Use of amplatzer® device for closure of bronchopleural fistulas, a hybrid procedure using bronchoscopy and radiology. Rev Esp Cardiol. 2011;64:1065–6.
42. West D, Togo A, Kirk AJB. Are bronchoscopic approaches to post-pneumonectomy bronchopleural fistula an effective alternative to repeat thoracotomy? Interact Cardiovasc Thorac Surg. 2007;6:547–50.
43. Stamatis G, Freitag L, Wencker M, Greschuchna D. Omentopexy and muscle transposition: two alternative methods in the treatment of pleural empyema and mediastinitis. Thorac Cardiovasc Surg. 1994;42:225–32.
44. Høier-Madsen K, Schulze S, Møller Pedersen V, Halkier E. Management of bronchopleural fistula following pneumonectomy. Scand J Thorac Cardiovasc Surg. 1984;18:263–6.
45. Ricci ZJ, Haramati LB, Rosenbaum AT, Liebling MS. Role of computed tomography in guiding the management of peripheral bronchopleural fistula. J Thorac Imaging. 2002;17:214–8.
46. Hsu JT, Bennett GM, Wolff E. Radiologic assessment of bronchopleural fistula with empyema. Radiology. 1972;103:41–5.
47. Alifano M, Sepulveda S, Mulot A, Schussler O, Regnard J-F. A new method for detection of postpneumonectomy bronchopleural fistulas. Ann Thorac Surg. 2003;75:1662–4.
48. Kim EA, Lee KS, Shim YM, et al. Radiographic and CT findings in complications following pulmonary resection. Radiographics. 2002;22:67–86.
49. Misthos P, Konstantinou M, Kokotsakis J, Skottis I, Lioulias A. Early detection of occult bronchopleural fistula after routine standard pneumonectomy. Thorac Cardiovasc Surg. 2006;54: 264–7.
50. Roksvaag H, Skalleberg L, Nordberg C, Solheim K, Høivik B. Endoscopic closure of bronchial fistula. Thorax. 1983;38:696–7.
51. Regel G, Sturm JA, Neumann C, Schueler S, Tscherne H. Occlusion of bronchopleural fistula after lung injury—a new treatment by bronchoscopy. J Trauma. 1989;29:223–6.
52. Lan RS, Lee CH, Tsai YH, Wang WJ, Chang CH. Fiberoptic bronchial blockade in a small bronchopleural fistula. Chest. 1987;92:944–6.

53. Pace R, Rankin RN, Finley RJ. Detachable balloon occlusion of bronchopleural fistulae in dogs. Invest Radiol. 1983;18:504–6.
54. Ratliff JL, Hill JD, Tucker H, Fallat R. Endobronchial control of bronchopleural fistulae. Chest. 1977;71:98–9.
55. Ferguson JS, Sprenger K, Van Natta T. Closure of a bronchopleural fistula using bronchoscopic placement of an endobronchial valve designed for the treatment of emphysema. Chest. 2006;129:479–81.
56. Cooper WA, Miller JI. Management of bronchopleural fistula after lobectomy. Semin Thorac Cardiovasc Surg. 2001;13:8–12.
57. Baldwin JC, Mark JB. Treatment of bronchopleural fistula after pneumonectomy. J Thorac Cardiovasc Surg. 1985;90:813–7.
58. Phillips YY, Lonigan RM, Joyner LR. A simple technique for managing a bronchopleural fistula while maintaining positive pressure ventilation. Crit Care Med. 1979;7:351–3.
59. Powner DJ, Grenvik A. Ventilatory management of life-threatening bronchopleural fistulae. A summary. Crit Care Med. 1981;9:54–8.
60. Hazerian TE, Berrezueta R, Pittokopitis K, Buckle FG, Robinson L. Technical consideration of synchronized chest tube occlusion in bronchopleural fistula. Crit Care Med. 1983;11:484.
61. Bishop MJ, Benson MS, Sato P, Pierson DJ. Comparison of high-frequency jet ventilation with conventional mechanical ventilation for bronchopleural fistula. Anesth Analg. 1987;66:833–8.
62. Sabanathan S, Richardson J. Management of postpneumonectomy bronchopleural fistulae. A review. J Cardiovasc Surg. 1994;35:449–57.
63. Hollaus PH, Huber M, Lax F, et al. Closure of bronchopleural fistula after pneumonectomy with a pedicled intercostal muscle flap. Eur J Cardiothorac Surg. 1999;16:181–6.
64. Stefani A, Jouni R, Alifano M, et al. Thoracoplasty in the current practice of thoracic surgery: a singleinstitution 10-year experience. Ann Thorac Surg. 2011;91:263–8.
65. Walsh MD, Bruno AD, Onaitis MW, et al. The role of intrathoracic free flaps for chronic empyema. Ann Thorac Surg. 2011;91:865–8.
66. Snell GI, Holsworth L, Fowler S, et al. Occlusion of a broncho-cutaneous fistula with endobronchial oneway valves. Ann Thorac Surg. 2005;80:1930–2.
67. Sedrakyan A, van der Meulen J, Lewsey J, Treasure T. Video assisted thoracic surgery for treatment of pneumothorax and lung resections: systematic review of randomised clinical trials. BMJ (Clinical research ed). 2004;329(7473):1008.
68. Nosotti M, Cioffi U, De Simone M, et al. Omentoplasty and thoracoplasty for treating postpneumonectomy bronchopleural fistula in a patient previously submitted to aortic prosthesis implantation. J Cardiothorac Surg. 2009;4:38.
69. Molnar TF. Current surgical treatment of thoracic empyema in adults. Eur J Cardiothorac Surg. 2007; 32:422–30.
70. Glover W, Chavis TV, Daniel TM, Kron IL, Spotnitz WD. Fibrin glue application through the flexible fiberoptic bronchoscope: closure of bronchopleural fistulas. J Thorac Cardiovasc Surg. 1987;93:470–2.
71. Hollaus PH, Lax F, Janakiev D, et al. Endoscopic treatment of postoperative bronchopleural fistula: experience with 45 cases. Ann Thorac Surg. 1998;66:923–7.
72. Chowdhury JK. Percutaneous use of fiberoptic bronchoscope to investigate bronchopleurocutaneous fistula. Chest. 1979;75:203–4.
73. Hartmann W, Rausch V. New therapeutic application of the fiberoptic bronchoscope. Chest. 1977;71:237.
74. García-Polo C, León-Jiménez A, López-Campos JL, et al. Endoscopic sealing of bronchopleural fistulas with submucosal injection of a tissue expander: a novel technique. Can Respir J. 2010;17:e23–4.
75. Baumann WR, Ulmer JL, Ambrose PG, Garvey MJ, Jones DT. Closure of a bronchopleural fistula using decalcified human spongiosa and a fibrin sealant. Ann Thorac Surg. 1997;64:230–3.
76. Sivrikoz CM, Kaya T, Tulay CM, et al. Effective approach for the treatment of bronchopleural fistula: application of endovascular metallic ring-shaped coil in combination with fibrin glue. Ann Thorac Surg. 2007;83:2199–201.
77. Keckler SJ, Spilde TL, St Peter SD, Tsao K, Ostlie DJ. Treatment of bronchopleural fistula with small intestinal mucosa and fibrin glue sealant. Ann Thorac Surg. 2007;84:1383–6.
78. Andreetti C, D'Andrilli A, Ibrahim M, et al. Submucosal injection of the silver-human albumin complex for the treatment of bronchopleural fistula. Eur J Cardiothorac Surg. 2010;37:40–3.
79. Varoli F, Roviaro G, Grignani F, et al. Endoscopic treatment of bronchopleural fistulas. Ann Thorac Surg. 1998;65:807–9.
80. Andreetti C, D'Andrilli A, Ibrahim M, et al. Effective treatment of post-pneumonectomy bronchopleural fistula by conical fully covered self-expandable stent. Interact Cardiovasc Thorac Surg. 2012;14:420–3.
81. Paul S, Talbot SG, Carty M, Orgill DP, Zellos L. Bronchopleural fistula repair during Clagett closure utilizing a collagen matrix plug. Ann Thorac Surg. 2007;83:1519–21.
82. Tao H, Araki M, Sato T, et al. Bronchoscopic treatment of postpneumonectomy bronchopleural fistula with a collagen screw plug. J Thorac Cardiovasc Surg. 2006;132:99–104.
83. Ranu H, Gatheral T, Sheth A, Smith EEJ, Madden BP. Successful endobronchial seal of surgical bronchopleural fistulas using BioGlue. Ann Thorac Surg. 2009;88:1691–2.
84. Bellato V, Ferraroli GM, De Caria D, et al. Management of postoperative bronchopleural fistula with a tracheobronchial stent in a patient requiring mechanical ventilation. Intensive Care Med. 2010;36:721–2.
85. Chae EY, Shin JH, Song H-Y, et al. Bronchopleural fistula treated with a silicone-covered bronchial occlusion stent. Ann Thorac Surg. 2010;89:293–6.
86. Fruchter O, Kramer MR, Dagan T, et al. Endobronchial closure of bronchopleural fistulae using amplatzer devices: our experience and literature review. Chest. 2011;139:682–7.
87. Eckersberger F, Moritz E, Klepetko W, Müller MR, Wolner E. Treatment of postpneumonectomy empyema. Thorac Cardiovasc Surg. 1990;38:352–4.
88. Matthew TL, Spotnitz WD, Kron IL, et al. Four years' experience with fibrin sealant in thoracic and cardiovascular surgery. Ann Thorac Surg. 1990;50:40–3; discussion 43-4.
89. Takaoka K, Inoue S, Ohira S. Central bronchopleural fistulas closed by bronchoscopic injection of absolute ethanol. Chest. 2002;122:374–8.
90. Martin WR, Siefkin AD, Allen R. Closure of a bronchopleural fistula with bronchoscopic instillation of tetracycline. Chest. 1991;99:1040–2.
91. Watanabe S, Watanabe T, Urayama H. Endobronchial occlusion method of bronchopleural fistula with metallic coils and glue. Thorac Cardiovasc Surg. 2003;51:106–8.
92. Kanno R, Suzuki H, Fujiu K, Ohishi A, Gotoh M. Endoscopic closure of bronchopleural fistula after pneumonectomy by submucosal injection of polidocanol. Jpn J Thorac Cardiovasc Surg. 2002;50:30–3.
93. Watanabe Y, Matsuo K, Tamaoki A, Komoto R, Hiraki S. Bronchial occlusion with endobronchial Watanabe spigot. J Bronchol. 2003;10:264–7.
94. Roukema JA, Verpalen MC, Lobach HJ, Palmen FM. Bronchopleural fistula: the use of tissue glue. J Thorac Cardiovasc Surg. 1992;103:167.
95. Fujisawa T, Hongo H, Yamaguchi Y, et al. Intratumoral ethanol injection for malignant tracheobronchial lesions: a new bronchofiberscopic procedure. Endoscopy. 1986;18:188–91.

96. Jessen C, Sharma P. Use of fibrin glue in thoracic surgery. Ann Thorac Surg. 1985;39:521–4.
97. Jones DP, David I. Gelfoam occlusion of peripheral bronchopleural fistulas. Ann Thorac Surg. 1986;42:334–5.
98. Mathisen DJ, Grillo HC, Vlahakes GJ, Daggett WM. The omentum in the management of complicated cardiothoracic problems. J Thorac Cardiovasc Surg. 1988;95:677–84.
99. Salmon CJ, Ponn RB, Westcott JL. Endobronchial vascular occlusion coils for control of a large parenchymal bronchopleural fistula. Chest. 1990;98:233–4.
100. Ponn RB, D'Agostino RS, Stern H, Westcott JL. Treatment of peripheral bronchopleural fistulas with endobronchial occlusion coils. Ann Thorac Surg. 1993;56:1343–7.
101. Menard JW, Prejean CA, Tucker WY. Endoscopic closure of bronchopleural fistulas using a tissue adhesive. Am J Surg. 1988;155:415–6.
102. Wood RE, Lacey SR, Azizkhan RG. Endoscopic management of large, postresection bronchopleural fistulae with methacrylate adhesive (Super Glue). J Pediatr Surg. 1992;27(2):201–2.
103. Chawla RK, Madan A, Bhardwaj PK, Chawla K. Bronchoscopic management of bronchopleural fistula with intrabronchial instillation of glue (N-butyl cyanoacrylate). Lung India. 2012;29:11–4.
104. Chang C-C, Hsu H-H, Kuo S-W, Lee Y-C. Bronchoscopic gluing for post-lung-transplant bronchopleural fistula. Eur J Cardiothorac Surg. 2007;31:328–30.
105. Keller FS, Rösch J, Barker AF, Dotter CT. Percutaneous interventional catheter therapy for lesions of the chest and lungs. Chest. 1982;81:407–12.
106. Scappaticci E, Ardissone F, Ruffini E, Baldi S, Mancuso M. Postoperative bronchopleural fistula: endoscopic closure in 12 patients. Ann Thorac Surg. 1994;57:119–22.
107. Hamid UI, Jones JM. Closure of a bronchopleural fistula using glue. Interact Cardiovasc Thorac Surg. 2011;13:117–8.
108. Belda-Sanchís J, Serra-Mitjans M, Iglesias Sentis M, Rami R. Surgical sealant for preventing air leaks after pulmonary resections in patients with lung cancer. Cochrane Database Syst Rev (Online). 2010;(1):CD003051.
109. Onotera RT, Unruh HW. Closure of a post-pneumonectomy bronchopleural fistula with fibrin sealant (Tisseel). Thorax. 1988;43:1015–6.
110. York EL, Lewall DB, Hirji M, Gelfand ET, Modry DL. Endoscopic diagnosis and treatment of postoperative bronchopleural fistula. Chest. 1990;97:1390–2.
111. Kinoshita T, Miyoshi S, Katoh M, et al. Intrapleural administration of a large amount of diluted fibrin glue for intractable pneumothorax. Chest. 2000;117:790–5.
112. Vietri F, Tosato F, Passaro U, et al. The use of human fibrin glue in fistulous pathology of the lung. G Chir. 1991;12(6):399–402.
113. McCarthy PM, Trastek VF, Bell DG, et al. The effectiveness of fibrin glue sealant for reducing experimental pulmonary air leak. Ann Thorac Surg. 1988;45:203–5.
114. Potaris K, Mihos P, Gakidis I. Preliminary results with the use of an albumin-glutaraldehyde tissue adhesive in lung surgery. Med Sci Mon Int Med J Exp Clin Res. 2003;9:PI79–83.
115. Lin J, Iannettoni MD. Closure of bronchopleural fistulas using albumin-glutaraldehyde tissue adhesive. Ann Thorac Surg. 2004;77:326–8.
116. Sakamaki Y, Kido T, Fujiwara T, Kuwae K, Maeda M. A novel procedure using a tissue expander for management of persistent alveolar fistula after lobectomy. Ann Thorac Surg. 2005;79:2130–2.
117. Heffner JE, Standerfer RJ, Torstveit J, Unruh L. Clinical efficacy of doxycycline for pleurodesis. Chest. 1994;105:1743–7.
118. Asaki S. Tissue solidification in coping with digestive tract bleeding: hemostatic effect of local injection of 99.5 % ethanol. Tohoku J Exp Med. 1981;134:223–7.
119. Otani T, Tatsuka T, Kanamaru K, Okuda S. Intramural injection of ethanol under direct vision for the treatment of protuberant lesions of the stomach. Gastroenterology. 1975;69:123–9.
120. Aynaci E, Kocatürk CI, Yildiz P, Bedirhan MA. Argon plasma coagulation as an alternative treatment for bronchopleural fistulas developed after sleeve pneumonectomy. Interact Cardiovasc Thorac Surg. 2012;14:912–4.
121. Kiriyama M, Fujii Y, Yamakawa Y, et al. Endobronchial neodymium:yttrium-aluminum garnet laser for noninvasive closure of small proximal bronchopleural fistula after lung resection. Ann Thorac Surg. 2002;73:945–8; discussion 948-9.
122. Kodama H, Yamakado K, Murashima S, et al. Intractable bronchopleural fistula caused by radiofrequency ablation: endoscopic bronchial occlusion with silicone embolic material. Br J Radiol. 2009;82:e225–7.
123. Shen H-N, Lu FL, Wu H-D, Yu C-J, Yang P-C. Management of tension pneumatocele with highfrequency oscillatory ventilation. Chest. 2002; 121:284–6.
124. Uchida T, Wada M, Sakamoto J, Arai Y. Treatment for empyema with bronchopleural fistulas using endobronchial occlusion coils: report of a case. Surg Today. 1999;29:186–9.
125. Albes JM, Schäfers HJ, Gebel M, Ross UH. Tracheal stenting for malignant tracheoesophageal fistula. Ann Thorac Surg. 1994;57:1263–6.
126. Witt C, Ortner M, Ewert R, et al. Multiple fistulas and tracheobronchial stenoses require extensive stenting of the central airways and esophagus in squamous-cell carcinoma. Endoscopy. 1996;28:381–5.
127. Colt HG, Meric B, Dumon JF. Double stents for carcinoma of the esophagus invading the tracheo-bronchial tree. Gastrointest Endosc. 1992;38(4):485–9.
128. Freitag L, Tekolf E, Steveling H, Donovan TJ, Stamatis G. Management of malignant esophagotracheal fistulas with airway stenting and double stenting. Chest. 1996;110:1155–60.
129. Watanabe S, Shimokawa S, Yotsumoto G, Sakasegawa K. The use of a Dumon stent for the treatment of a bronchopleural fistula. Ann Thorac Surg. 2001;72:276–8.
130. Tayama K, Eriguchi N, Futamata Y, et al. Modified Dumon stent for the treatment of a bronchopleural fistula after pneumonectomy. Ann Thorac Surg. 2003;75:290–2.
131. Tsukada H, Osada H. Use of a modified Dumon stent for postoperative bronchopleural fistula. Ann Thorac Surg. 2005;80:1928–30.
132. Dutau H, Breen DP, Gomez C, Thomas PA, Vergnon J-M. The integrated place of tracheobronchial stents in the multidisciplinary management of large postpneumonectomy fistulas: our experience using a novel customised conical self-expandable metallic stent. Eur J Cardiothorac Surg. 2011;39:185–9.
133. Ferraroli GM, Testori A, Cioffi U, et al. Healing of bronchopleural fistula using a modified Dumon stent: a case report. J Cardiothorac Surg. 2006;1:16.
134. Takahashi M, Takahashi H, Itoh T, et al. Ultraflex expandable stents for the management of air leaks. Ann Thorac Cardiovasc Surg. 2006;12:50–2.
135. Dua J, Chessa M, Piazza L, et al. Initial experience with the new Amplatzer Duct Occluder II. J Invasive Cardiol. 2009;21:401–5.
136. Thanopoulos BD, Laskari CV, Tsaousis GS, et al. Closure of atrial septal defects with the Amplatzer occlusion device: preliminary results. J Am Coll Cardiol. 1998;31:1110–6.
137. Butera G, Chessa M, Carminati M. Percutaneous closure of ventricular septal defects. Cardiol Young. 2007;17(3):243–53.

138. Han YM, Gu X, Titus JL, et al. New self-expanding patent foramen ovale occlusion device. Catheter Cardiovasc Interv. 1999;47:370–6.
139. Scordamaglio PR, Tedde ML, Minamoto H, Pedra CAC, Jatene FB. Endoscopic treatment of tracheobronchial tree fistulas using atrial septal defect occluders: preliminary results. J Bras Pneumol. 2009;35:1156–60.
140. Gulkarov I, Paul S, Altorki NK, Lee PC. Use of Amplatzer device for endobronchial closure of bronchopleural fistulas. Interact Cardiovasc Thorac Surg. 2009;9:901–2.
141. Tedde ML, Scordamaglio PR, Minamoto H, et al. Endobronchial closure of total bronchopleural fistula with Occlutech Figulla ASD N device. Ann Thorac Surg. 2009;88:e25–6.
142. Passera E, Guanella G, Meroni A, et al. Amplatzer device and vacuum-assisted closure therapy to treat a thoracic empyema with bronchopleural fistula. Ann Thorac Surg. 2011;92:e23–5.
143. Sciurba FC, Ernst A, Herth FJF, et al. A randomized study of endobronchial valves for advanced emphysema. N Engl J Med. 2010;363:1233–44.
144. Feller-Kopman D, Bechara R, Garland R, Ernst A, Ashiku S. Use of a removable endobronchial valve for the treatment of bronchopleural fistula. Chest. 2006;130:273–5.
145. Levin AV, Tseĭmakh EV, Saĭmulenkov AM, et al. Use of endobronchial valve in postresection empyema and residual cavities with bronchopleural fistulas. Probl Tuberk Bolezn Legk. 2007;6:46–9.
146. Toma TP, Kon OM, Oldfield W, et al. Reduction of persistent air leak with endoscopic valve implants. Thorax. 2007;62:830–3.
147. Yu WC, Yeung YC, Chang Y, et al. Use of endobronchial one-way valves reveals questions on etiology of spontaneous pneumothorax: report of three cases. J Cardiothorac Surg. 2009;4:63.
148. Conforti S, Torre M, Fieschi S, Lomonaco A, Ravini M. Successful treatment of persistent postoperative air leaks following the placement of an endobronchial one-way valve. Monaldi Arch Chest Dis. 2010;73:88–91.
149. Schweigert M, Kraus D, Ficker JH, Stein HJ. Closure of persisting air leaks in patients with severe pleural empyema—use of endoscopic one-way endobronchial valve. Eur J Cardiothorac Surg. 2011;39:401–3.
150. Rosell A, López-Lisbona R, Cubero N, et al. Endoscopic treatment of persistent alveolar-pleural air leaks with a unidirectional endobronchial valve. Arch Bronconeumol. 2011;47:371–3.
151. Travaline JM, McKenna RJ, De Giacomo T, et al. Treatment of persistent pulmonary air leaks using endobronchial valves. Chest. 2009;136:355–60.
152. Gillespie CT, Sterman DH, Cerfolio RJ, et al. Endobronchial valve treatment for prolonged air leaks of the lung: a case series. Ann Thorac Surg. 2011;91:270–3.
153. El-Sameed Y, Waness A, Al Shamsi I, Mehta AC. Endobronchial valves in the management of broncho-pleural and alveolo-pleural fistulae. Lung. 2012;190:347–51.
154. FDA approves lung valve to control some air leaks after surgery. www.fda.gov/newsEvents/ newsroom/…2008/ ucm116970.hmt. Accessed 15 Jul 2012.

第 13 章
支气管镜异物移除

Erik Folch and Adnan Majid

本章提要 可疑气道异物吸入，是支气管镜检的一项重要指征。气道异物吸入的临床表现多样：可以是无症状并且偶然检查发现的，也可以是急性且威胁生命的中央气道阻塞。大多数异物吸入见于儿童和老年人。一些伴随情况，如酗酒、痴呆及其他慢性神经系统疾病，都会增加异物吸入的风险。为避免延误，必须重视可疑异物吸入的诊断。患者怀疑异物吸入时，支气管镜检是诊断治疗的金标准。大型气道异物移除，尤其儿科患者，硬质支气管镜优于纤维支气管镜。然而，目前对硬质支气管镜缺乏专门培训，所以气道异物移除，尤其成年人，常采用纤维支气管镜。用纤维支气管镜移除气道异物时，可用一些辅助设备。比如，近年来冷冻探针对于有机性异物的移除很有帮助。如今有经验、熟练的操作者使用软镜，可以移除大多数的气道异物。本章我们将讨论异物吸入的临床表现、辅助设备以及使用纤维支气管镜移除异物的技术要点。

关键词 气道异物，异物吸入，硬质支气管镜，儿科气道异物。

引 言

患者发生异物吸入时，使用硬质支气管镜或纤维支气管镜诊断及治疗已成为标准[1]。纤维支气管镜和硬质支气管镜的选择，常取决于当地的资源条件及专业水平。硬质支气管镜的优势在于：更好地保护气道，更利于使用工具移除异物。故硬质支气管镜移除异物更安全。若想成功移除儿科患者的气道异物，常需要使用硬质支气管镜，有时需要纤维支气管镜辅助。在美国，由于硬质支气管镜操作者分布差异较大[2-4]，而纤维支气管镜更普及，因此成人在适度镇静后常采用纤维支气管镜移除气道异物[5]。不过小型机构或者发展中国家的医疗中心甚至可能不具备纤维支气管镜操作的辅助设备及相关的熟练度和技巧。在这种情况下，为及时移除吸入异物，建议早期转诊至三级医疗中心。

异物吸入大多见于年轻人和老年人。表13.1 列出了一些气道异物吸入的危险因素。尽管无特殊症状的患者并不罕见，仍很有必要询问详细病史、进行细致的体格检查以及拍摄胸部平片（表13.2）。患者偶尔记不起病史，但若高度怀疑异物吸入，应及时做出诊断。不必惊讶，相当多的患者只有在支气管镜直视下才能做出异物吸入的诊断。进行支气管镜操作时，大多数吸入异物可同时移除。

应清楚认识到，每例异物吸入可产生不同的临床过程。可变性因素包括异物类型、异物在气道的位置、吸入到移除的时间间隔以及宿主对异物的反应。最终结果还取决于异物的物理特性、临床表现以及支气管镜操作者的熟练度。由于移除气道异物成功率高，并发症发生率低，所以不管是患者还是术者，手术操作价值很高。

表 13.1　成人异物吸入的危险因素

酗酒

使用镇静催眠药

牙列不齐

高龄

精神发育迟滞

帕金森病

原发神经系统疾病，伴吞咽障碍或精神状态异常

创伤，伴意识丧失

惊厥

全麻

咽食管憩室

表 13.2　异物吸入的体征及症状

哽咽史

长期咳嗽

单侧呼吸音减弱

肺不张

单侧过度充气

反复肺炎

单侧或双侧哮喘

咯血

气胸

纵隔气肿

皮下积气

支气管扩张

肺脓肿

胸膜疼痛

然而使用支气管镜移除气道异物的操作依然很困难。本章我们将讨论诊断及移除气道异物的原则，并提供适用于特殊情况、当地所具水平及技术的路径方法。

临床表现

成人的吞咽反射可保护气道免于异物吸入。若该保护机制失效，一旦发生了气道异物吸入，依赖强有力的咳嗽反射，大多数可自行缓解。

异物吸入的临床表现取决于异物位置及大小，其差异很大，可表现细微，也可威胁生命（表 13.2）。例如，如果异物位于声带附近，即使小物体也会导致强烈刺激、咳嗽，而若异物位于远端气道，可能只产生咳嗽和梗阻性肺炎。因此，患者高度怀疑有异物吸入风险非常关键。一旦存疑，先行支气管镜检将会避免严重远期并发症的发生[6]。哽咽发作后，大约 1/3 的异物位于声门附近。由于异物通常较大，很容易阻塞喉部。急性患者将表现为重度咳嗽、哽咽、声音嘶哑和不能发声。

观察报道称，哽咽发作是儿童最常见的临床表现。某些情况下，儿童异物吸入即告危急，X 线透视示不透明异物或单侧过度充气。另外，成人异物吸入无哽咽史，常表现为慢性咳嗽[7]。急性发作期表现为"渗透症状"（Baharloo 等报道），患者常表现为突发的哽咽及难治性咳嗽，可伴呕吐，较少咳嗽、发热、呼吸困难和哮喘[8]。值得一提的是，39% 的异物吸入患者无阳性体征发现[9]，6%~38% 的患者胸片可能显示正常[9-15]。相当一部分患者（具体数字不详），在送至医院前异物就咳出体外，有些甚至可将异物吞咽下肚。

一些提示有临床吸入情况伴哽咽史的儿童，约 50% 气道内并无异物。很难说上述患者是否曾吸入异物；或者确有吸入，但找不到异物，至于到底是自发咳出还是吞咽下肚，不得而知。

部　位

大部分成人吸入的异物位于右肺下叶。因

为儿童左主支气管大小不如成人宽，分支角不如成人锐利，故右下叶不常见[8,16]。

机制

有观点认为，用筷子吃饭、喝汤或吸入植物性物质时，常需借助吸气力。吸气力可能有助于将食物推至会厌，从而更易发生异物吸入[17-19]。儿童使用门牙可推动异物至咽后部。儿童异物吸入发生率之所以增高，可能与其口欲期的好奇天性及在吃饭时易哭闹、发笑和玩耍有关[5,18]。

时间轴

不同患者从吸入异物到医学评估之间的时间间隔多有差异。一些作者报道，成人相比儿童间隔较长。无机性异物吸入相比有机性异物吸入，临床表现及诊断间隔时间较短[8]。当然，诊断的时效性也取决于临床医师的经验和直觉。

放射性评估

一旦怀疑异物吸入，常先行胸片检查。吸入异物多透射线，所以X线透视的诊断作用有限。然而吸气期及呼气期X线平片可能显示一些细微征象，提示气道异物吸入，如空气潴留、肺不张、纵隔移位或肺浸润。在已发表的研究中，胸片检测气道异物的敏感性为70%~82%，特异性为44%~74%，阳性预测值为72%~83%，阴性预测值为41%~73%[11,12]。因此，若胸片示不透射线物体，可诊断异物吸入；但胸片正常或有细微改变时，则不能排除异物吸入诊断，而应根据相关临床背景谨慎解读胸片结果。实际上，一旦鉴别诊断考虑异物吸入，医师应放宽支气管镜指征，建议患者行支气管镜检。毕竟在此类患者中，支气管镜检查是诊断的基础。

儿童表现为纵隔气胸或皮下气肿时，临床医师应警惕异物吸入可能[20,21]。双侧颈部X线平片见声门下密度增加或水肿，提示喉气管异物存在可能[22]。X线平片见钙化异物，提示先前气道异物漏诊可能，因为植物性物质在气道内可逐渐钙化[23]；钙化也可能是支气管结石。

在慢性气道梗阻中，胸部CT可显示异物吸入的晚期并发症，比如支气管狭窄、支气管扩张、支气管内肿块或肉芽组织。另外已报道，MRI可用于花生吸入的诊断[24-26]。花生脂肪在T1加权上呈高信号。有时气道黏液可有类似气道异物的临床表现和放射学特征。然而，黏液在CT上表现为低衰减、起泡表现、附着相应气道，而且常随猛烈咳嗽移动位置[27]。

仿真支气管镜（VB）可用于可疑气道异物的诊断，最近有人使用VB调查了60例儿童[28]。在40例患者中，高分辨率的CT模拟出仿真支气管镜，然后显示可疑异物的缺损。33个异物得到确认，随后用支气管镜进行了移除。作者建议将仿真支气管镜用于异物的确认及定位，以辅助制定术前计划。在该系列研究中，7例仿真支气管镜阴性的患者，硬质支气管镜检查无一例有异物，这表明仿真支气管镜评价气道异物阴性预测值很高。不过仿真支气管镜不具治疗性，而且很多医院不具备该设备。同时，进行VB操作可能推迟必要的手术干预。Sudan的一份报告强调了CT气道重建的范围；在缺乏支气管镜的医疗中心，CT气道重建可作为异物吸入的诊断工具[29]。

值得一提的是，不论对于儿童还是成人，异物吸入常被误诊为哮吼、复发性咽炎、哮喘、复发性肺炎或原发性气道肿瘤，从而引起不必要及不适宜的诊治[30,31]。

儿童异物吸入

相比成人，儿童吸入事件及威胁生命的并发症发生率明显较高。婴儿在口欲期由于好奇心和独立探索的缘故，更易接触到小物体，所以1~3岁儿童异物吸入的发生率最高[8]。此外，还合并气道保护机制薄弱、门牙咬下物体后送至喉后部的推力过强的因素。而且儿童尝试吞咽异物时，可能还在哭泣、发笑及玩耍。儿童最常见的吸入异物为花生、种子、小型食品或者玩具。

成人异物吸入

成人吸入异物的种类差异很大，在很多情况下与文化、生活方式有关。肉类最常导致成人异物吸入[32]。然而有相当一部分病例异物颗粒潴留在声门位置，可被咳出或者被体位引流。成人其他常见的食物吸入颗粒包括坚果、南瓜子[33]、香瓜子[34,35]、西瓜子[35]、牙科装置、牙部填充物、硬币、扣针、耳坠、玻璃、气管切开插管碎片[36]和药丸[37]（图 13.1）。在美国，年轻健康男性可见钉和针的吸入[38,39]。在中东国家，吸入祷告珠、烦恼珠及针相对常见[35,40,41]。值得一提的是，成人全部年龄组都有异物吸入，但异物吸入最常见于有牙部疾病、吞咽困难、精神状态改变或痴呆的老年人（表 13.1）。不过，一些案例报道了相当多吸入食物中骨头的情况[42]。医疗操作或牙科操作也报道有异物吸入，如气道胃十二指肠镜进行套圈结扎时[43]。

成功率

支气管镜在取出气道异物方面，是一线治疗手段。一些研究表明支气管镜有很高的成功率，尤其联合使用硬质支气管镜和纤维支气管镜时成功率高达 97%~99%。表 13.3 简述了一些对硬质支气管镜和纤维支气管镜移除异物的研究。表单并不详尽，仅仅是目前已出版证据的代表性样本。

所有气道异物并非全能通过硬质支气管镜或纤维支气管镜取出。一些失败常与气道异物嵌入位置过深有关，当时无法进行球囊变位。其他失败原因为外在异物穿刺，如爆炸后遗留的金属残骸[42]。有趣的是，一些报道称，

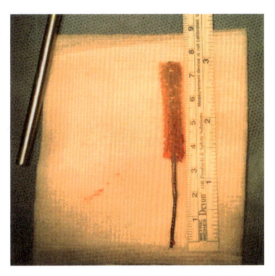

图 13.1 成功移除清洁时误吸的气管造口刷

虽然在外院行初始支气管镜失败或因操作者经验少失败，但后来却取得成功[8,42]。这些情况表明，在支气管镜操作中，经验和适时的训练很重要。

患者异物吸入的治疗方法

若怀疑患者异物吸入，需密切观察，直至确诊或排除诊断或异物被移除。患者即使临床状态稳定，但由于异物迁移或出血、气胸等并发症的发生[44,45]，其临床条件甚至会突然发生改变。

组织反应的可能性及程度增加了异物留存气道的时间[13,46,47]。以下情况才能推迟手术：协调必要人员及设备，为了将患者快速转移到可处理异物吸入的医院。值得一提的是，在第一个 24 小时内，支气管内黏膜常有轻度炎症、红斑和肉芽组织形成[13]。然而，炎症反应程度取决于吸入异物的成分。坚果、花生和青菜最具刺激性。我们团队移除过花生等坚果，术中见不同程度的肉芽组织形成（图 13.2）。然而，气道湿润环境增加了花生碎裂、阻塞远端气道的可能。

患者的全部处理方法可分为体位引流、硬

表 13.3 纤维支气管镜和硬质支气管镜移除气管异物的案例

作者	纤维支气管镜（F），硬质支气管镜（R），或联合（B）	患者总数	成功移除数	成功率（%）
Hiller[91]	F	7	6	86
Cunanan[92]	F	300	267	89
Clark[93]	F	3	3	100
Nunez[94]	F	17	12	71
Lan[95]	F	33	32	97
Limper[50]	F	23	14	61
Chen[18]	F	43	32	97
Moura e sa[96]	F	2[a]	2[a]	100
Ali Ali[41]	F	16	9	57
Gencer[40]	F	23	21	91
Debeljak[42]	B	63	61	97
Donado Una[97]	F	56	53	95
Baharloo[8]	R	112	103	92
Kalyanappagol[98]	R	206	206	100
Lima[99]	?	83	83	100
Blanco-Ramos[100]	B	32	24	75
Saki[87]	R	967	967	100
Oguzkaya[101]	R	500	498	99
Rahbarimanesh[102]	R	44	44	100
Metrangelo[103]	R	70	70	100
Martinot[11]	R	40	40	100
Chik[104]	R	27	27[b]	100
Yetim[105]	R	38	37	97
Tang[106]	F	1 027	938	91
Boyd[107]	F	20	18	90
Weissberg[108]	R	66	55	83
Zhijun[109]	R	1 428	1 424	99
Pasaoglu	R	639	639	100
Skoulakis[110]	R	130	130	100
Maddali[111]	R	140	140	100
Kiyan[112]	R	153	153	100

注：a. 77 例患者有 2 例异物不能用硬质支气管镜或联合方法移除；b. 4 例患者有异物残片，需反复行支气管镜检

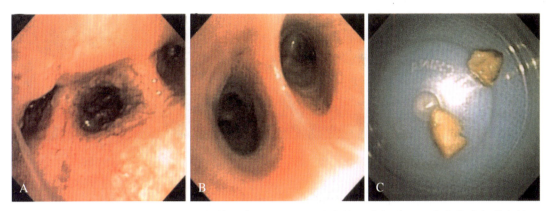

图 13.2　A. 花生吸入后的局限性支气管内炎症；B. 同一患者的正常气道；C. 成功移除气道内的两颗花生

质支气管镜和纤维支气管镜三部分。有很多专门设计的辅助装置帮助取出气道异物。冷冻探针技术作为近些年最适合移除有机性异物的方法，将在下面介绍。

非内镜性治疗

小部分患者异物向近端迁移可致心跳呼吸骤停，所以开始处理异物吸入时，不推荐吸入支气管扩张剂或体位引流[48]。推迟支气管镜检会增加并发症的风险，如肺炎、肺不张和心跳呼吸骤停，同时还降低了支气管镜移除异物的成功率。至少有一例临床试验，用吸入支气管扩张剂及体位引流来治疗气道异物，患者出现了心跳呼吸骤停。也有其他作者指出使用非内镜治疗方法会延长异物吸入的住院时间，产生更多并发症[46,48,49]。

还有一种极少使用的方法：当患者咳嗽时，进行治疗性叩诊。尽管有个别成功的报道，然而却不能因此耽搁更安全有效的治疗方法，如纤维支气管镜或硬质支气管镜。

对于口咽部异物，可伸入麦氏钳帮助取出[5]。

硬质支气管镜

近期大多数研究报道称，使用硬质支气管镜取出吸入的异物，成功率为95%~99%[33-35,44,47,50,51]。硬质支气管镜有诸多优势，包括可保持适宜通气、拥有更好的视野和更强劲的吸引力。全麻下若操作得当，患者可感受最大的舒适度，安全并且有效。硬质支气管镜取异物时，可使用多种器械，如光学钳、鳄牙钳、四叉钩、筐、冷冻治疗探针和一些型号的球囊。异物种类及位置决定使用器械的类型。在一些情况下，要成功移除气道异物，可能需要多种设备。尤其移除尖锐异物，硬质支气管镜很有帮助。然而也有一些报道纤维支气管镜成功移除气道内针头的案例[40,41]。

不过在美国，硬质支气管镜还不够普及，只有4%~8%的呼吸科医师会操作[2-4]。

纤维支气管镜

纤维支气管镜是评估成人异物吸入的常用初始诊断工具。一旦怀疑异物吸入，纤维支气管镜可经口探查。因为检查者有时不能立即发现明显异物，所以对每个病例都有必要进行全面检查。有些病例中，异物包裹在血液或肉芽组织中，增加了诊断难度。还有稍不常见的异物碎裂，异物分散在多个远端气道。

一旦异物类型、大小及位置确定，就可以尝试移除。尝试移除时，最好准备一些可用设备，最理想的当然是硬质支气管镜。通过纤维支气管镜移除异物，已开发的设备包括软钳、有齿镊、勒除器、输尿管取石网、渔网篮、冷

介入支气管镜临床指南

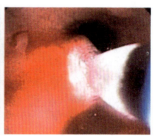

图 13.3　冷冻探针及其在良性气道疾病中的应用

冻治疗探针（图 13.3）、球囊导管和磁力吸引器。

若纤维支气管镜成功移除了异物，患者可免除随后的硬质支气管镜操作，节省了相关费用。一些报道证明，软镜可成功移除异物，熟练者可有 > 90% 的成功率[42,52,53]。纤维支气管镜可移除异物的种类广泛，包括牙齿、挡风玻璃、耳塞、大头针、钉子、鱼骨、花生、硬币和牙髓针[40,41,54-59]。

使用纤维支气管镜移除某些异物时，一些文献作者推荐使用气管导管以尽可能减少上呼吸道损伤的风险[42]。

目前文献中关于支气管镜的激烈争论围绕选择硬镜还是选择软镜来移除异物。个人偏好及个人专长、纤维支气管镜和硬质支气管镜各自的可用设备及可用技术使争议部分升级。有作者认为纤维支气管镜在诊断及移除成人气道异物方面有重要意义。不过，在打算移除异物时，硬质支气管镜也应准备，可起重要的补充作用[2,42,60]。所有纤维支气管镜操作者均应了解移除气道异物时操作失败后可能的结果。一旦操作失败，并不是每个操作纤维支气管镜的呼吸科医师都能轻松处理随后的结果。一旦决定操作纤维支气管镜时存疑，最好稳定住患者病情，并推荐患者到硬质支气管镜和纤维支气管镜都很专业的医疗机构诊治。

麻醉及镇痛

与硬质支气管镜不同，纤维支气管镜在适度镇静局麻下就可取出异物，而硬质支气管镜要在全麻下才能操作。适度镇静取出异物的优势在于可保留咳嗽反射，这样可进一步促进异物的移除。先通过支气管镜将异物带至气管，然后嘱咐患者咳嗽，多可咳出异物。

纤维支气管镜不建立安全气道，在适度镇静下就可移除异物，这反而引起了很多批评。有些人认为，纤维支气管镜操作时，在声门下的狭窄区域可能会丢失异物，有潜在窒息的风险。不过就我们所知，在医学文献里还未有窒息报道。虽然窒息的发生罕见，但一旦发生，通过支气管镜引导或在喉镜直视下紧急插管往往可保护气道。为此，大多数支气管镜中心最好配备不同型号的气管插管及喉镜。这样，一旦发生窒息，可接着通过气管内插管进行取出异物的操作。不过，也可采用其他方法（除了紧急插管），如再次使用纤维支气管镜，把异物推至远端气道，从而解除上呼吸道梗阻。

对于一些复杂病例，适度镇静不能很好地达到效果。此时全麻下使用硬质支气管镜是最佳选择。当异物过远、不能通过硬质支气管镜移除时，可在纤维支气管镜内引入气管导管或硬管来移除异物。当异物直径大于导管直径时，气管插管或硬管可与支气管镜、完整异物一起取出[61,62]。不过取出后，仍需即刻再次插管、反复气道探查。全麻下气管插管可用喉罩代替[63]。深度镇静下，只要气道条件控制适宜，甚至就可行纤维支气管镜检[64,65]。磷丙泊酚是丙泊酚的前体。最近的实践经验表明，在纤维支气管镜操作中使用磷丙泊酚安全有效[66]。有意思的是，磷丙泊酚并不是全麻药，它有特别的药代动力学及药效学特点，因而不需要麻醉监控[67]。然而，磷丙泊酚在支气管镜临床治疗操作中的应用，还未有人报道。

目前在儿童麻醉上还未达成共识。然而，一项对 12 979 例患儿的大型综述研究发现，维持连续通气可使远端部分梗阻转变成完全梗阻的风险最小化。那么，在合理通气的同时，联合静脉药物和肌肉松弛药物，可达到所需麻醉水平，从而创造出适宜硬质支气管镜操作的条件[68]。

纤维支气管镜的附件

使用纤维支气管镜移除异物，可用的辅助装置有多种类型。装置的选择多取决于异物位置、种类以及伴随的宿主组织反应。

抓钳

钳子是使用最广泛的器械，有多种类型，包括不同的杯口杯形、旋转机制、有齿或无齿以及多种附件装置，比如有中央窗或配备针头。抓钳又分弯钳、鳄齿钳、鼠齿钳、鲨齿钳以及包头钳。

应选择钳齿够大的钳子，以足够包绕异物全径。推荐鼠齿或鲨齿钳，因为鳄齿钳为防止坚硬物体滑脱，常需紧握。对于更精细的操作，可能需要弯钳或包头钳。一般情况下，抓钳在尝试移除易碎有机性异物时，会导致异物碎裂，从而解离和扩散到远端气道，所以抓钳仅适用于取出平、薄的无机性异物（如硬币、大头针、螺钉、夹子）或坚硬的有机性异物（如骨头）。

球囊导管

为移除气道异物，可充气球囊导管可能是最佳、最实用的方法（图 13.4）。尽管仅有部分型号有售，但 Fogarty 管仍最常用。Fogarty 管有不同的型号（4-7F），均可以通过纤维支气管镜的工作通道。它由导管引导至远端异物，然后用 1~3 ml 的盐水扩张球囊。牵拉球囊导管，直至异物送至利于移除的近端。

输尿管取石网

胃肠病学家和泌尿学家常用改进的输尿管取石网移除胆总管结石和膀胱结石。不过，输尿管取石网也可用于支气管镜气道异物移除。网翼可以在直径 1.6 mm 的 Teflon 导管内正常撤回。取石网在气道内打开，通过操纵两翼张开包绕并卡住异物。输尿管取石网最适用于大型异物移除。

渔网筐

渔网筐是息肉切除术中套索的改进装置。

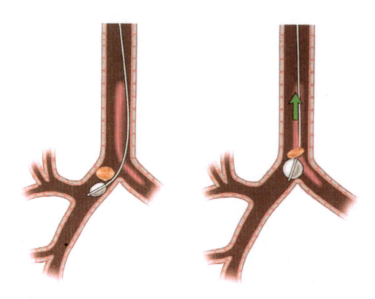

图 13.4 Fogarty 导管帮助将异物移至近端

为了更利于折叠、展开，术中常把粗线织成的网附着于套索的电线上（图13.5）。纤维支气管镜工作通道创造出简易的导管内路径供网筐通过，而网筐通常就在该路径中撤回。勒除器前进时，渔网缓慢释放，包绕异物，然后围成的陷阱缓慢收缩，在筐内困住异物。上述操作一旦完成，渔网筐、捕获的异物和支气管镜将作为整体一起退出。渔网筐也最适用于大型异物移除。

三叉套索或四叉套索

套索常一起挤压进导管。一旦布置好设备，释放套索，包绕异物。操作者按压设备柄，叉子远端合拢，进而捕获异物。确认捕获异物后，异物、套索和纤维支气管镜一起，整体小心撤出。因为叉子很脆弱，移除坚硬固体异物时不用套索。

磁力吸引器

磁力吸引器含有弹性探针，探针头端常有磁性圆筒。吸引器经过专门设计，可以通过纤维支气管镜的工作通道。该设备可轻易移除小型可移动的金属异物，如损坏的钳子或细胞刷[69,70]。

冷冻治疗导管

冷冻探针有黏合的特性，最适合移除富含水性介质的异物。该系统含有冷冻剂水槽（如氮氧化物或氮气）。水槽通过快速气体解压或焦耳-汤姆孙效应，在专门设计的冷冻探针头部（图13.3）创造出极度低温的环境（-40~-15℃）。冷冻探针与异物直接接触后，两者会连接在一起，然后操作者将冷冻探头、异物及纤维支气管镜一起撤出。该项技术特别适用于血凝块、黏膜球、有机物和小型无机物的移除[71]。

据我们的经验，冷冻治疗导管非常适用于有机物的移除。最近我们联合使用硬质支气管镜、儿童用纤维支气管镜和儿童用冷冻探针，移除了一例2岁儿童气道内的一枚花生碎。

为防止接触周围黏膜、不小心移除粘连的正常组织，支气管镜学家应注意保持视野清晰。

纤维支气管镜异物移除

一旦怀疑异物吸入，纤维支气管镜最好避过狭窄鼻腔，经口操作[72]。不过，首先健侧肺须做全套气道检查。可疑异物吸入区域最后检查。做全套细致检查，是为了保证仅有1个异

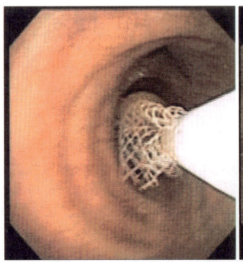
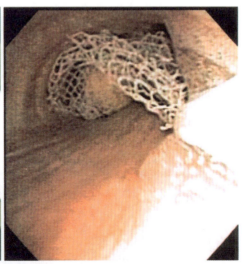

图13.5　内镜下使用渔网筐移除异物

物,或即使异物碎裂,也没有分散到其他气道。若观察到异物,在尝试取出异物前,应仔细检查异物及其周围区域的形状结构。支气管镜下可能看不完全整个异物,这时可能需行 X 线平片检查,判断不可视部分的方位。根据异物的大小、形状、位置和密度,选择合适的支气管镜附件。

使用纤维支气管镜时,务必小心:不要把异物推下气道!一般在尝试取出异物前,我们会使用 Fogarty 球囊带动异物靠近气管[54]。Fogarty 球囊管先放置于异物远端,然后扩张球囊,拉动异物远离支气管段或肺叶气道,到达气管(图 13.4)。一旦异物位于气管,就很容易移除了。异物推至上段气管时,我们会吩咐患者坐起,咳出异物。我们常使用这种技术处理柔软小型异物,成功率约 90%。

成功移除异物的关键在于:使用支气管镜附件抓取或者环套时,要合理保护好异物,保证异物完整。一旦异物被套扎或捕获,三个装置(支气管镜、抓钳和异物)作为整体同时撤出。撤出时,支气管镜操作者必须时刻保证异物可视,使异物一直处于气道中央。移除尖锐异物极具挑战。移除这种类型的异物,关键在于定位好异物的尖端,然后尝试变动尖端位置。一旦异物尖端游离,异物即可抓取并移除。抓取突起物品的体部或对侧端,会增加移除难度,因为这很有可能导致异物卡在黏膜。

同样,若异物周围组织反应干扰了移除过程,也会增加操作难度。有时在移除异物前,需要清除周围的肉芽组织。在上述一些患者中,支气管镜移除异物可能很有必要在全麻下进行。有时消融治疗有助于蒸发掉周围肉芽组织,比如激光切除。也可用激光破坏较大的异物,使其变小,变得更好处理,易于支气管镜移除[73-75]。其他方式,类似的有支气管镜电烙术,也可用于蒸发周围肉芽组织。一些专家建议在移除气道异物前使用短疗程的激素。不过,激素的效用还未获得验证[14,76]。

大量咯血是异物移除的罕见并发症,最好用硬质支气管镜控制[74]。咯血确定发生时,我们的经验是:经支气管镜缓慢滴入肾上腺素液(1:10 000~1:12 000),使局部血管收缩、血流降低,直至出血血管栓塞;对于止血,缓慢滴入冷盐水(4℃)也很有效。冷盐水导致低温性血管收缩,最终出血血管栓塞。

不明异物吸入

几乎每个异物移除经验丰富的医师都会提到这样的情况:异物移至口腔却发生丢失,怎么也找不到;或者放射显影有异物,实际探查却没有找到。最常见的原因是,患者无意识、自发咳出了异物。不过,若怀疑原异物遗留有小碎片或异物丢失,最好行全套气道检查。据一些人报道,病理标本偶然发现有相伴的恶性病变。所以移除异物时,最好同时送标本去病理分析[18]。接下来介绍吸入药片溶解的案例。Lee 等报道了一例铁离子药丸吸入的病例,吸入发生后 2 个月时支气管镜也没有发现吸入的异物,不过内镜活组织检查确认有铁残留,而残留导致了严重的肉芽组织形成[37]。最近,Parry 等报道了异物从右边迁移到了左边的案例[77]。

关于多学科团队

我们的经验同其他团队一样[11,42]:呼吸科、耳鼻喉科和胸科手术的专家之间的优秀工作关系,可以改善气道异物吸入的治疗结果。

异物遗留的罕见病例

医学文献报道了一些病例。因为不能移除异物或由于临床症状恶化阻碍了异物移除,所以异物遗留在体内[78]。尽管这些情况可能发生,我们依然强调:由于气道异物可引起长期并发症,故每一步都必须尽全力,保证异物安全移除,包括尽早送至专病中心。有一些罕见病例,患者咳出了遗留异物[79]。同时也有罕见病例,

呼吸设备故障导致异物吸入

不幸的是，采用呼吸治疗和机械通气时，常伴有异物吸入病例增多。案例包括吸入插管探丝[81]、吸引管[81,82]和气管切开刷（图 13.1）。

药片吸入

发生气道药片吸入，相对较常见。吸入药片可以有很突兀的结果。潮湿后，药片快速膨胀，据称若和硫糖铝一同服用，可致急性气道梗阻[83]。有其他案例报道：金属药片迅速溶解后，因为炎症和纤维化，产生了不良的长期结果[37]。我们团队近期报道了 2 例二甲双胍和石榴异物吸入案例[84]。

异物吸入的并发症

异物吸入有很高的发生短期和长期并发症的风险。这些并发症，文献中有广泛报道，包括急性呼吸衰竭、窒息[72]、肺炎、脓胸[85]、肺不张、心搏骤停、咯血、肉芽组织形成、喉头水肿、气胸、纵隔气肿、气管支气管破裂、气管食管瘘、支气管狭窄、局部肺不张[86]、纵隔炎、肺扭曲[18]和缺氧性脑损伤[87]。Aziz[85]展示了一则有趣的报道：异物吸入可以导致一连串事件，如气道梗阻、梗阻后肺炎和脓胸。

体外膜肺案例和异物吸入

医学文献有报道 ECMO 治疗近致死的异物吸入案例[88,89]。因为化脓性分泌物吸入和严重感染导致呼吸衰竭加重，近期一例复杂支气管镜移除异物操作寻求了 ECMO 的支持[90]。尽管很少采用这种方法，这些案例仍支持一点：只要临床可行，尽快送至专科气道中心更有利。

结 论

异物吸入的临床表现各异，从无症状到偶然发现，再到威胁生命的气道梗阻。不管怎样，为解除当前病症，防止远期并发症的发生，异物必须尝试移至气管支气管树后再取出。对于异物吸入患者，支气管镜仍是首位考虑的诊断性和治疗性选择。大部分专家同意，在移除大型气道异物方面，硬质支气管镜比纤维支气管镜更有效。而且，在儿科群体中，更推荐使用硬质支气管镜。然而，硬质支气管镜因为缺少训练、缺乏经验，实用性很低。因此在临床团队中，取出成人气道异物，纤维支气管镜仍然是最常使用的工具。假于有经验、专业操作者之手，纤维支气管镜技术可以移除大多数气道异物。同时，操作者必须熟悉多种附属器械，促进气道异物取出。若纤维支气管镜移除异物失败，即行硬质支气管镜检。如果当地不具备治疗设备，应尽早送至三级治疗中心。

参考文献

1. Rafanan AL, Mehta AC. Adult airway foreign body removal. What's new? Clin Chest Med. 2001;22:319–30.
2. Prakash UB, Offord KP, Stubbs SE. Bronchoscopy in North America: the ACCP survey. Chest. 1991;100:1668–75.
3. Tape TG, Blank LL, Wigton RS. Procedural skills of practicing pulmonologists. A national survey of 1,000 members of the American College of Physicians. Am J Respir Crit Care Med. 1995;151:282–7.
4. Colt HG, Prakash UBS, Offord KP. Bronchoscopy in North America: survey by the American Association for Bronchology, 1999. J Bronchol. 2000;7:8–25.
5. Marquette CH, Martinot A. Interventional bronchoscopy. Basel: Karger; 2000.
6. Paksu S, Paksu MS, Kilic M, et al. Foreign body aspiration in childhood: evaluation of diagnostic parameters. Pediatr Emerg Care. 2012;28:259–64.
7. al-Majed SA, Ashour M, al-Mobeireek AF, al-Hajjaj MS, Alzeer AH, al-Kattan K. Overlooked inhaled foreign bodies: late sequelae and the likelihood of recovery. Respir Med. 1997;91:293–6.
8. Baharloo F, Veyckemans F, Francis C, Biettlot MP, Rodenstein

DO. Tracheobronchial foreign bodies: presentation and management in children and adults. Chest. 1999;115:1357–62.
9. McGuirt WF, Holmes KD, Feehs R, Browne JD. Tracheobronchial foreign bodies. Laryngoscope. 1988;98:615–8.
10. Mantor PC, Tuggle DW, Tunell WP. An appropriate negative bronchoscopy rate in suspected foreign body aspiration. Am J Surg. 1989;158:622–4.
11. Martinot A, Closset M, Marquette CH, et al. Indications for flexible versus rigid bronchoscopy in children with suspected foreign-body aspiration. Am J Respir Crit Care Med. 1997;155:1676–9.
12. Hoeve LJ, Rombout J, Pot DJ. Foreign body aspiration in children. The diagnostic value of signs, symptoms and pre-operative examination. Clin Otolaryngol Allied Sci. 1993;18:55–7.
13. Wiseman NE. The diagnosis of foreign body aspiration in childhood. J Pediatr Surg. 1984;19:531–5.
14. Banerjee A, Rao KS, Khanna SK, et al. Laryngotracheo-bronchial foreign bodies in children. J Laryngol Otol. 1988;102:1029–32.
15. Pasaoglu I, Dogan R, Demircin M, Hatipoglu A, Bozer AY. Bronchoscopic removal of foreign bodies in children: retrospective analysis of 822 cases. Thorac Cardiovasc Surg. 1991;39:95–8.
16. Cleveland RH. Symmetry of bronchial angles in children. Radiology. 1979;133:89–93.
17. Casson AG, Guy JR. Foreign-body aspiration in adults. Can J Surg. 1987;30:193–4.
18. Chen CH, Lai CL, Tsai TT, Lee YC, Perng RP. Foreign body aspiration into the lower airway in Chinese adults. Chest. 1997;112:129–33.
19. Case records of the Massachusetts General Hospital. Weekly clinicopathological exercises. Case 33-1997. A 75-year-old man with chest pain, hemoptysis, and a pulmonary lesion. N Engl J Med. 1997;337:1220–6.
20. Burton EM, Riggs Jr W, Kaufman RA, Houston CS. Pneumomediastinum caused by foreign body aspiration in children. Pediatr Radiol. 1989;20:45–7.
21. Nimrey-Atrash N, Bentur L, Elias N. Subcutaneous emphysema and pneumomediastinum due to foreign body aspiration in children with asthma. Pediatr Pulmonol. 2012;47:88–90.
22. Esclamado RM, Richardson MA. Laryngotracheal foreign bodies in children. A comparison with bronchial foreign bodies. Am J Dis Child. 1987;141:259–62.
23. Shepard JA. The bronchi: an imaging perspective. J Thorac Imaging. 1995;10:236–54.
24. Imaizumi H, Kaneko M, Nara S, Saito H, Asakura K, Akiba H. De finitive diagnosis and location of peanuts in the airways using magnetic resonance imaging techniques. Ann Emerg Med. 1994;23:1379–82.
25. Kitanaka S, Mikami I, Tokumaru A, O'Uchi T. Diagnosis of peanut inhalation by MRI. Pediatr Radiol. 1992;22:300–1.
26. O'Uchi T, Tokumaru A, Mikami I, Yamasoba T, Kikuchi S. Value of MR imaging in detecting a peanut causing bronchial obstruction. AJR Am J Roentgenol. 1992;159:481–2.
27. Marom EM, Goodman PC, McAdams HP. Focal abnormalities of the trachea and main bronchi. AJR Am J Roentgenol. 2001;176:707–11.
28. Cevizci N, Dokucu AI, Baskin D, et al. Virtual bronchoscopy as a dynamic modality in the diagnosis and treatment of suspected foreign body aspiration. Eur J Pediatr Surg. 2008;18:398–401.
29. Salah MT, Hamza S, Murtada M, Salma M. Delayed diagnosis of foreign body aspiration in children. Sudanese J of Public Health. 2007;2:48–50.
30. Atmaca S, Unal R, Sesen T, Kilicarslan H, Unal A. Laryngeal foreign body mistreated as recurrent laryngitis and croup for one year. Turk J Pediatr. 2009;51:65–6.
31. Barben J, Berkowitz RG, Kemp A, Massie J. Bronchial granuloma—where's the foreign body? Int J Pediatr Otorhinolaryngol. 2000;53:215–9.
32. Mittleman RE, Wetli CV. The fatal cafe coronary. Foreign-body airway obstruction. JAMA. 1982;247:1285–8.
33. Daniilidis J, Symeonidis B, Triaridis K, Kouloulas A. Foreign body in the airways: a review of 90 cases. Arch Otolaryngol. 1977;103:570–3.
34. Abdulmajid OA, Ebeid AM, Motaweh MM, Kleibo IS. Aspirated foreign bodies in the tracheobronchial tree: report of 250 cases. Thorax. 1976;31:635–40.
35. Elhassani NB. Tracheobronchial foreign bodies in the Middle East. A Baghdad study. J Thorac Cardiovasc Surg. 1988;96:621–5.
36. Yapici D, Atici S, Birbicer H, Oral U. Manufacturing defect in an endotracheal tube connector: risk of foreign body aspiration. J Anesth. 2008;22:333–4.
37. Lee P, Culver DA, Farver C, Mehta AC. Syndrome of iron pill aspiration. Chest. 2002;121:1355–7.
38. Clancy MJ. Bronchoscopic removal of an inhaled, sharp, foreign body: an unusual complication. J Laryngol Otol. 1999;113:849–50.
39. Vander Salm TJ, Ellis N. Blowgun dart aspiration. J Thorac Cardiovasc Surg. 1986;91:930–2.
40. Gencer M, Ceylan E, Koksal N. Extraction of pins from the airway with flexible bronchoscopy. Respiration. 2007;74:674–9.
41. Al-Ali MA, Khassawneh B, Alzoubi F. Utility of fiberoptic bronchoscopy for retrieval of aspirated headscarf pins. Respiration. 2007;74:309–13.
42. Debeljak A, Sorli J, Music E, Kecelj P. Bronchoscopic removal of foreign bodies in adults: experience with 62 patients from 1974–1998. Eur Respir J. 1999;14:792–5.
43. Betancourt M, Bekteshi E, Toth J, Alam S. Foreign body aspiration during esophagogastroduodenoscopy with band ligation. J Bronchol Intervento Pulmonol. 2008;15:204–5.
44. Kosloske AM. Bronchoscopic extraction of aspirated foreign bodies in children. Am J Dis Child. 1982;136:924–7.
45. Kosloske AM. Tracheobronchial foreign bodies in children: back to the bronchoscope and a balloon. Pediatrics. 1980;66:321–3.
46. Law D, Kosloske AM. Management of tracheobronchial foreign bodies in children: a reevaluation of postural drainage and bronchoscopy. Pediatrics. 1976;58:362–7.
47. Steen KH, Zimmermann T. Tracheobronchial aspiration of foreign bodies in children: a study of 94 cases. Laryngoscope. 1990;100:525–30.
48. Bose P, El Mikatti N. Foreign bodies in the respiratory tract. A review of forty-one cases. Ann R Coll Surg Engl. 1981;63:129–31.
49. Cotton EK, Abrams G, Vanhoutte J, Burrington J. Removal of aspirated foreign bodies by inhalation and postural drainage. A survey of 24 cases. Clin Pediatr (Phila). 1973;12:270–6.
50. Limper AH, Prakash UB. Tracheobronchial foreign bodies in adults. Ann Intern Med. 1990;112:604–9.
51. Hsu W, Sheen T, Lin C, Tan C, Yeh T, Lee S. Clinical experiences of removing foreign bodies in the airway and esophagus with a rigid endoscope: a series of 3217 cases from 1970 to 1996. Otolaryngol Head Neck Surg. 2000;122:450–4.
52. Surka AE, Chin R, Conforti J. Bronchoscopic myths and legends: airway foreign bodies. Clin Pulm Med. 2006;13:209–11.
53. Swanson KL, Prakash UB, MdCougall JC, Midthun DE, Edell ES, Brutinel MW, et al. Airway foreign bodies in adults. J Bronchol. 2003;10:107–11.
54. Heinz 3rd GJ, Richardson RH, Zavala DC. Endobronchial foreign body removal using the bronchofiberscope. Ann Otol Rhinol Laryngol. 1978;87:50–2.
55. Mehta AC, Grimm M. Breakage of Nd-YAG laser sapphire contact probe inside the endobronchial tree. Chest. 1988;93:1119.
56. Fieselmann JF, Zavala DC, Keim LW. Removal of foreign bodies (two teeth) by fiberoptic bronchoscopy. Chest. 1977;72:241–3.

57. Klayton RJ, Donlan CJ, O'Neil TJ, Foreman DR. Letter: foreign body removal via fiberoptic bronchoscopy. JAMA. 1975;234:806.
58. Lee M, Fernandez NA, Berger HW, Givre H. Wire basket removal of a tack via flexible fiberoptic bronchoscopy. Chest. 1982;82:515.
59. Rohde FC, Celis ME, Fernandez S. The removal of an endobronchial foreign body with the fiberoptic bronchoscope and image intensifier. Chest. 1977; 72:265.
60. Prakash UB, Midthun DE, Edell ES. Indications for flexible versus rigid bronchoscopy in children with suspected foreign-body aspiration. Am J Respir Crit Care Med. 1997;156:1017–9.
61. Downey RJ, Libutti SK, Gorenstein L, Mercer S. Airway management during retrieval of the very large aspirated foreign body: a method for the flexible bronchoscope. Anesth Analg. 1995;81:186–7.
62. Verea-Hernando H, Garcia-Quijada RC, Ruiz de Galarreta AA. Extraction of foreign bodies with fiberoptic bronchoscopy in mechanically ventilated patients. Am Rev Respir Dis. 1990;142:258.
63. Rodrigues AJ, Scussiatto EA, Jacomelli M, et al. Bronchoscopic techniques for removal of foreign bodies in children's airways. Pediatr Pulmonol. 2012;47:59–62.
64. Hirai T, Yamanaka A, Fujimoto T, Shiraishi M, Fukuoka T. Bronchoscopic removal of bronchial foreign bodies through the laryngeal mask airway in pediatric patients. Jpn J Thorac Cardiovasc Surg. 1999;47:190–2.
65. McGrath G, Das-Gupta M, Clarke G. Bronchoscopy via continuous positive airway pressure for patients with respiratory failure. Chest. 2001;119:670–1.
66. Silvestri GA, Vincent BD, Wahidi MM, Robinette E, Hansbrough JR, Downie GH. A phase 3, randomized, double-blind study to assess the efficacy and safety of fospropofol disodium injection for moderate sedation in patients undergoing flexible bronchoscopy. Chest. 2009;135:41–7.
67. Jantz MA. The old and the new of sedation for bronchoscopy. Chest. 2009;135:4–6.
68. Fidkowski CW, Zheng H, Firth PG. The anesthetic considerations of tracheobronchial foreign bodies in children: a literature review of 12,979 cases. Anesth Analg. 2010;111:1016–25.
69. Saito H, Saka H, Sakai S, Shimokata K. Removal of broken fragment of biopsy forceps with magnetic extractor. Chest. 1989;95:700–1.
70. Mayr J, Dittrich S, Triebl K. A new method for removal of metallic-ferromagnetic foreign bodies from the tracheobronchial tree. Pediatr Surg Int. 1997;12:461–2.
71. De Weerdt S, Noppen M, Remels L, Vanherreweghe R, Meysman M, Vincken W. Successful removal of a massive endobronchial blood clot by means of cryotherapy. J Bronchol. 2005;12:23–4.
72. Mehta AC. Nasal versus oral insertion of the flexible bronchoscope. J Bronchol. 1996;3:224–8.
73. Boelcskei PL, Wagner M, Lessnau KK. Laser-assisted removal of a foreign body in the bronchial system of an infant. Lasers Surg Med. 1995;17:375–7.
74. Rees JR. Massive hemoptysis associated with foreign body removal. Chest. 1985;88:475–6.
75. Hayashi AH, Gillis DA, Bethune D, Hughes D, O'Neil M. Management of foreign-body bronchial obstruction using endoscopic laser therapy. J Pediatr Surg. 1990;25:1174–6.
76. Bolliger CT, Mathur PN. Interventional bronchoscopy. Basel: Karger; 2000.
77. Parray T, Abraham E, Apuya JS, Ghafoor AU, Saif Siddiqui M. Migration of a foreign body from right to left lung. Internet J Anesthesiol. 2010;24.
78. Mohnssen SR, Greggs D. Iatrogenic aspiration of components of respiratory care equipment. Chest. 1993;103:964–5.
79. Pinals M, Pinals D, Tracy JD, Brandstetter RD. Expectoration of an occult foreign body six asymptomatic years after aspiration. Chest. 1993;103:1930–1.
80. Karapolat S. Foreign-body aspiration in an adult. Can J Surg. 2008;51:411; author reply -2.
81. Mohnssen SR. Iatrogenic aspiration. Follow-up. Chest. 1994;105:976.
82. Iannuzzi M, De Robertis E, Rispoli F, Piazza O, Tufano R. A complication of a closed-tube endotracheal suction catheter. Eur J Anaesthesiol. 2009;26:974–5.
83. Overdahl MC, Wewers MD. Acute occlusion of a mainstem bronchus by a rapidly expanding foreign body. Chest. 1994; 105:1600–2.
84. Kinsey CM, Folch E, Majid A, Channick C. Evaluation and management of pill aspiration: case discussion. In:17th World Congress for bronchology and interventional pulmonology, Cleveland, OH; 2012.
85. Aziz F. Natural history of an aspirated foreign body. J Bronchol. 2006;13:161–2.
86. James P, Christopher DJ, Balamugesh T, Thomas R. Multiple foreign body aspiration and bronchiectasis. J Bronchol. 2006;13:218–20.
87. Saki N, Nikakhlagh S, Rahim F, Abshirini H. Foreign body aspirations in infancy: a 20-year experience. Int J Med Sci. 2009;6: 322–8.
88. Brown KL, Shefler A, Cohen G, DeMunter C, Pigott N, Goldman AP. Near-fatal grape aspiration with complicating acute lung injury successfully treated with extracorporeal membrane oxygenation. Pediatr Crit Care Med. 2003;4:243–5.
89. Ignacio Jr RC, Falcone Jr RA, Brown RL. A case report of severe tracheal obstruction requiring extracorporeal membrane oxygenation. J Pediatr Surg. 2006;41:E1–4.
90. Isherwood J, Firmin R. Late presentation of foreign body aspiration requiring extracorporeal membrane oxygenation support for surgical management. Interact Cardiovasc Thorac Surg. 2011;12:631–2.
91. Hiller C, Lerner S, Varnum R, et al. Foreign body removal with the flexible fiberoptic bronchoscope. Endoscopy. 1977;9:216–22.
92. Cunanan OS. The flexible fiberoptic bronchoscope in foreign body removal. Experience in 300 cases. Chest. 1978;73:725–6.
93. Clark PT, Williams TJ, Teichtahl H, Bowes G, Tuxen DV. Removal of proximal and peripheral endobronchial foreign bodies with the flexible fibreoptic bronchoscope. Anaesth Intensive Care. 1989;17:205–8.
94. Nunez H, Perez Rodriguez E, Alvarado C, et al. Foreign body aspirate extraction. Chest. 1989;96:698.
95. Lan RS, Lee CH, Chiang YC, Wang WJ. Use of fiberoptic bronchoscopy to retrieve bronchial foreign bodies in adults. Am Rev Respir Dis. 1989;140:1734–7.
96. Moura e Sa J, Oliveira A, Caiado A, et al. Tracheobronchial foreign bodies in adults—experience of the Bronchology Unit of Centro Hospitalar de Vila Nova de Gaia. Rev Port Pneumol. 2006;12:31–43.
97. Donado Una JR, de Miguel Poch E, Casado Lopez ME, Alfaro Abreu JJ. Fiber optic bronchoscopy in extraction of tracheo-bronchial foreign bodies in adults. Arch Bronconeumol. 1998;34:76–81.
98. Kalyanappagol VT, Kulkarni NH, Bidri LH. Management of tracheobronchial foreign body aspirations in paediatric age group—a 10 year retrospective analysis. Indian J Anaesth. 2007;51:20–3.
99. Lima AG, Santos NA, Rocha ER, Toro IF. Bronchoscopy for foreign body removal: where is the delay? Jornal Brasileiro de Pneumologia: Publicacao Oficial da Sociedade Brasileira de Pneumologia e Tisilogia. 2008;34:956–8.

100. Ramos MB, Fernandez-Villar A, Rivo JE, et al. Extraction of airway foreign bodies in adults: experience from 1987–2008. Interact Cardiovasc Thorac Surg. 2009;9:402–5.
101. Oguzkaya F, Akcali Y, Kahraman C, Bilgin M, Sahin A. Tracheobronchial foreign body aspirations in childhood: a 10-year experience. Eur J Cardiothorac Surg. 1998;14:388–92.
102. Rahbarimanesh A, Noroozi E, Molaian M, Salamati P. Foreign body aspiration: a five-year report in a children's hospital. Iran J Pediatr. 2008;18:191–2.
103. Metrangelo S, Monetti C, Meneghini L, Zadra N, Giusti F. Eight years' experience with foreignbody aspiration in children: what is really important for a timely diagnosis? J Pediatr Surg. 1999;34:1229–31.
104. Chik KK, Miu TY, Chan CW. Foreign body aspiration in Hong Kong Chinese children. Hong Kong Med J. 2009;15:6–11.
105. Yetim DT, Bayarogullari H, Arica V, Akcora B, Arica SG, Tutanc M. Foreign body aspiration in children; analysis of 42 cases. J Pulmon Resp Med. 2012;2:121–5.
106. Tang LF, Xu YC, Wang YS, et al. Airway foreign body removal by flexible bronchoscopy: experience with 1027 children during 2000–2008. World J Pediatr. 2009;5:191–5.
107. Boyd M, Watkins F, Singh S, et al. Prevalence of flexible bronchoscopic removal of foreign bodies in the advanced elderly. Age Ageing. 2009;38:396–400.
108. Weissberg D, Schwartz I. Foreign bodies in the tracheobronchial tree. Chest. 1987;91:730–3.
109. Zhijun C, Fugao Z, Niankai Z, Jingjing C. Therapeutic experience from 1428 patients with pediatric tracheobronchial foreign body. J Pediatr Surg. 2008;43:718–21.
110. Skoulakis CE, Doxas PG, Papadakis CE, et al. Bronchoscopy for foreign body removal in children. A review and analysis of 210 cases. Int J Pediatr Otorhinolaryngol. 2000;53:143–8.
111. Maddali MM, Mathew M, Chandwani J, Alsajwani MJ, Ganguly SS. Outcomes after rigid bronchoscopy in children with suspected or confirmed foreign body aspiration: a retrospective study. J Cardiothorac Vasc Anesth. 2011;25:1005–8.
112. Kiyan G, Gocmen B, Tugtepe H, Karakoc F, Dagli E, Dagli TE. Foreign body aspiration in children: the value of diagnostic criteria. Int J Pediatr Otorhinolaryngol. 2009;73:963–7.

第 14 章
支气管镜在咯血中的作用

Santhakumar Subramanian, Arvind H. Kate, and Prashant N. Chhajed

本章提要 咯血是一种常见症状，且是一种危险的征兆。非大咯血与大咯血之间没有具体的定义。实际上，大咯血是指咯血的规模而不是咯血量。急性支气管炎是引起非大咯血的主要原因。而大咯血常见的原因包括支气管扩张、肺结核、肺癌、足分支菌病。支气管镜在咯血的诊断与治疗中发挥重要的作用。它可以直接检查出咯血部位，并能防止血液流向其他肺叶引起窒息。在处理大咯血时，硬质支气管镜要优于纤维支气管镜，因大部分医疗中心缺乏训练有素的医师而使它的作用受限。在没有硬质支气管镜的条件下，先进行气管插管，开放气道，用纤维支气管镜在早期进行检查，并进行积极的抢救。支气管镜技术包括球囊填塞术，而局部使用冰盐水、血管收缩剂以及促凝剂均有利于暂时性控制出血。支气管介入技术包括对病灶进行激光切除或氩离子凝固。暂时性地控制出血有利于对特定患者做支气管动脉栓塞术或者进行手术。

关键词 咯血，支气管镜，硬质支气管镜，大咯血，支气管动脉栓塞术。

引 言

咯血是有潜在危险的症状之一，它可表现为少量的痰血。中度的大咯血可能会阻塞气道，引起血流动力学变化，甚至危及生命。据估计，6.8% 的胸外科门诊患者和 11% 的住院患者因咯血入院[1]。大咯血的死亡率高达 80%，而一般咯血的死亡率约为 7%~30%[2-4]。窒息是致死的主要原因，而不是出血[5]，且窒息经常同时伴有心力衰竭。像其他危及生命的情况一样，处理咯血的首要原则是开放气道，从而获得稳定的血流动力学。一旦气道开放，支气管镜可在对腔内出血病变确定位置，隔离气道，以及控制出血中起到重要作用[6]。在本章节当中，我们着重讨论对支气管镜在治疗大咯血中的研究，以及回顾咯血的定义、血供、病因、评估以及处理。

定 义

咯血可分为非大咯血与大咯血，虽然对大咯血的定义还没有共识，对咯血量与质的定义已经用于不同研究。在咯血量上，大咯血是指 24 小时咯血量在 100~1 000 ml，而非大咯血是指 24 小时咯血量 < 100 ml[6]。基于 Crocco 等[7] 的研究，现在广泛接受的大咯血定义是指 24 小时内咯血量超过 600 ml。4 小时内咯血量 > 600 ml 的咯血的死亡率为 71%，而 < 60 ml 的咯血在 24~48 小时内的死亡率只有 5%。据估计，肺泡腔中累积超过 400 ml 的血液就会导致缺氧[8]。以上定义对咯血量缺乏统一指标，同时没有考虑其他的因素，如出血速度，患者的心肺功能，气道保护能力。因此更加合理的定义可基于咯血对患者的整体影响，包括以下参数：输血量、住院天数、气管插管、吸痰、气道梗阻、氧合

（PaO_2 <8 kPa 或 60 mmHg）、死亡。

血 供

呼吸系统有两种不同来源的血供：一是高压（体）循环，提供支气管到终末支气管的血液供应；另一种是低压（肺）循环，提供肺泡内外的血液供应[9]。支气管动脉起源于降主动脉，常在 T5、T6 水平，最常见的情况为右侧支气管动脉为单支，左侧为双支。其中约 20% 患者的支气管动脉异常起源于其他动脉。在 5% 的患者中，支气管动脉还会发出一支脊柱动脉[10]。

病 因

医师要有一个重要的意识，即鼻咽部的出血，以及胃肠道的呕血与咯血很像。引起咯血的重要病因列于表 14.1。慢性炎性疾病如支气管扩张、肺结核、肺脓肿、肺癌，是大咯血的常见原因。咯血也可发生于足分支菌病形成的空洞[12]。

在老年患者当中，73% 的患者咯血的原因是肺结核[7]。这包括新老患者。肺结核在咯血中的病理生理机制包括①直接引起支气管动脉的感染以及炎症。②支气管扩张导致慢性炎症，使血管扩张，曲折，变脆导致自发出血。③足分支菌病导致肉芽组织和新生血管形成的巨大空洞（Rasmussen 动脉瘤）。④结核性感染导致肺动脉扩张，引起破裂。

各种原因引起的支气管扩张如慢性支气管炎、肺囊性变、去纤毛运动、免疫缺陷在咯血中占了相当的比例[13]。这些患者中潜在的病理生理机制是扩大、扩张、屈曲的支气管动脉形成。累及支气管的原发性或者继发性肺恶性肿瘤常具有丰富血供，动脉易自发性破裂出血，偶尔可引起大咯血。尽管支气管循环的破裂出血在大咯血病例中占多数，但也有为数不少的患者为肺动脉出血。其他因素，如坏死性的肺感染，恶性肿瘤，脉管炎，Swan-Gan 插管术引

表 14.1 咯血原因

感染	血管
• 分枝杆菌特别是结核感染	• 肺栓塞和肺梗死
• 真菌感染足菌肿	• 二尖瓣狭窄
• 肺脓肿	• 动脉支气管瘘
• 坏死性肺炎（肺炎克雷伯菌，金色葡萄球菌，军团菌）	• 动静脉畸形
医源性的创伤	• 支气管扩张
• 支气管镜检查	• 左心衰竭
• Swan-Ganz 导管置入术	凝血功能障碍
• 支气管活检术	• 血管性血友病
• 支气管镜吸痰术	• 血友病
寄生虫	• 抗凝治疗
• 包虫囊肿	• 血小板减少症
• 并殖吸虫病	• 血小板功能异常
创伤	• 弥散性血管内凝血
• 贯穿伤	• 血管炎
• 吸入性溃疡	• 白塞氏综合征
• 支气管血管瘘	
肿瘤	肺部疾病
• 支气管癌	• 支气管扩张（包括囊肿扩张）
• 支气管腺瘤	• 慢性支气管炎
• 肺转移瘤	• 肺大疱
• 肺肉瘤	其他
小儿咯血	• 淋巴结缔组织增生
• 异物吸入	• 月经（肺子宫内膜异位症）
• 支气管腺瘤	• 尘肺
• 血管异常	• 支气管结石
	• 特发性的肺疾病
	误诊
	• 鼻出血
	• 吐血

起的损伤，肺动静脉畸形等来自肺循环的出血也可引起大咯血。尽管肺泡出血也能引起咯血，但它极少表现为大咯血，因为肺泡腔内能容纳大量的血液。有趣的是，根据最近的文献报道，尽管现在检查设施齐全，仍有11%~19%的患者有隐源性的大咯血[14]。肺静脉栓塞，肺子宫内膜异位症，肺动静脉畸形，支气管血管瘘是其他罕见大咯血的原因。

诊 断

当气道开放，血压稳定后，在小、中度的咯血之初用支气管镜检查可能会引起大咯血，以往的经验和临床检查可用于区分咯血、呕血和上呼吸道出血。咯血没有统一的诊断标准。这需要胸片，胸部CT与支气管镜检查来明确诊断。凝血谱和血管炎谱像将有助于诊断。33%~82%的患者仅用胸片就能确定出血部位[15]，并可揭示35%患者的病因。胸部CT在确定出血部位以及明确病因、指导后续治疗方面优于胸片。88%的出血能用CT定位[16]。对咯血患者而言，先做CT还是支气管镜争论已久。一些医者认为CT可以代替支气管镜作为咯血患者的首要诊断性检查，因为它有更高的诊断率[17]，而其他人认为它只能作为支气管镜的补充[18]。目前，薄层CT能很精确地显示支气管动静脉与肺血管[19,20]。然而它也有局限性，比如对于双侧肺部疾病的患者，纤维支气管镜能更好地发现与定位病灶。支气管镜检查也能用于血压相对不稳定，不能转运至CT室检查的患者。

纤维支气管镜用于大咯血定位的诊断率是73%~79%，在轻、中度咯血中的诊断率较低[21,22]。对纤维支气管镜检查的最佳时机（早期或晚期）仍有争议，在非大咯血患者中行早期或者晚期支气管镜检查的结果没有区别[23,24]。在危及生命的大咯血患者中不可使用纤维支气管镜。它在开放气道和通气方面具有局限性，相比之下硬质支气管镜更能有效地开放气道，保持通气，清洁气道和有更好的可视度[25]。

咯血的处理原则

非大咯血

咯血患者的处理目标有如下3点：止血，防止误吸，以及治疗病因。急性支气管炎是急性轻度咯血的常见病因，这种咯血往往具有自限性。临床上，胸片正常的低危患者可在门诊予以密切观察以及口服抗生素治疗。胸片提示有异常肿块时，门诊需行支气管镜检查。对于一个存在肺癌或咯血复发风险的正常胸片患者，应首选高分辨率CT检查，除非紧急情况下行支气管镜检查。

大咯血的处理原则

大咯血患者不能行常规的诊疗，需要紧急处理以维持心肺系统稳定。开放气道与保持血流动力学稳定是首要任务。如果明确出血侧，需使患者保持同向的侧卧位。加强患者护理，根据需要进行紧急补液与输血。如凝血功能异常应及时纠正。硬质支气管镜能有效地清除气道分泌物与血凝块，开放气道与保护其他肺叶，从而防止窒息，保持通气正常。然而，硬质支气管镜并非总是可行的，特别是当紧急情况下无法立即配备熟练的气管镜医师和准备妥当的操作室时。这种情况下需气管插管，维持气道稳定，防止窒息。

气道的保护与复苏

如果不能立即用硬质支气管镜检查，需用大号导管（最好是8号或者更大）紧急气管插管（ET），并用纤维支气管镜通过气管导管进行吸取清洁气道。选择性非出血侧的气管插管，可以考虑在纤维支气管镜的引导下进行（图14.1）。但是，应尽量避免右主支气管插管，因其容易引起右上肺叶的通气障碍。在这种情况下，可先行气管插管，待一个球囊导管可通过 ET 管边或者从 ET 管直接进入左主支气管后，使球囊充气（图 14.2）。在极少数情况下，使用双腔气管插管可以隔离出血的肺叶，并保证正常肺叶的通气（图 14.3），标准的液体复苏应与上述支气管镜操作同步进行。按需给予晶体液，升压药，血制品等。必要时进行实验室与血清学检查，根据具体诊断，对血管炎、结缔组织疾病、韦格纳肉芽肿进行特异性的免疫抑制治疗。Goodpasture 综合征可使用糖皮质激素和血浆置换术处理。一旦心肺系统稳定，可予以血管内治疗。在大咯血时，早期可进行胸外科会诊，紧急情况下可行肺叶切除术来控制出血。

支气管镜介入治疗

在适当情况下，应用纤维支气管镜能停止咯血，并能通过止血暂时稳定病情或者能在特定情况下长期有效地控制大咯血。虽然使用纤维支气管镜还是硬质支气管镜还长期存在争论，

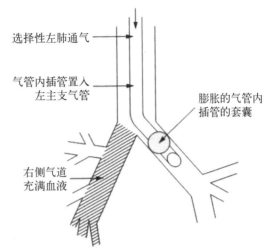

图 14.1 选择性左主支气管插管对右肺出血的处理 [转自 Lordan JL, Gascoigne A, Corris PA. The Pulmonary physician in critical care-illustrative case7: assessment and management of massive haemoptysis, Thorax.2003; 58（9）: 814–9. With permission from BMJ Publishing Group Ltd.]

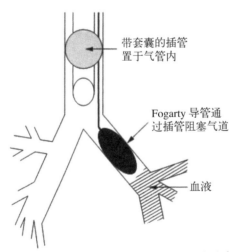

图 14.2 放置一个充气球囊导管隔离左主支气管出血 [转自 Lordan JL, Gascoigne A, Corris PA. The Pulmonary physician in critical care-illustrative case7: assessment and management of massive haemoptysis, Thorax.2003; 58（9）: 814–9. With permission from BMJ Publishing Group Ltd.]

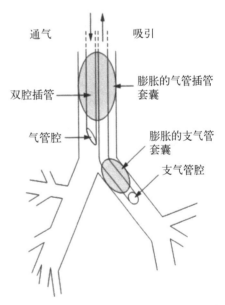

图 14.3 支气管和支气管开口运用双腔气管插管 [转自 Lordan JL, Gascoigne A, Corris PA. The Pulmonary physician in critical care-illustrative case7:assessment and management of massive haemoptysis, Thorax.2003; 58（9）: 814–9. With permission from BMJ Publishing Group Ltd.]

但没有一个随机对照试验支持其中一方。可以确定的是支气管镜的选择取决于是否供应，以及操作者的喜好和技术特点。现有的纤维支气管镜与硬质支气管镜各有优缺点（表14.2）。然而，对于一个熟练的操作者来说，硬质支气管镜更高效安全。相比纤维支气管镜其优势具体如下：硬质支气管镜具有气管支气管的通气口，能在正常肺通气的同时接受治疗。硬质镜头连接独立的吸引管和治疗管，能分别清洁气道和进行电凝及激光治疗。还有一个重要的组件是通气孔侧孔，这个能进行一般的表面麻醉。光源和镜头能使其直接在电视屏幕上显示。不同的内窥镜仪器和药物可以通过大孔进入支气管内。因此硬质支气管镜可先用于稳定患者心肺系统，再行进一步的诊断和治疗。但硬质支气管镜只能看见主支气管的情况。可通过在支气管镜腔放置一个纤维支气管镜进行远端支气管检查从而克服这个限制。文献里有阐述各种腔内支气管镜的检查方法。

局部用药

内镜下局部使用血管收缩剂或促凝剂可在施行最终的咯血治疗方案以前保证暂时安全。这些药物还包括冰生理盐水、肾上腺素、血管加压素及相似物，以取得收缩血管的效果，另外包括纤维蛋白原和凝血酶-氨甲环酸，其主要有促凝作用。

冰生理盐水的作用

局部应用冰生理盐水可产生低温从而使血管收缩以减少出血。1980年Conlan等首先报道了冰生理盐水的使用。在这个报道中，23例大咯血患者使用冰生理盐水灌注后，在最终的手术进行之前终止出血[25]。该报道采用硬质支气管镜取50~500 ml 4℃的生理盐水冲洗支气管从而实现止血。硬质支气管镜可改善视野和气道清洁度，这些患者没有明显的并发症，除了1例患者出现短暂的心动过缓。

肾上腺素和血管加压素的作用

支气管镜活检术或刷检术后使用稀释后的肾上腺素进行局部冲洗已经被证实对轻中度的出血有暂时性的止血效果[26]。然而使用肾上腺素和更高浓度的肾上腺素进行支气管冲洗会导致一些患者出现心律失常或者心动过速[27,28]。一些学者发现如特利加压素和鸟氨酸加压素之类的加压素也有类似肾上腺素的止血作用，但没有太多的心血管副作用。然而该发现没有随机实验加以证实[29-31]。

局部使用促凝药物

在黏膜出血、术后出血或出血性疾病患者中使用抗纤溶剂-氨甲环酸能达到长时间的止血效果。全身静脉滴注或者口服氨甲环酸能有效控制肺囊性纤维化以及支气管动脉异常患者的复发性咯血[32-34]。现已证实用氨甲环酸（500~1 000 ml）进行局部冲洗支气管能有效止血[35]。

局部联合使用纤维蛋白-凝血酶在不能手术或者有手术禁忌证的中到大咯血患者中可能成为更有效的方法。即使以前有少数病例报

表14.2 纤维支气管镜与硬质支气管镜在处理咯血时的优缺点

	纤维支气管镜	硬质支气管镜
优点	技术上易于操作，能通过更小的肺段，可以在ICU床边操作	气道保护通气良好，更好吸引，更多治疗选择
缺点	吸引能力差，治疗手段较少	需要操作室，技术含量更高

道[37,38]提示这类药物疗效良好，但该结论仍需要大量临床研究加以证实。

支气管封堵装置

对于上述局部药物无效的中到大度咯血，在出血段或亚段支气管放置堵塞装置可有效止血（图 14.4）。在某些情况下，可使用气囊对患者的支气管动脉进行封堵。下面对各种不同的封堵技术做一简介。

各种球囊装置能实现临时止血。这些装置能安置长达 48~72 小时，如果持续超过 5 天，患者可能在阻塞性肺段或肺叶处出现阻塞性肺炎，声带与导管长时间接触可形成肉芽肿，甚至可能因装置脱位引起反复的出血。Frietag 等人研制出一种双腔二囊管，通过纤维支气管镜工作管道插入，用第二腔室施用局部药物。26/27 的中度咯血患者使用此导管填塞成功[38]。Dutau 等人发明了一种能在纤维或硬质支气管镜直视下放置在支气管上的树脂胶套管，它能放置在出血段数小时，直到支气管动脉闭塞[39]。最近 Valipour 和他的同事通过纤维支气管镜使用一种氧化再生纤维素网在 56/58 例咯血患者当中取得立即止血的疗效[40]。

气管内生物胶封堵

在最新报道中采用 N-乙酰-氰基丙烯酸盐黏合剂封堵支气管，这一种生物黏合剂在一定湿度下能自行凝固，是一种有效、安全和简单的方法。Bhattacharyya[41]等报道了对 67 例经纤维支气管镜使用该材料的患者为期 6 个月的随访。长期随访显示的成功率是 79%。21% 的患者操作失败，原因是定位错误（46%）、生物胶放置不当（31%）和插管困难（23%）。

支气管镜激光术

1970 年，Strong 和他的同事率先使用了支气管镜下 CO_2 激光术[42]，1985 年 Dumon 等首次报道使用钇铝石榴石激光（Nd:YAG laser）在支气管镜下进行电凝，1 064 nm 波长的钇铝

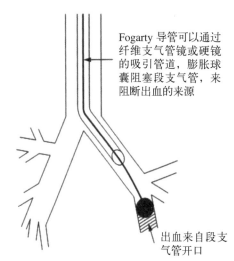

图 14.4 经纤维支气管镜引导在支气管导管放置球囊导管阻塞支气管 [转自 Lordan JL, Gascoigne A, Corris PA. The Pulmonary physician in critical care-illustrative case7: assessment and management of massive haemoptysis, Thorax.2003; 58（9）：814-9. With permission from BMJ Publishing Group Ltd.]

石榴石激光器最适于支气管镜下应用，Nd:YAG 激光吸收系数低于散热系数，允许更深的切割和更广泛的凝固，是对支气管镜下可见的咯血进行有效治疗的方法。它能对出血的黏膜进行电凝止血，并能对深部组织进行切除汽化，从而获得确切疗效。通过纤维支气管镜或者硬质支气管镜，激光探头应超出气管镜末端，并保持在病灶近端 5 mm 处。首先将 FiO_2 降到 40% 以下，采用脉冲式低功率激光（20 W）。根据组织的反应，缓慢地增加激光的强度。通过电凝，病变部位组织可分离和钳取。各项研究表明，激光电凝术是一种有效控制肿瘤血管出血和切除病变组织的方法。Han 等报道了运用 Nd:YAG 激光进行治疗后，94% 的癌症患者的咯血症状能得到改善，74% 患者的出血能完全停止[44]。在另一项研究中，Hetzel 和 Smith 发现对不能手术切除的肿瘤运用激光电凝止血，1 个月内没有再次出血[45]。近些年，钇铝石榴石激光（Nd:YAG laser）可作为肺部介入治疗的医

疗设备。1 340 nm 波长 Nd:YAG 激光水中吸收率是 1 064 nm 波长的 20 倍，因此具有更高效的功率比。理论上它应该对支气管病变部位产生更高效的电凝。这种新型激光仪器的应用正日趋成熟。

氩离子凝固术

氩离子凝固术（APC）相比传统电刀和 Nd:YAG 激光有若干个优点（表 14.3）。它是一种非接触式电凝刀，采用高频电流而不是热能，更容易到达复杂的解剖位置，比激光器的能量分布更为均匀。血液是良好的电导体，一旦出血的支气管凝固，其导电性能就会变差，这能防止电流穿透到更深的组织[46,47]。一些研究表明，APC 能有效地处理支气管病变引起的咯血，同时对止血和切除肿瘤病变都非常有效。Morice 和他的同事已经证明 31/31 例腔内出血使用 APC 能立即止血，随访观察发现，97 天内未见复发出血[47]。Keller 等报道了 1 例心脏移植患者支气管黏膜息肉摘除术后使用 APC 止血，10 个月后都没有复发咯血[46]。

电凝术

通过纤维支气管镜进行电凝术，Homasson 报道了用电凝术对 56 例中晚期恶性或者良性肿瘤患者的咯血进行止血，其中 75% 的患者有效[48]。

其他方法

冷冻术能使血管收缩，形成动静脉微小血栓，从而达到止血效果[49,50]。因此，支气管镜下冷冻术能控制一些支气管肿瘤患者的慢性咯血。同样，虽然施行放疗能有效姑息性治疗晚期肺癌患者的咯血，但并不能作为大咯血的治疗选择[51]。

光动力疗法（PDT）可用于咯血的治疗，但由于在非热能激光术前 48 小时需注射原卟啉，它并不能用于大咯血的治疗。然而它可用于一些支气管肿瘤患者的低度慢性咯血的控制。

非支气管镜介入治疗

虽然支气管镜技术的发展开发出了针对所有类型咯血患者的技术和方法，但对难治性出血或者反复咯血的患者来说，血管内介入治疗如采用支气管动脉栓塞术止血是必要的。如上所述，支气管动脉通常是出血的来源。支气管动脉造影术能显示这些动脉的形态是扩张膨大的，并且常有侧支循环，一旦破裂易引起大咯血。通过造影术找到出血的部位，并且放置明胶海绵、可吸收明胶海绵、氰基丙烯酸酯、弹簧圈、聚乙烯醇等其他硬化剂，可堵塞出血的血管。这种技术对于支气管镜盲区的出血非常有用，特别是在支气管扩张、肺结核、曲菌球感染的患者以及其他支气管镜疗效不足的情况[52,53]。

总结和结论

咯血是非常普遍且十分危险的症状。大咯血与非大咯血之间并无严格的定义。实际上，用危险程度定义大咯血比用咯血量更好，急性支气管炎是非大咯血的常见原因。引起咯血的常见原因包括支气管扩张、肺结核、肺癌、足分支菌病。支气管镜检查术在咯血的诊断以及处理上有重要的作用。它能明确出血部位，隔

表 14.3　氩离子凝固术（APC）和 Nd:YAG 激光比较

Nd:YAG 激光	氩离子凝固术
非接触激光	无触点凝固
热能	电能
深层组织穿透	表面和侧向传播
高温	能到达远端以及边缘组织
	均匀组织脱水

离出血，防止血液流向非出血部位，防止窒息。在处理大咯血上硬质支气管镜要优于纤维支气管镜，但它的应用往往受限于大多数中心医疗机构中专业人员的不足。

在没有硬质支气管镜的条件下，首先用气管插管开放气道，再进行支气管检查术，然后进行液体复苏。一些支气管镜技术，比如气囊填塞，局部使用冰冻生理盐水，以及血管收缩剂、促凝药物，可临时控制出血。一些合适的患者能使用支气管镜介入术如激光切除术和APC。暂时性的止血对后续的支气管动脉栓塞术或者对一些合适患者的手术治疗能有帮助。

参考文献

1. Stoller JK. Diagnosis and management of massive hemoptysis: a review. Respir Care. 1992;32:564–81.
2. Conlan AA, Hurwitz SS, Krige L, et al. Massive hemoptysis. Review of 123 cases. J Thorac Cardiovasc Surg. 1983;85:120–4.
3. Yeoh CB, Hubaytar RT, Ford JM, et al. Treatment of massive hemorrhage in pulmonary tuberculosis. J Thorac Cardiovasc Surg. 1967;54:503–10.
4. Holsclaw DS, Grand RJ, Shwachman H. Massive hemoptysis in cystic fibrosis. J Pediatr. 1970;76:829–38.
5. Marshall TJ, Jackson JE. Vascular intervention in the thorax: bronchial artery embolization for hemoptysis. Eur Radiol. 1997;7:1221–7.
6. Sakr L, Dutau H. Massive hemoptysis: an update on the role of bronchoscopy in diagnosis and management. Respiration. 2010;80:38–58.
7. Crocco JA, Rooney JJ, Fankushen DS, DiBenedetto JR, Lyons HA. Massive hemoptysis. Arch Intern Med. 1968;121:495–8.
8. Corder R. Hemoptysis. Emerg Med Clin North Am. 2003;21:421–35.
9. Levitzky MG. Pulmonary physiology. Blood flow to the lung. McGraw-Hill 1995;4:87–114.
10. Cauldwell EW, Sickert RG, Lininger RE, et al. The bronchial arteries: an anatomic study of 150 human cadavers. Surg Gynecol Obstet. 1948;86:395–412.
11. Hirshberg B, Biran I, Glazer M, et al. Hemoptysis: etiology, evaluation, and outcome in a tertiary referral hospital. Chest. 1997;112:440–4.
12. Rumbak M, Kohler G, Eastrige C, et al. Topical treatment of life threatening hemoptysis from aspergillomas. Thorax. 1996;51:253–5.
13. Ong TH, Eng P. Massive hemoptysis requiring intensive care. Intensive Care Med. 2003;29:317–20.
14. Savale L, Parrot A, Khalil A, et al. Cryptogenic hemoptysis: from a benign to a life threatening pathologic vascular condition. Am J Respir Crit Care Med. 2007;175:1181–5.
15. Marshall TJ, Flower CD, Jackson JE. The role of radiology in the investigation and management of patients with hemoptysis. Clin Radiol. 1996;51:391–400.
16. Haponik EF, Britt EJ, Smith PL, Bleecker ER. Computed chest tomography in the evaluation of hemoptysis: impact on diagnosis and treatment. Chest. 1987;91:80–5.
17. Revel MP, Fournier LS, Hennebicque AS, Cuenod CA, Meyer G, Reynaud P, et al. Can CT replace bronchoscopy in the detection of the site and cause of bleeding in patients with large or massive hemoptysis? Am J Roentgenol. 2002;179:1217–24.
18. Khalil A, Soussan M, Mangiapan G, Fartoukh M, Parrot A, Carette MF. Utility of high-resolution chest CT scan in the emergency management of hemoptysis in the intensive care unit: severity, localization and etiology. Br J Radiol. 2007;80:21–5.
19. RemyJardin M, Bouaziz N, Dumont P, Brillet PY, Bruzzi J, Remy J. Bronchial and non-bronchial systemic arteries at multi-detector row CT angiography: comparison with conventional angiography. Radiology. 2004;233:741–9.
20. Khalil A, Parrot A, Nedelcu C, Fartoukh M, Marsault C, Carette MF. Severe hemoptysis of pulmonary arterial origin: signs and role of multidetector row CT. Chest. 2008;133:212–9.
21. Hsiao EI, Kirsch CM, Kagawa FT, Wehner JH, Jensen WA, Baxter RB. Utility of fiberoptic bronchoscopy before bronchial artery embolization for massive hemoptysis. Am J Roentgenol. 2001;177:861–7.
22. Naidich DP, Funt S, Ettenger NA, Arranda C. Hemoptysis: CT-bronchoscopic correlations in 58 cases. Radiology. 1990;177:357–62.
23. Gong Jr H, Salvatierra C. Clinical efficacy of early and delayed fiberoptic bronchoscopy in patients with hemoptysis. Am Rev Respir Dis. 1981;124:221–5.
24. Dweik R, Stoller JK. Role of bronchoscopy in massive hemoptysis. Clin Chest Med. 1999;20:89–105.
25. Conlan AA, Hurwitz SS. Management of massive hemoptysis with the rigid bronchoscope and cold saline lavage. Thorax. 1980;35:901–4.
26. Zavala DC. Pulmonary hemorrhage in fibreoptic transbronchial biopsy. Chest. 1976;70:584–8.
27. Mazkereth R, Paret G, Ezra D, et al. Epinephrine blood concentrations after peripheral bronchial versus endotracheal administration of epinephrine in dogs. Crit Care Med. 1992;20:1582–7.
28. Kalyanaraman M, Carpenter RL, McGlew MJ, Guertin SR. Cardiopulmonary compromise after use of topical and submucosal α agonists: possible added complication by the use of β-blocker therapy. Otolaryngol Head Neck Surg. 1997;117:56–61.
29. Breuer HW, Charchut S, Worth H, Trampisch HJ, Gläzer K. Endobronchial versus intravenous application of the vasopressin derivative glypressin during diagnostic bronchoscopy. Eur Respir J. 1989;2:225–8.
30. Sharkey AJ, Brennen MD, O'Neill MP, et al. A comparative study of the haemostatic properties and cardiovascular effects of adrenaline and ornipressin in children using enflurane anaesthesia. Acta Anaesthesiol Scand. 1982;26:368–70.
31. Tuller C, Tuller D, Tamm M, Brutsche MH. Hemodynamic effects of endobronchial application of ornipressin versus terlipressin. Respiration. 2004;71:397–401.
32. Wong LT, Lillquist YP, Culham G, DeJong BP, Davidson AG. Treatment of recurrent hemoptysis in a child with cystic fibrosis by repeated bronchial artery embolizations and long-term tranexamic acid. Pediatr Pulmonol. 1996;22:275–9.
33. Chang AB, Ditchfield M, Robinson PJ, Robertson CF. Major hemoptysis in a child with cystic fibrosis from multiple aberrant bronchial arteries treated with tranexamic acid. Pediatr Pulmonol.

1996;22:416–20.
34. Graff GR. Treatment of recurrent severe hemoptysis in cystic fibrosis with tranexamic acid. Respiration. 2001;68:91–4.
35. Solomonov A, Fruchter O, Zuckerman T, Brenner B, Yigla M. Pulmonary hemorrhage: a novel mode of therapy. Respir Med. 2009;103:1196–200.
36. Tsukamoto T, Sasaki H, Nakamura H. Treatment of hemoptysis patients by thrombin and fibrinogenthrombin infusion therapy using a fiberoptic bronchoscope. Chest. 1989;96:473–6.
37. Bense L. Intrabronchial selective coagulative treatment of hemoptysis. Chest. 1990;97:990–6.
38. Freitag L, Tekolf E, Stamatis G, Montag M, Greschuchna D. Three years experience with a new balloon catheter for the management of hemoptysis. Eur Respir J. 1994;7:2033–7.
39. Dutau H, Palot A, Haas A, Decamps I, Durieux O. Endobronchial embolization with a silicone spigot as a temporary treatment for massive hemoptysis. Respiration. 2006;73:830–2.
40. Valipour A, Kreuzer A, Koller H, Koessler W, Burghuber OC. Bronchoscopy-guided topical hemostatic tamponade therapy for the management of lifethreatening hemoptysis. Chest. 2005;127:2113–8.
41. Sarkar BP, Ghosh D, Nag S, Chowdhury S, et al. Evaluation of the technical details of bronchoscopic endobronchial sealing: review of 67 patients. Indian J Chest Dis Allied Sci. 2007;49:137–42.
42. Strong MS, Jako GJ. Laser surgery in the larynx. Early clinical experience with CO_2 laser. Ann Otol Rhinol Laryngol. 1972;86:791–8.
43. Dumon JF, Meric B, Surpas P, Ragni J. Endoscopic resection in bronchology using the YAG laser. Evaluation of a five year experience. Schweiz Med Wochenschr. 1985;115:1336–44.
44. Han CC, Prasetyo D, Wright GM. Endobronchial palliation using Nd-YAG laser is associated with improved survival when combined with multimodal adjuvant treatments. J Thorac Oncol. 2007;2:59–64.
45. Hetzel MR, Smith SGT. Endoscopic palliation of tracheobronchial malignancies. Thorax. 1991;46:325–33.
46. Keller CA, Hinerman R, Singh A, Alvarez F. The use of endoscopic argon plasma coagulation in airway complications after solid organ transplantation. Chest. 2001;119:1968–75.
47. Morice RC, Ece T, Ece F, Keus L. Endobronchial argon plasma coagulation for treatment of hemoptysis and neoplastic airway obstruction. Chest. 2001;119:781–7.
48. Homasson JP. Endobronchial electrocautery. Semin Respir Crit Care Med. 1997;18:535–43.
49. Mathur PN, Wolf KM, Busk MF, Briete WM, Datzman M. Fiberoptic bronchoscopic cryotherapy in the management of tracheobronchial obstruction. Chest. 1996;110:718–23.
50. Maiwand MO, Asimakopoulos G. Cryosurgery for lung cancer: clinical results and technical aspects. Technol Cancer Res Treat. 2004;3:143–50.
51. Cardona AF, Reveiz L, Ospina EG, Ospina V, Yepes A. Palliative endobronchial brachytherapy for nonsmall cell lung cancer. Cochrane Database Syst Rev. 2008; 16:CD004284.
52. Cremaschi P, Nascimbene C, Vitulo P, et al. Therapeutic embolization of bronchial artery: a successful treatment in 209 cases of relapse hemoptysis. Angiology. 1993;44:295–9.
53. Yu-Tang Goh P, Lin M, Teo N, En SWD. Embolization for hemoptysis: a six year review. Cardiovasc Intervent Radiol. 2002;25:17–25.